Atlas of Anatomic Pathology

Series Editor

Liang Cheng
Indianapolis, Indiana, USA

This Atlas series is intended as a "first knowledge base" in the quest for diagnosis of usual and unusual diseases. Each atlas will offer the reader a quick reference guide for diagnosis and classification of a wide spectrum of benign, congenital, inflammatory, nonneoplastic, and neoplastic lesions in various organ systems. Normal and variations of "normal" histology will also be illustrated. Each atlas will focus on visual diagnostic criteria and differential diagnosis. It will be organized to provide quick access to images of lesions in specific organs or sites. Each atlas will adapt the well-known and widely accepted terminology, nomenclature, classification schemes, and staging algorithms. Each volume in this series will be authored by nationally and internationally recognized pathologists. Each volume will follow the same organizational structure. The first Section will include normal histology and normal variations. The second Section will cover congenital defects and malformations. The third Section will cover benign and inflammatory lesions. The fourth Section will cover benign tumors and benign mimickers of cancer. The last Section will cover malignant neoplasms. Special emphasis will be placed on normal histology, gross anatomy, and gross lesion appearances since these are generally lacking or inadequately illustrated in current textbooks. The detailed figure legends will concisely summarize the critical information and visual diagnostic criteria that the pathologist must recognize, understand, and accurately interpret to arrive at a correct diagnosis. This book series is intended chiefly for use by pathologists in training and practicing surgical pathologists in their daily practice. The atlas series will also be a useful resource for medical students, cytotechnologists, pathologist assistants, and other medical professionals with special interest in anatomic pathology. Trainees, students, and readers at all levels of expertise will learn, understand, and gain insights into the complexities of disease processes through this comprehensive resource. Macroscopic and histological images are aesthetically pleasing in many ways. This new series will serve as a virtual pathology museum for the edification of our readers.

More information about this series at http://www.springer.com/series/10144

Hector H. Li-Chang • Richard Kirsch
James Conner • Aysegul Sari • Aaron Pollett
Hala El-Zimaity • Dhanpat Jain • Romulo Celli
Stephanie L. Reid • Robert H. Riddell

Atlas of Intestinal Pathology

Volume 1: Neoplastic Diseases of the Intestines

Springer

Hector H. Li-Chang
Pathology and Laboratory Medicine
University of British Columbia
Royal Victoria Regional Health Centre
Barrie, ON
Canada

James Conner
Department of Pathology and Laboratory
Medicine, Mount Sinai Hospital
University of Toronto
Toronto, ON
Canada

Aaron Pollett
Department of Laboratory Medicine
and Pathobiology, Mount Sinai Hospital
University of Toronto
Toronto, ON
Canada

Dhanpat Jain
Department of Pathology
Yale New Haven Hospital
New Haven, CT
USA

Stephanie L. Reid
Discipline of Laboratory Medicine
Health Sciences Centre, Memorial University
of Newfoundland
St. John's, NL
Canada

Richard Kirsch
Department of Pathology and Laboratory
Medicine, Mount Sinai Hospital
University of Toronto
Toronto, ON
Canada

Aysegul Sari
Department of Pathology and Laboratory
Medicine, Mount Sinai Hospital
University of Toronto
Toronto, ON
Canada
İzmir Katip Celebi University Ataturk Training
and Research Hospital
İzmir, Turkey

Hala El-Zimaity
Dynacare Laboratories
Brampton, ON
Canada

Romulo Celli
Department of Pathology
Yale New Haven Hospital
New Haven, CT
USA

Robert H. Riddell
Department of Laboratory
Medicine and Pathobiology
University of Toronto
Toronto, ON
Canada
Pathology and Laboratory Medicine
Mount Sinai Hospital
Toronto, ON
Canada

ISSN 2625-3372 ISSN 2625-3380 (electronic)
Atlas of Anatomic Pathology
ISBN 978-3-030-12377-2 ISBN 978-3-030-12379-6 (eBook)
https://doi.org/10.1007/978-3-030-12379-6

This Springer imprint is published by the registered company Springer Nature Switzerland AG.
The registered company address is: Gewerbestrasse 11, 6330 Cham, Switzerland

Series Preface

One Picture Is Worth Ten Thousand Words

— Frederick Barnard, 1927

Remarkable progress has been made in anatomic and surgical pathology during the last 10 years. The ability of surgical pathologists to reach a definite diagnosis is now enhanced by immunohistochemical and molecular techniques. Many new clinically important histopathologic entities and variants have been described using these techniques. Established diagnostic entities are more fully defined for virtually every organ system. The emergence of personalized medicine has also created a paradigm shift in surgical pathology. Both promptness and precision are required of modern pathologists. Newer diagnostic tests in anatomic pathology, however, cannot benefit the patient unless the pathologist recognizes the lesion and requests the necessary special studies. An up-to-date atlas encompassing the full spectrum of benign and malignant lesions, their variants, and evidence-based diagnostic criteria for each organ system is needed. This atlas is not intended as a comprehensive source of detailed clinical information concerning the entities shown. Clinical and therapeutic guidelines are served admirably by a large number of excellent textbooks. This atlas, however, is intended as a "first knowledge base" in the quest for definitive and efficient diagnosis of both usual and unusual diseases.

The *Atlas of Anatomic Pathology* is presented to the reader as a quick reference guide for diagnosis and classification of benign, congenital, inflammatory, nonneoplastic, and neoplastic lesions organized by organ systems. Normal and variations of "normal" histology are illustrated for each organ. The atlas focuses on visual diagnostic criteria and differential diagnosis. The organization is intended to provide quick access to images and confirmatory tests for each specific organ or site. The atlas adopts the well-known and widely accepted terminology, nomenclature, classification schemes, and staging algorithms.

This book series is intended chiefly for use by pathologists in training and practicing surgical pathologists in their daily practice. It is also a useful resource for medical students, cytotechnologists, pathologist assistants, and other medical professionals with special interest in anatomic pathology. We hope that our trainees, students, and readers at all levels of expertise will learn, understand, and gain insight into the pathophysiology of disease processes through this comprehensive resource. Macroscopic and histological images are aesthetically pleasing in many ways. We hope that the new series will serve as a virtual pathology museum for the edification of our readers.

Indianapolis, IN, USA

Liang Cheng

Preface

Intestinal neoplasia comprises a large part of a surgical pathologist's workload. Pathologists play a key role not only in the classification of malignancies but also in assisting screening programs, identifying incidental neoplasms, and guiding treatment by providing essential prognostic features for individual entities. A large variety of neoplasms affect the intestines, and there is ongoing discovery of new entities and prognostic features for known diseases. Pathologists and trainees should have a solid understanding of key morphologic features, pitfalls, and differential diagnoses. Importantly, pathologists should recognize and communicate features that will help their clinical colleagues in making treatment decisions, with the ultimate goal of benefiting the patient first and foremost.

This atlas provides a comprehensive yet concise, primarily visual review of intestinal neoplasms. It should also serve as a useful resource primarily for pathologists and trainees in pathology by providing a concise yet comprehensive summary of the morphology of intestinal neoplasia. Clinical practitioners and trainees will also benefit from an understanding of the pathologic correlates to the diseases they manage.

Barrie, ON, Canada — Hector H. Li-Chang
Toronto, ON, Canada — Richard Kirsch
Toronto, ON, Canada — James Conner
Toronto, ON, Canada — Aysegul Sari
Toronto, ON, Canada — Aaron Pollett
Brampton, ON, Canada — Hala El-Zimaity
New Haven, CT, USA — Dhanpat Jain
New Haven, CT, USA — Romulo Celli
St. John's, NL, Canada — Stephanie L. Reid
Toronto, ON, Canada — Robert H. Riddell

Acknowledgment

We would like to acknowledge the hard work and contribution of our colleagues, trainees, and support staff, especially those at Mount Sinai Hospital (Toronto, Ontario).

Contents

Contributors

Romulo Celli, MD Department of Pathology, Yale New Haven Hospital, New Haven, CT, USA

James Conner, MD, PhD Department of Pathology and Laboratory Medicine, Mount Sinai Hospital, University of Toronto, Toronto, ON, Canada

Hala El-Zimaity, MD Dynacare Laboratories, Brampton, ON, Canada

Dhanpat Jain, MD Department of Pathology, Yale New Haven Hospital, New Haven, CT, USA

Richard Kirsch, MBChB, PhD Department of Pathology and Laboratory Medicine, Mount Sinai Hospital, University of Toronto, Toronto, ON, Canada

Hector H. Li-Chang, MD Pathology and Laboratory Medicine, University of British Columbia, Royal Victoria Regional Health Centre, Barrie, ON, Canada

Aaron Pollett, MD, FRCPC Department of Laboratory Medicine and Pathobiology, Mount Sinai Hospital, University of Toronto, Toronto, ON, Canada

Stephanie L. Reid, MD, FRCPC Discipline of Laboratory Medicine, Health Sciences Centre, Memorial University of Newfoundland, St John's, NL, Canada

Robert H. Riddell, MD Department of Laboratory Medicine and Pathobiology, University of Toronto, Toronto, ON, Canada

Pathology and Laboratory Medicine, Mount Sinai Hospital, Toronto, ON, Canada

Aysegul Sari, MD Department of Pathology and Laboratory Medicine, Mount Sinai Hospital, University of Toronto, Toronto, ON, Canada

İzmir Katip Celebi University Ataturk Training and Research Hospital, İzmir, Turkey

1 Epithelial Polyps

Hector H. Li-Chang

The vast majority of polyps arising in the small and large intestines are derived from epithelial cells. These are routinely sampled by endoscopists during screening and diagnostic procedures, and hence they comprise a large proportion of the work done by pathologists. The proper diagnosis of intestinal polyps is required to gauge the risk of subsequent intestinal malignancy, either through the enumeration and classification of premalignant polyps, or less commonly through the identification of polyps that may alert clinicians to an underlying neoplastic syndrome. Although polyps from the small bowel are relatively rare specimens, most of the principles from the colorectum can be extended to this site.

Our understanding of the significance of epithelial polyps continues to evolve. For example, the malignant potential of sessile serrated adenomas/polyps (SSA/Ps) often went unrecognized in the relatively recent past, as they were often diagnosed as hyperplastic polyps. Recent studies suggest a relationship between at least some hyperplastic polyps, SSA/Ps, and traditional serrated adenomas.

Despite their frequency in daily practice, certain diagnostic challenges persist even in the diagnosis of the most commonly encountered types of polyps. There continues to be some uncertainty on occasion in distinguishing hyperplastic polyps from SSA/Ps. There is also disagreement on the architectural classification of adenomas and dysplasia grading. The high amount of interobserver variability that exists in this space has led some pathologists to suggest that these qualifiers not be reported. More than occasionally, benign submucosal epithelial misplacement of adenomatous epithelium is difficult to distinguish from invasive adenocarcinoma. Finally, abnormal findings are sometimes not initially appreciated in initial sections because of specimen orientation, requiring deeper levels to arrive at adequate diagnoses.

This chapter attempts to describe and illustrate diagnostic features of epithelial polyps, with special attention paid to highlighting helpful features in challenging situations.

1.1 Inflammatory Polyps

Inflammatory polyps in the small intestine arise as a result of a variety of conditions, most commonly NSAID injury, gastric *Helicobacter* infection, and inflammatory bowel disease [1]. The example in Fig. 1.1 is characterized by abundant gastric foveolar-type metaplasia, lamina propria expansion by a chronic inflammatory infiltrate, and architectural distortion (villous blunting and crypt elongation/branching). A neutrophilic infiltrate may be present, and the foveolar metaplasia may harbor an ectopic *Helicobacter* infection.

Foveolar metaplasia is not always readily identified by beginners. Note that the native duodenal epithelium on the left side of Fig. 1.2 is composed of absorptive cells with abundant eosinophilic cytoplasm, and goblet cells whose cytoplasm is composed of a large mucin droplet. In contrast, the metaplastic foveolar cells on the right contain a cap of mucin with pink cytoplasm in between this droplet and the nucleus.

Colonic inflammatory polyps may arise from a wide range of conditions, and they are occasionally solitary idiopathic findings. They are characterized by irregularly shaped crypts, a variably mixed chronic and neutrophilic inflammatory infiltrate, and expansion of the lamina propria by edema and inflammatory cells [2]. Figure 1.3 shows marked expansion of the lamina propria by a mixed infiltrate rich in plasma cells. The crypts are elongated and irregular in their shape and distribution, and the surface has begun to acquire an undulating, villous-like appearance. In severe conditions, inflammatory polyps may reach large sizes and have such villous-like architectures.

H. H. Li-Chang et al., *Atlas of Intestinal Pathology*, Atlas of Anatomic Pathology,
https://doi.org/10.1007/978-3-030-12379-6_1

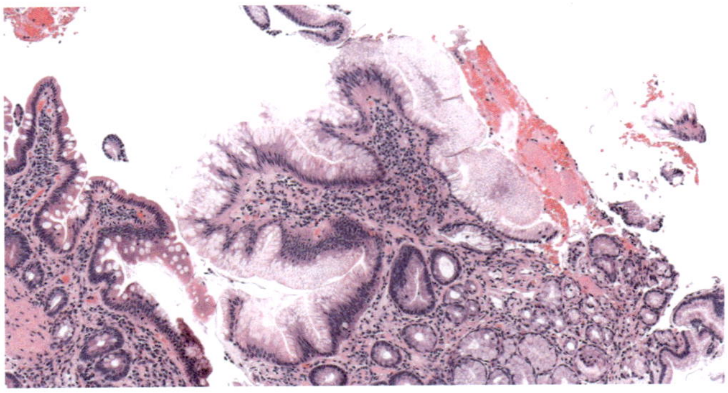

Fig. 1.1 Duodenal inflammatory polyp

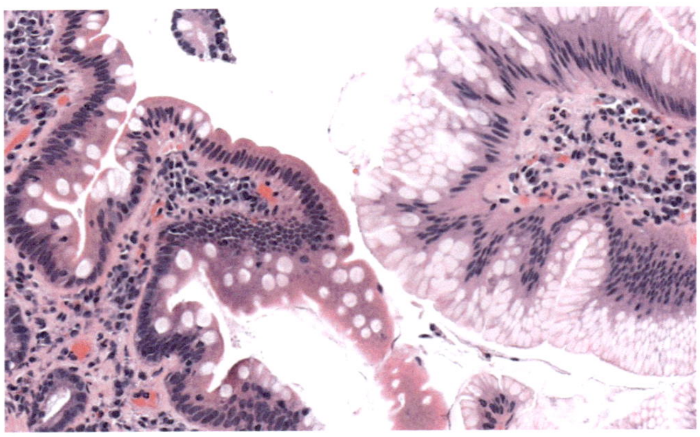

Fig. 1.2 Duodenal inflammatory polyp

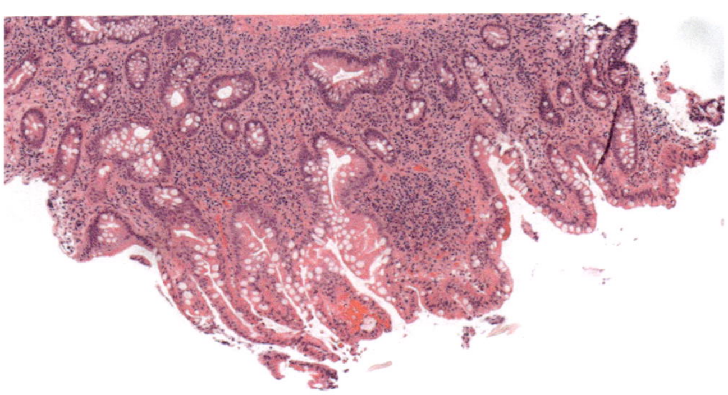

Fig. 1.3 Colonic inflammatory polyp

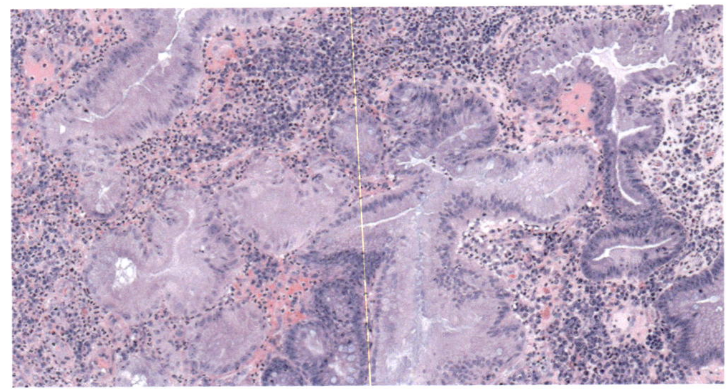

Fig. 1.4 Colonic inflammatory polyp

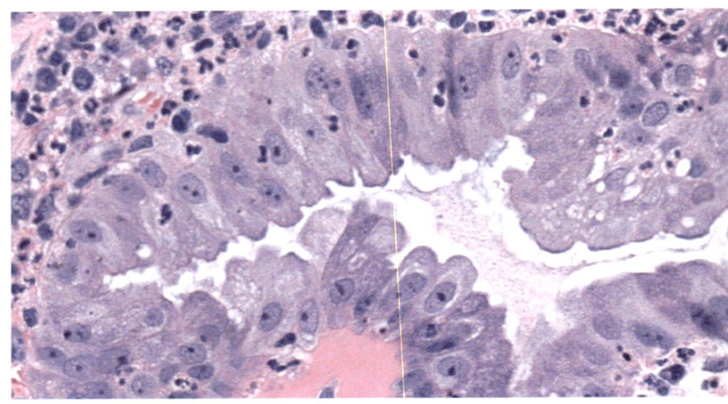

Fig. 1.5 Colonic inflammatory polyp

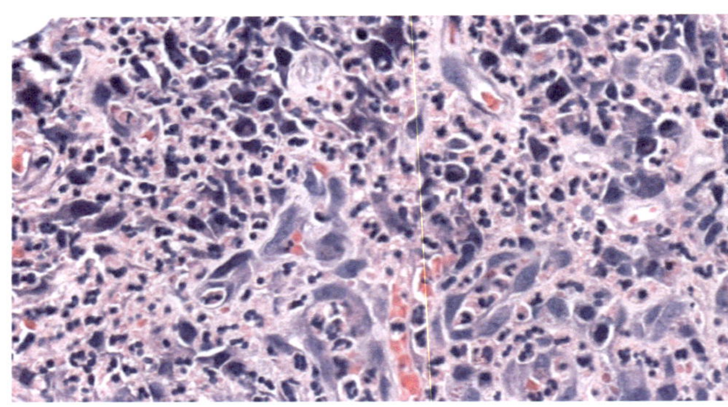

Fig. 1.6 Colonic inflammatory polyp

Inflammatory polyps may occasionally show ongoing active inflammation, often in the setting of an overlying or adjacent erosion. Figure 1.4 shows prominent neutrophilic inflammation in an example associated with inflammatory bowel disease; the architectural changes can also be striking.

The epithelial changes associated with active inflammation can be significant, as in Fig. 1.5, which shows enlarged nuclei and markedly prominent nucleoli. Within intestinal epithelium, a vesicular chromatin pattern with prominent nucleoli is usually, but not always, a reactive phenomenon rather than a neoplastic one. The association with neutrophils, gradual changing to merge with the surrounding epithelium, and association with other inflammatory changes in the polyp and background mucosa help in distinguishing such changes from those of dysplasia.

Erosions and ulcers in the gastrointestinal tract, including those occurring within inflammatory polyps, can result in marked reactive changes within the fibroblasts and endothelial cells (Fig. 1.6). Such cells (humorously referred to by some as "ulcerocytes") are characterized by nucleomegaly, multinucleation, anisocytosis, smudgy chromatin, mitotic

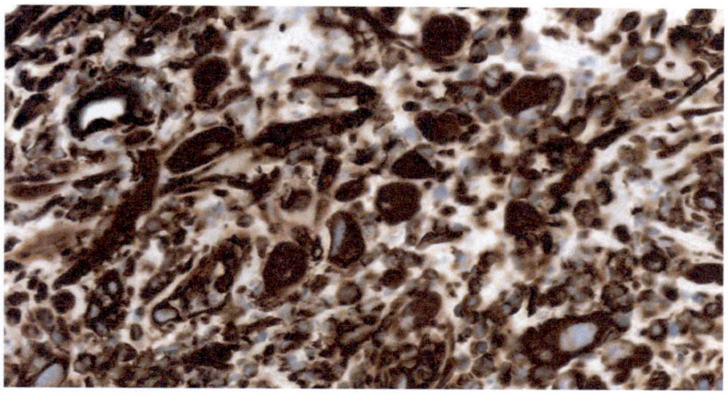

Fig. 1.7 Colonic inflammatory polyp (vimentin stain)

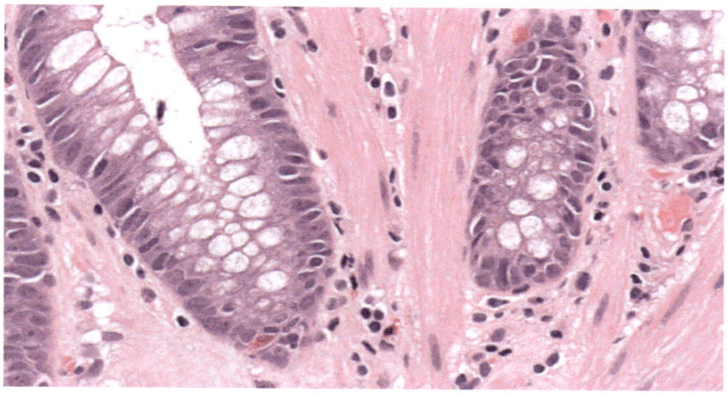

Fig. 1.9 Mucosal prolapse polyp

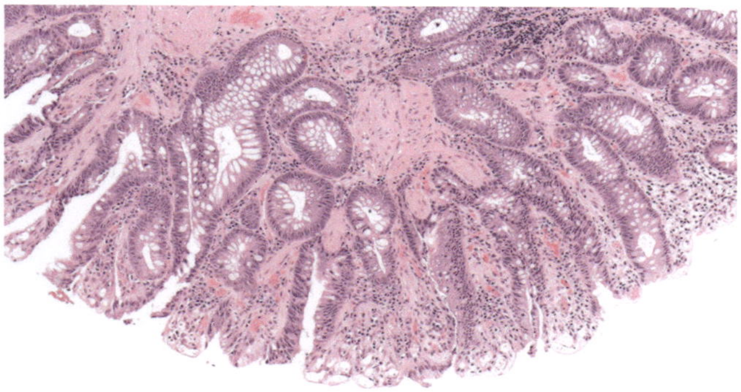

Fig. 1.8 Mucosal prolapse polyp

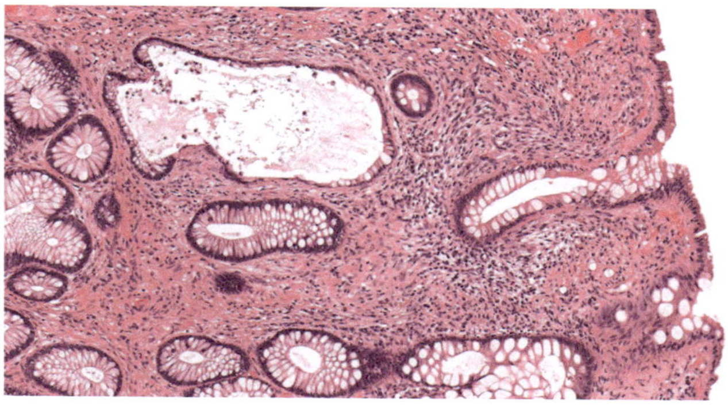

Fig. 1.10 Inflammatory myoglandular polyp

figures, and prominent nucleoli. Such marked reactive changes should not be confused with those of malignancy, and a high threshold for diagnosing malignancy should be employed in the setting of ulcers.

A vimentin stain highlights the reactive, atypical fibroblasts in Fig. 1.7. In contrast, a broad-spectrum cytokeratin stain and melanoma stains are completely negative. This helps to confirm the fibroblastic and reactive nature of these atypical cells in cases where there is concern for malignancy.

Mucosal prolapse polyps can be considered a subtype of inflammatory polyps, seen almost exclusively in the distal colon and rectum (Fig. 1.8). They are thought to result from trauma to the mucosa being dragged into the colonic lumen. They are characterized by a hamartoma-like admixture of thickened, disorganized smooth muscle and crypts, particularly at the crypt bases, with a variable degree of ischemia-like surface epithelial attenuation, erosion, and granulation tissue. Other terms applied to variants of this polyp include "inflammatory cap polyp" (depending on the prominence of surface erosion) and "inflammatory cloacogenic polyp" (depending on the prominence of hamartoma-like features).

The smooth muscle fibers in prolapse polyp splay perpendicularly and superficially to form a cup under the crypt bases (Fig. 1.9). The epithelium in these polyps usually shows regenerative atypia, with hyperchromasia and increased mitotic activity mimicking those of an adenoma. In contrast to adenomas, the nuclear features are most marked at the bases and dissipate superficially, whereas adenomas are characterized by top-down atypia, as described below [3].

Inflammatory myoglandular polyps are rare polyps seen in the ileum and distal colon; they are usually solitary and pedunculated. They are characterized by variable amounts of granulation tissue, irregular and branching dilated glands, and a smooth muscle proliferation in the lamina propria (Fig. 1.10). They may be confused with Peutz-Jeghers polyps, but in contrast to Peutz-Jeghers polyps, inflammatory myoglandular polyps lack villous architecture and arborizing smooth muscle [4].

1.2 Hamartomatous Polyps

Juvenile polyps are the most common type of hamartomatous polyp arising in the colorectum (Fig. 1.11). These are characterized by expansion of the lamina propria by edema and a mixed inflammatory infiltrate, along with dilatation and branching of the crypts. In many cases, a definitive distinction between juvenile polyps and inflammatory polyps is

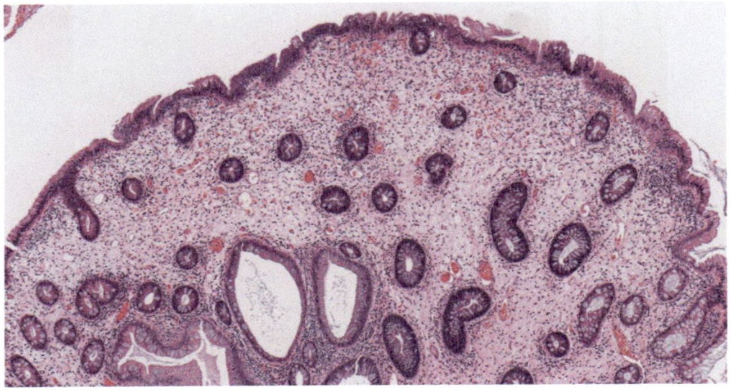

Fig. 1.11 Hamartoma (juvenile polyp and *PTEN* hamartoma tumor syndrome)

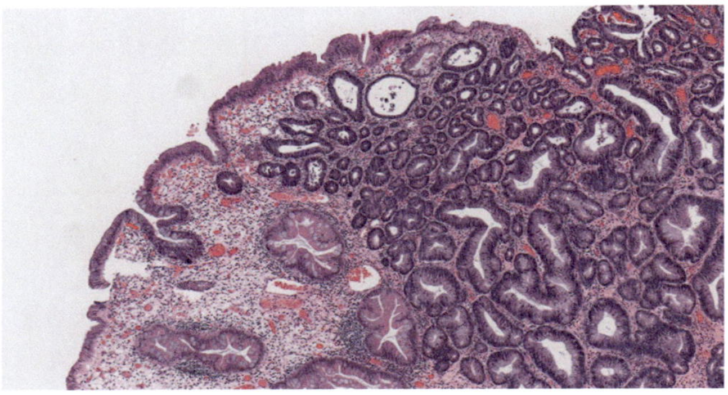

Fig. 1.12 Hamartoma (juvenile polyp and *PTEN* hamartoma tumor syndrome)

not possible. Juvenile polyps such as this one are essentially indistinguishable from those identified in *PTEN* hamartoma tumor syndrome (Cowden syndrome and related syndromes). Subtle histologic differences have been described that may allow pathologists to diagnose *PTEN* hamartoma syndrome, juvenile polyposis, or nonsyndromic polyps [5] but these are difficult to implement in practice.

When multiple hamartomatous polyps are identified, or when a mix of hamartomas and adenomas are present simultaneously, pathologists may play a role in raising the possibility of an underlying tumor predisposition syndrome. Occasionally hamartomatous polyps develop dysplasia in such settings, as in this case of suspected Cowden syndrome in Fig. 1.12, though frank malignancies directly arising from hamartomas are rare.

Cronkhite-Canada syndrome is a rare sporadic condition that can result in multiple polyps very similar to those seen in juvenile polyposis and *PTEN* hamartoma tumor syndrome [6]. Figure 1.13 demonstrates that the nonpolypoid mucosa in such cases can also show identical changes of edema and lamina propria chronic inflammation, so that correlation with clinical endoscopic findings is required to correctly classify such changes.

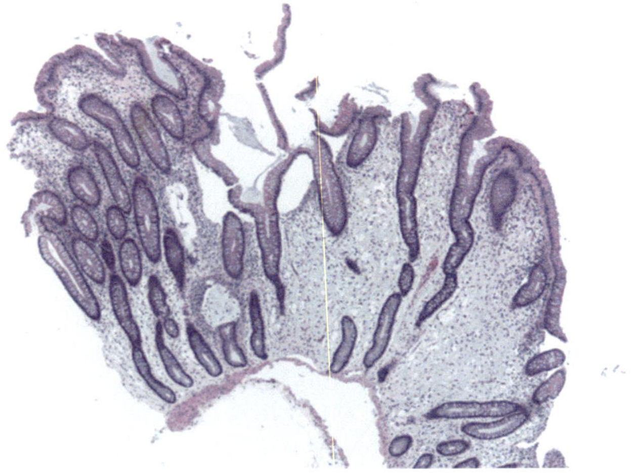

Fig. 1.13 Cronkhite-Canada syndrome (*Image courtesy of* Dr. Rish Pai)

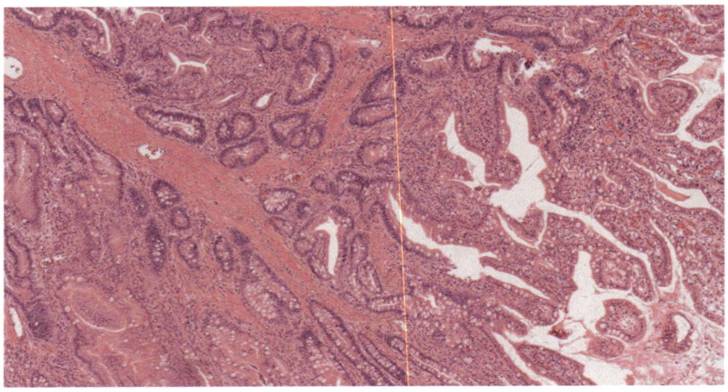

Fig. 1.14 Peutz-Jeghers polyp from the jejunum

The other major subtype of hamartomatous polyps is Peutz-Jeghers (PJ) polyps, which are most commonly found in the jejunum. A genetic predisposition to mucosal prolapse may underlie their development [7]. Some data suggest that *bona fide* PJ polyps may occur only in the small bowel, with gastric and colorectal instances perhaps representing examples of sporadic mucosal prolapse. The polyps are characterized by a tree-like hierarchical branching ("arborizing") pattern of smooth muscle lined by otherwise normal native mucosa. Figure 1.14, an example from the jejunum, demonstrates the presence of normal villi and crypts along the mucosa.

The suspected example of a colonic PJ polyp in Fig. 1.15 is lined by architecturally distorted and inflamed colonic mucosa. A diagnosis of mucosal prolapse polyp (inflammatory cloacogenic polyp) is also a consideration. Such polyps in the colorectum have not been shown to be associated with an increased systemic risk of malignancy, in contrast to *bona fide* PJ polyps arising in the small bowel. As such, a diagnosis of Peutz-Jeghers syndrome should be made with caution, if ever, in patients with colorectal PJ polyps.

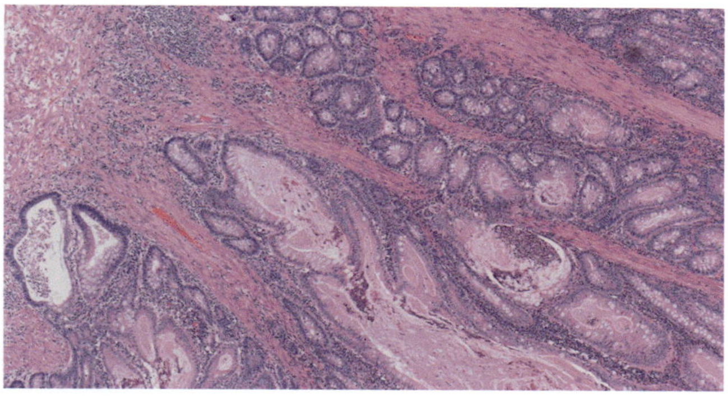

Fig. 1.15 Peutz-Jeghers polyp from the colon

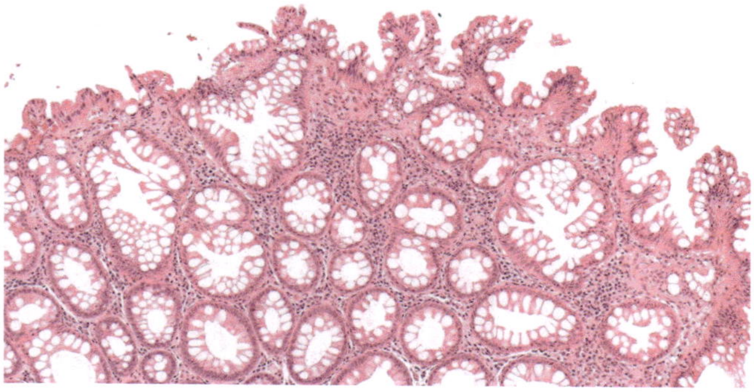

Fig. 1.16 Goblet-cell rich hyperplastic polyp

1.3 Hyperplastic Polyps

Three histologic subtypes of hyperplastic polyps are described (goblet-cell rich, microvesicular, and mucin-depleted), though a distinction between these is not necessary on pathology reports. Goblet-cell rich hyperplastic polyps, such as in Fig. 1.16, are usually easy to recognize from the serrated/stellate appearance of the surface and crypt epithelium on the right, which contrasts with the more flat and regular normal epithelium on the left. Occasionally this distinction can be subtle, however, and these hyperplastic polyps are frequently a cause of endoscopically but not histologically apparent polyps [8].

Figure 1.17 is another example of a goblet-cell rich hyperplastic polyp. Low-power recognition of serrations, as well as architecture and nuclear distribution, are usually sufficient to diagnose hyperplastic polyps with ease. In contrast to sessile serrated adenomas (SSAs, see below), the crypts in hyperplastic polyps are most narrow at the base, and open up superficially. The darkest nuclei are present at the base of the crypts, where the proliferation occurs (bottom-up growth), in contrast to tubular adenomas (see below).

The microvesicular subtype (Fig. 1.18) is the most common type of hyperplastic polyp. Microvesicular cytoplasm is also seen in SSAs, and a distinction between the two entities can sometimes be difficult. Hyperplastic polyps lack the basal serrations and basally differentiated cells of SSAs (see below). Though most hyperplastic polyps should have narrow crypt bases, an underrecognized confounding effect is seen in cases of hyperplastic polyps associated with mucosal prolapse changes, wherein smooth muscle proliferation and crypt architectural distortion, including a degree of dilatation, can impart an appearance reminiscent of SSA/Ps.

The surface of both microvesicular hyperplastic polyps and SSA/Ps contains foamy, pale cytoplasm with many small bubbles, and is somewhat reminiscent of secretory changes in the endometrium (Fig. 1.19). Mitotic figures and nuclear atypia are absent from the surface in both cases. The morphologic similarities between microvesicular hyperplastic polyps and SSA/Ps are also reflected in the increasingly recognized association between the two polyps as components along a spectrum of serrated polyps, with increasing size, number, and architectural abnormalities being associated with an increased risk of malignancy.

When dilated crypts are present in hyperplastic polyps with prolapse changes, they are typically accompanied by abnormal migration of muscularis mucosae fibers superficially into the lamina propria, as in Fig. 1.20. Other features of SSAs, such as basally located serrations and basally located differentiated cells, are absent.

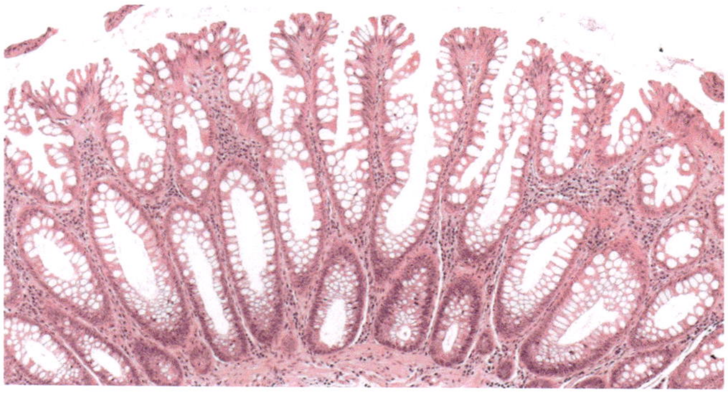

Fig. 1.17 Goblet-cell rich hyperplastic polyp

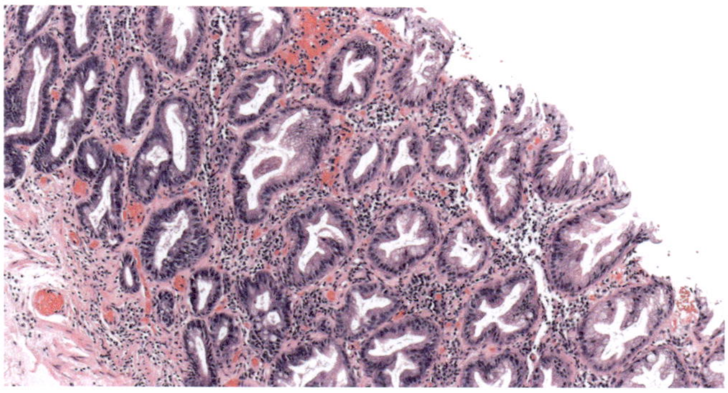

Fig. 1.18 Microvesicular hyperplastic polyp

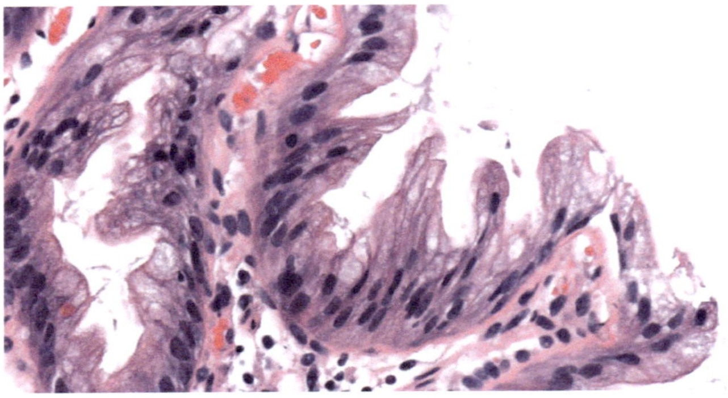

Fig. 1.19 Microvesicular hyperplastic polyp

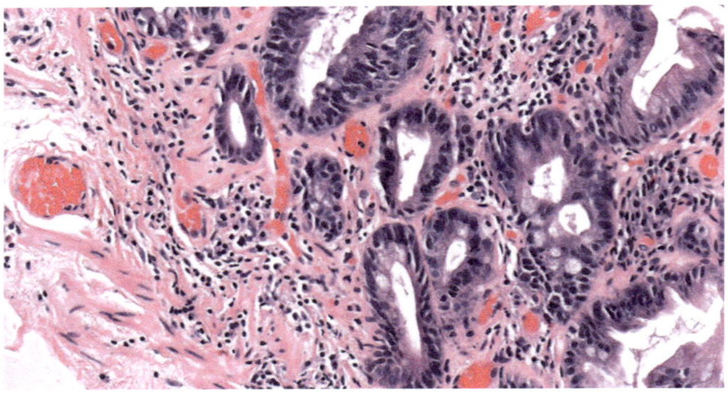

Fig. 1.20 Microvesicular hyperplastic polyp

1.4 Sessile Serrated Adenomas

Sessile serrated adenomas (SSAs) were until relatively recently unrecognized precursors to right-sided colonic carcinomas [9]. They share some histologic similarities with hyperplastic polyps, but in SSAs the epithelial serrations extend to the basal half of the crypt, there are terminally differentiated cells in the crypt bases, and (most importantly) there is dilatation of the crypt bases, resulting in the formation of boot, L, or inverted T shapes at the base of the crypts (Fig. 1.21).

SSAs may sometimes show very subtle histologic features. In some cases, abnormalities at the base of the crypts may be minimal. Recent guidelines recommend that only one abnormal crypt is necessary for the diagnosis of an SSA. This is especially true in large, proximally located polyps [10–21]. Figure 1.22 shows a large polyp with minimal architectural changes at the base of the crypts. Deeper levels may be of assistance in revealing diagnostic crypt shapes.

In other cases, sessile serrated adenomas are difficult to diagnose because of misorientation of the specimen, wherein the crypt bases are not in the plane of section. In such cases, an admixture of stellate and round crypts are a helpful clue to the diagnosis (Fig. 1.23).

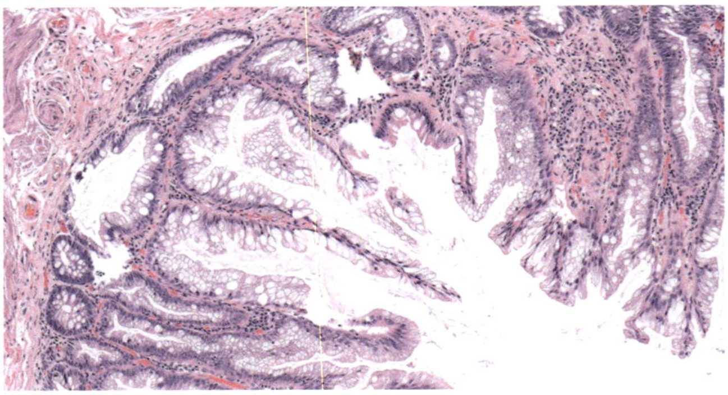

Fig. 1.21 Sessile serrated adenoma

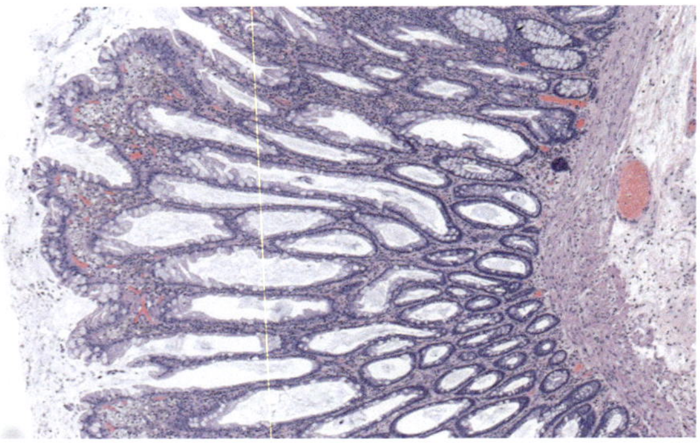

Fig. 1.22 Sessile serrated adenoma

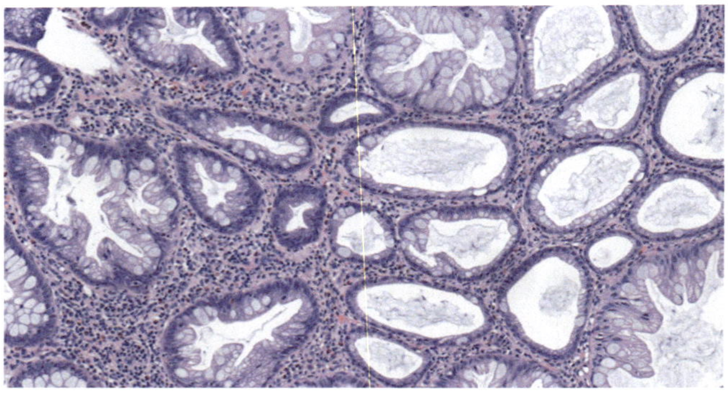

Fig. 1.23 Sessile serrated adenoma

SSAs that begin to advance towards malignancy often reflect this progression through morphologic features of dysplasia. In such "advanced SSAs," dysplasia may either be of conventional type, as in Fig. 1.24, or the "serrated" form of dysplasia. The presence of dysplasia should prompt a careful exclusion of invasive carcinoma at the base of the polyp, with deeper sections being obtained if necessary. Conventional dysplasia is characterized by nuclear hyperchromasia, crowding, and pseudostratification, essentially identical to that seen in adenomas.

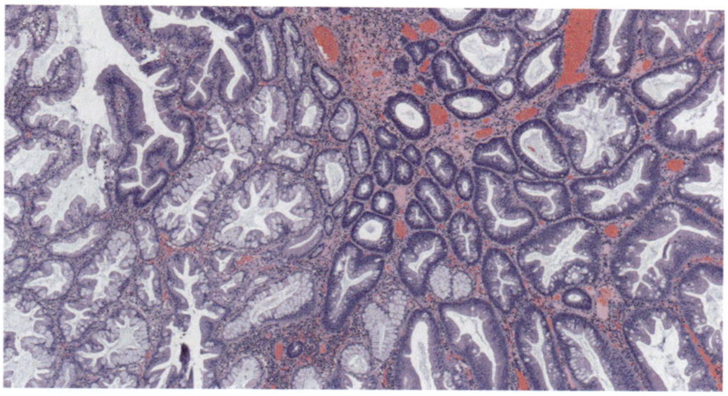

Fig. 1.24 Sessile serrated adenoma with conventional dysplasia

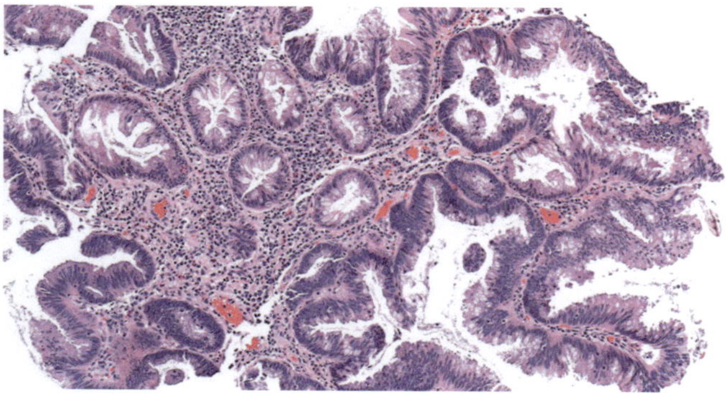

Fig. 1.25 Features of sessile serrated adenoma and cytologic dysplasia in the same tissue fragment

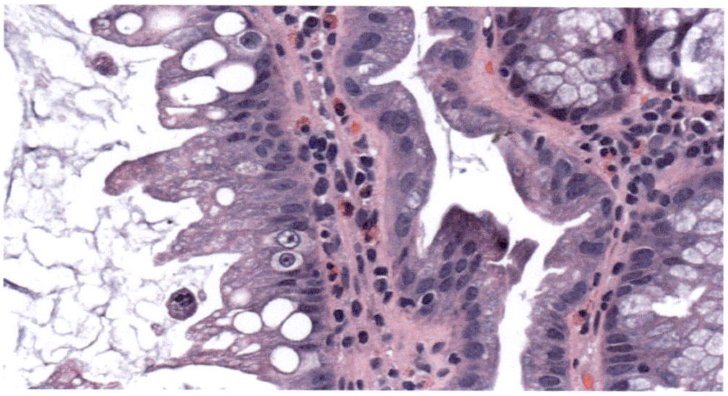

Fig. 1.26 Cytologic abnormalities in serrated dysplasia

Advanced sessile serrated adenomas/polyps (SSA/Ps) will show features of SSA and cytologic dysplasia within the same tissue fragment, as in Fig. 1.25. In cases where separate fragments of SSA and conventional adenoma are present, we report that the sample may represent either an advanced SSA or separate fragments of tubular adenoma and SSA.

In the serrated form of dysplasia, cytologic abnormalities manifest themselves not through hyperchromasia and crowding, as in conventional dysplasia. Instead, there are enlarged round vesicular nuclei with prominent nucleoli as in this case (Fig. 1.26).

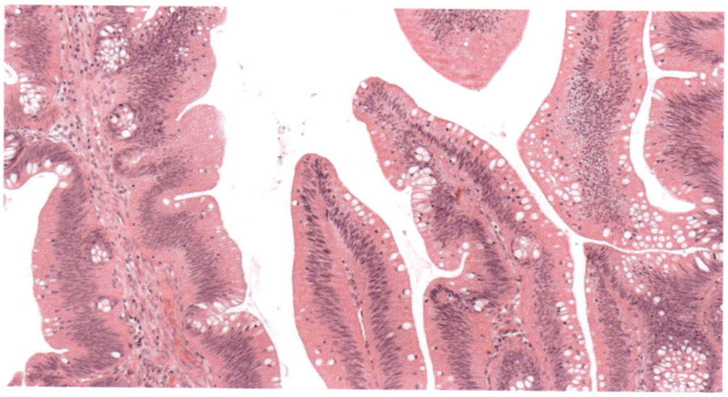

Fig. 1.27 Traditional serrated adenoma

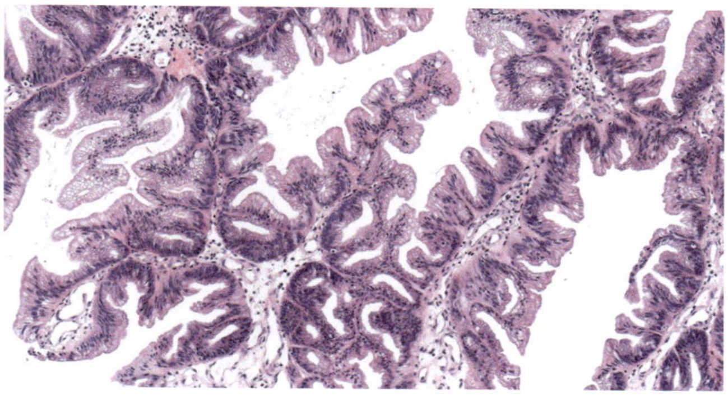

Fig. 1.28 Traditional serrated adenoma

1.5 Traditional Serrated Adenomas

Traditional serrated adenomas (TSAs) are typically large, villous, distally located polyps (Fig. 1.27). They characteristically have a very eosinophilic appearance imparted by abundant pink cytoplasm. Serrations can be more subtle than those in SSAs [22]. The most characteristic feature is the development of "ectopic crypts," which arise along the lengths of the villi and crypts. The nuclei are typically elongated (pencillate), though conventional dysplasia is often present (albeit of no clinical significance).

Occasionally serrated adenomas defy conventional classification. Figure 1.28 contains abundant gastric metaplasia, but has features otherwise typical of TSA in the form of ectopic crypt foci and elongated nuclei.

1.6 Duodenal/Periampullary Adenomas

Duodenal adenomas (Fig. 1.29) are histologically indistinguishable from their colorectal counterparts, though they are much rarer. They are often present in patients with familial adenomatous polyposis and can result in periampullary carcinomas when they progress.

An interesting phenomenon seen in some duodenal adenomas (and rarely in adenomas elsewhere) is the presence of pale cytoplasm in the neoplastic enterocytes (Fig. 1.30); this is believed by some to represent aberrant lipid resorption.

Dysplasia of the periampullary region may be of the intestinal type, which is similar to colorectal neoplasia, or of the pancreaticobiliary type (Fig. 1.31), which shares morphologic and molecular features with premalignant conditions of the exocrine pancreas and biliary tree. In this example, the neoplastic cells are more cuboidal than they are columnar, and there are complex, branching micropapillae with a greater degree of anisocytosis than in intestinal-type dysplasia.

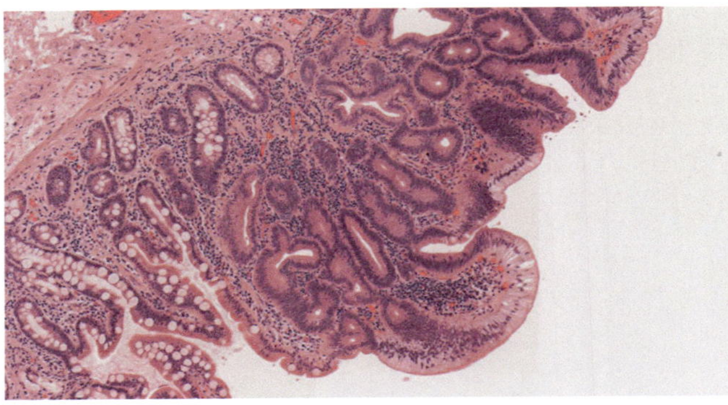

Fig. 1.29 Duodenal/periampullary adenoma

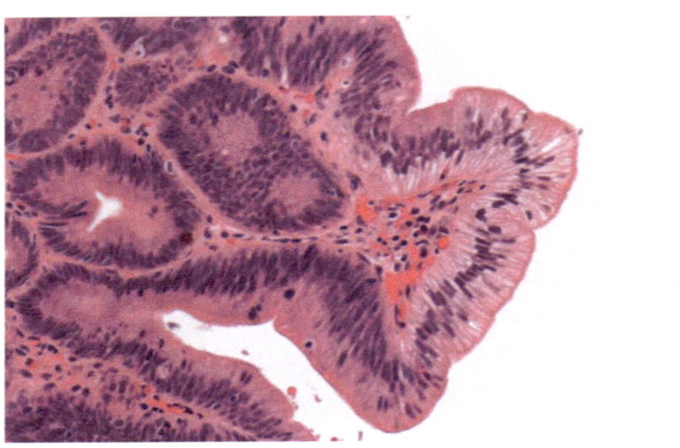

Fig. 1.30 Duodenal adenoma with pale cytoplasm in the neoplastic enterocytes

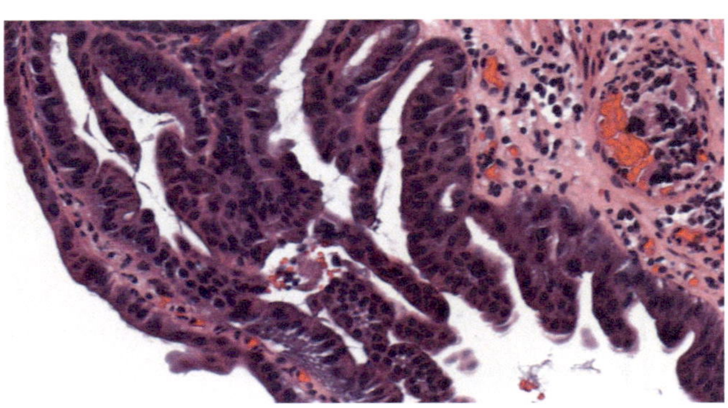

Fig. 1.31 Pancreaticobiliary high-grade dysplasia in a periampullary adenoma

1.7 Tubular Adenomas

Adenomas are one of the most common diagnoses seen by surgical pathologists. The diagnosis is typically straightforward, and is made at low power through the identification of epithelial cells with increased N:C ratios and nuclear hyperchromasia and pseudostratification. The dysplasia arises as a "top-down" process, such that the diagnostic changes of increased proliferation are more prominent superficially, and are more likely to be absent basally (Fig. 1.32). In contrast, nuclear hyperchromasia in normal mucosa and hyperplastic polyps is most prominent at the basal aspect of the epithelium. Dysplasia grade is primarily based on a low-power assessment of gland architecture [23, 24]. Low-grade dysplasia is characterized by the absence of cribriform and micropapillary architecture, dirty necrosis, and the absence of lamina propria invasion by small glands or single cells.

Low-grade dysplasia usually comprises hyperchromatic and pseudostratified cells that nevertheless maintain their nuclear polarity and show relative uniformity with one another (Fig. 1.33). Increased apoptotic activity and mitotic figures are also common findings in low-grade dysplasia.

Occasionally the pathologist will encounter only normal mucosa in specimens submitted as polyps. In most of these cases, deeper sectioning of the tissue in the block is recommended, as small adenomas may be located deeper in the tissue in up to 70% of cases, and are initially unsampled because of the tissue orientation. In Fig. 1.34, the inset shows the initial section; the deeper sections revealed a single dysplastic crypt at the surface of the tissue.

Along with polyp size, number and architecture, dysplasia grade is a variable used to stratify the risk of subsequent colorectal neoplasia, and thus helps to determine surveil-

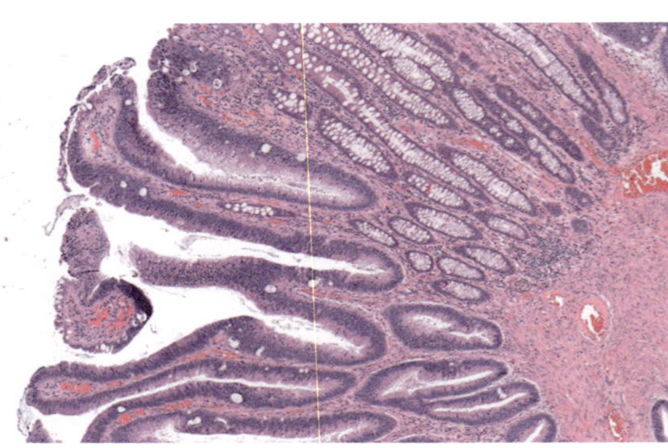

Fig. 1.32 Tubular adenoma

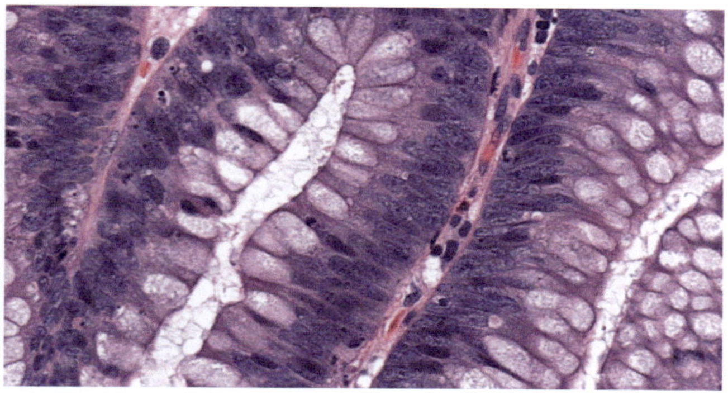

Fig. 1.33 Tubular adenoma (low-grade dysplasia)

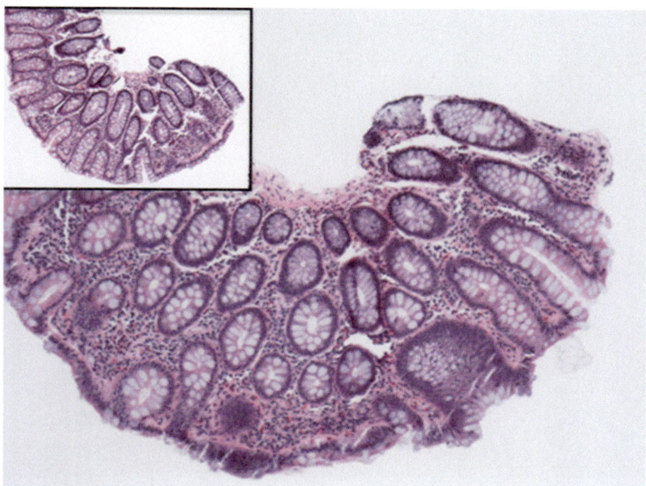

Fig. 1.34 Initial section (*inset*) and deeper section revealing a dysplastic crypt

lance intervals (5–10 years for low-grade dysplasia *versus* 3 years for high-grade dysplasia) [15, 16].

Colonic high-grade dysplasia is typically a low-power diagnosis. An emphasis should be placed on recognizing its architectural features to improve interobserver agreement, as the cytologic features of high-grade dysplasia are more likely to be subject to intraobserver and interobserver variability. The architectural features of high-grade dysplasia include cribriform formations with back-to-back glands, prominent glandular budding, and intraluminal papillary tufting. Glandular crowding alone is not a feature of high-grade dysplasia. In Fig. 1.35, cribriform crypts are readily recognized at low power to render a diagnosis of high-grade dysplasia.

Prominent intraluminal tufting, variability in nuclear size and orientation, and increased N:C ratios in high-grade dysplasia impart a blue and "dirty" appearance when compared with cases having only low-grade dysplasia (Fig. 1.36). More than one or two crypts should show the required high-grade features to avoid overinterpretation of occasionally tangentially sectioned branching crypts.

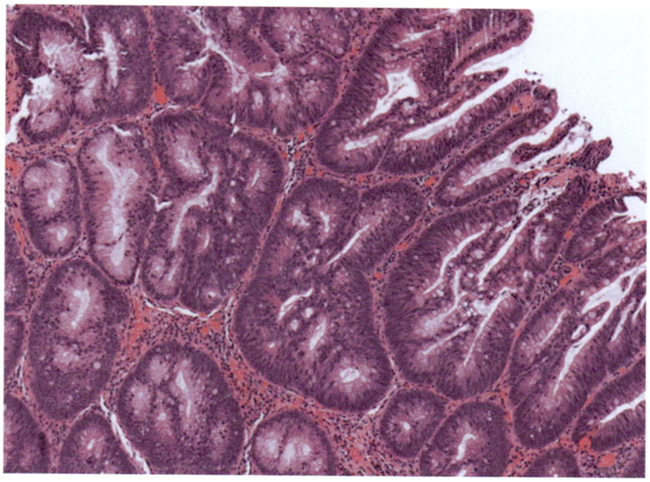

Fig. 1.35 Tubular adenoma (high-grade dysplasia)

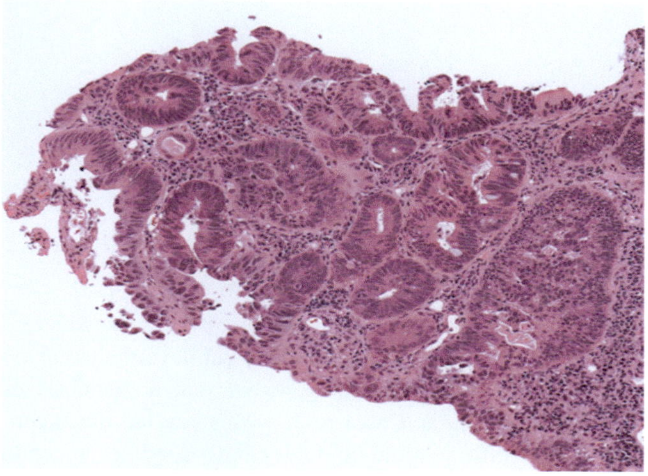

Fig. 1.36 Tubular adenoma (high-grade dysplasia)

Even when the crowded pattern of admixed, dissimilarly sized glands and single cells suggests a diagnosis of lamina propria invasion, the term "intramucosal carcinoma" should be avoided, as there is no risk of metastasis. Local excision suffices as treatment, as would be the case for high-grade dysplasia. Using the "high-grade dysplasia" term in such cases appropriately reflects the biologic potential of the lesion, while helping to prevent overtreatment. Some take this idea a step further, by commenting on the absence of metastatic potential, when a diagnosis of high-grade dysplasia is made.

The cytologic features of high-grade dysplasia that complement the architectural features include loss of cell polarity, nuclear stratification through the entire thickness of the epithelium, markedly enlarged nuclei with prominent nucleoli, atypical mitotic figures, dystrophic goblet cells, and prominent apoptosis (Fig. 1.37).

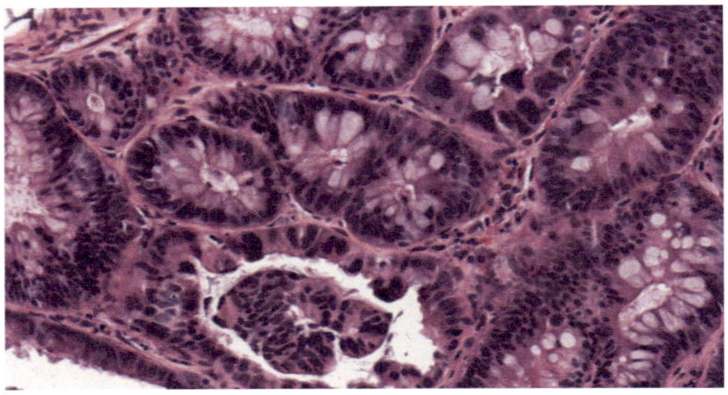

Fig. 1.37 Tubular adenoma (high-grade dysplasia)

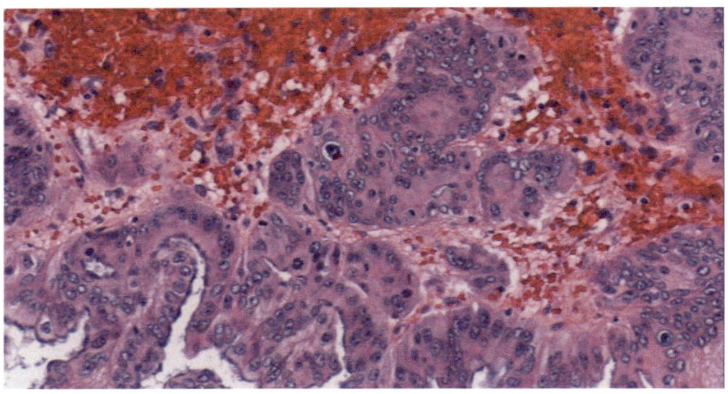

Fig. 1.38 Tubular adenoma (high-grade dysplasia)

Occasional cases of high-grade dysplasia show architectural features of low-grade dysplasia, but nevertheless show severe nuclear changes and likely warrant a diagnosis of high-grade dysplasia. Cases such as this one are the exception, and an effort should be made not to overinterpret mild to moderate cytologic changes, as they can inappropriately alter surveillance intervals.

High-grade dysplasia in other cases is present in the form of round, vesicular nuclei with prominent nucleoli, and is possibly related to "serrated dysplasia" which is seen in some advanced SSAs (Fig. 1.38). When there is extensive high-grade dysplasia or when the high-grade dysplasia is close to the muscularis mucosae, deeper sections of the tissue may be considered to exclude invasive carcinomas [25–28].

1.8 Villous and Tubulovillous Adenomas

Adenoma architecture is another one of the variables assessed when estimating the risk of subsequent colorectal neoplasia, which thus helps to determine surveillance intervals. Villi are leaf-like or finger-like projections of adenoma that extend from the polyp base into the lumen (Fig. 1.39).

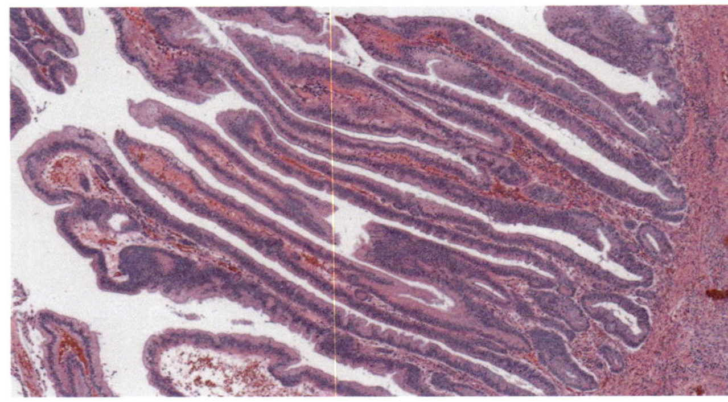

Fig. 1.39 Villous adenoma

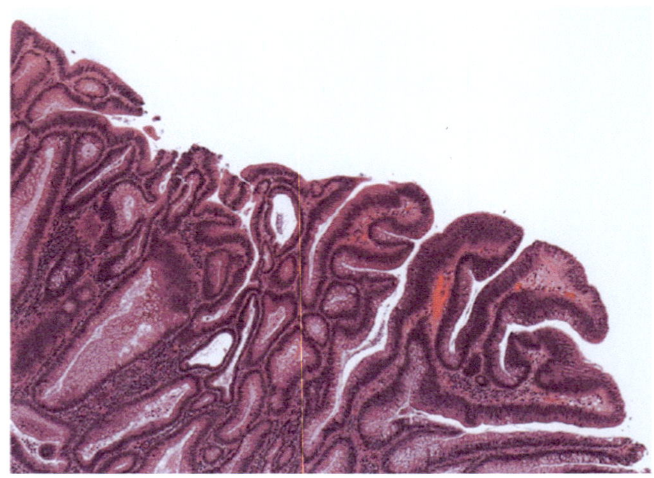

Fig. 1.40 Tubulovillous adenoma

Polyps in which less than 20–25% of the polyp is villous are classified as *tubular*. Polyps containing villi in 75–80% of their area are classified as *villous*. All other polyps are *tubulovillous* adenomas (Fig. 1.40). In practice, it is only important to distinguish between tubular *versus* tubulovillous or villous adenomas, as both tubulovillous and villous adenomas are treated similarly. (A screening interval of 3 years is recommended, compared with 5–10 years for tubular adenomas.)

It may be difficult to distinguish "true" villi from elongated and separated, axially sectioned crypts. Some arbitrarily define *villi* as structures that are more the twice the thickness of the normal colorectal mucosa, as in Fig. 1.41. In general, it is better to err on the side of under-diagnosis of villous changes, especially in small (<1 cm) adenomas. The term "at least tubulovillous" may be employed for small biopsies of a large polyp when at least one well-formed villus is present.

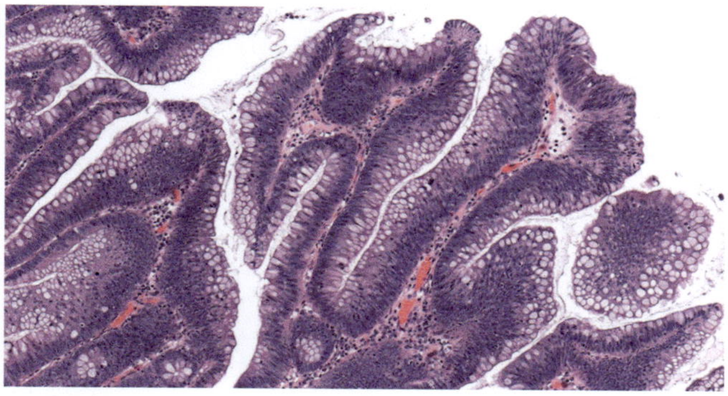

Fig. 1.41 Tubulovillous adenoma

1.9 Adenoma Variants

1.9.1 Clear Cell Changes

Clear cell changes are seen in less than 1% of adenomas, and have an endometrioid appearance (Fig. 1.42). They have been demonstrated to show aberrant MUC protein profiles compared with the background epithelium, and may evolve into adenocarcinomas that also demonstrate clear cell changes [29].

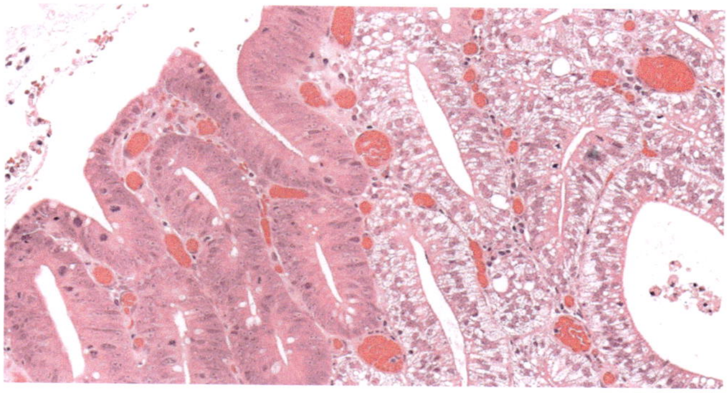

Fig. 1.42 Adenoma showing clear cell change

1.9.2 Paneth Cells

Paneth cells may be variably present in colorectal adenomas (Fig. 1.43). In some recent studies, their presence has been more frequent in males, and is associated with increased adenoma burden, as well as with a *decreased* risk of subsequent advanced neoplasia in distally located adenomas [30].

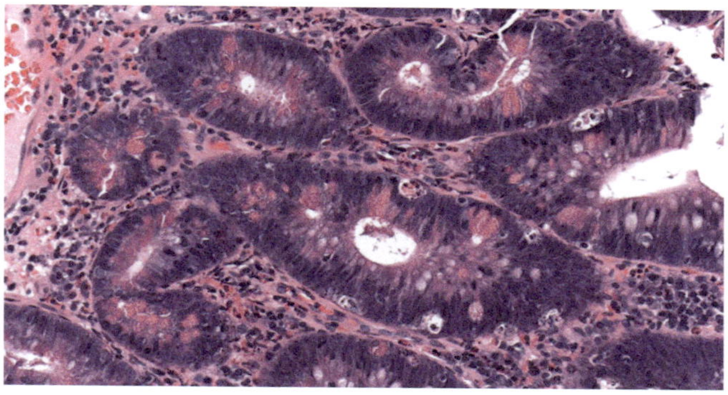

Fig. 1.43 Abundant Paneth cells in adenoma

1.9.3 Composite Adenoma-Microcarcinoid

Another rare variant of adenoma is the composite intestinal adenoma-microcarcinoid (Fig. 1.44). In these polyps, there is an intimate admixture of adenoma cells with a low-grade neuroendocrine proliferation. Typically the neuroendocrine component lacks significant nuclear pleomorphism, necrosis, and mitotic activity. Most cases behave in an indolent manner. Exceptionally, the neuroendocrine component may evolve into a neuroendocrine carcinoma [31].

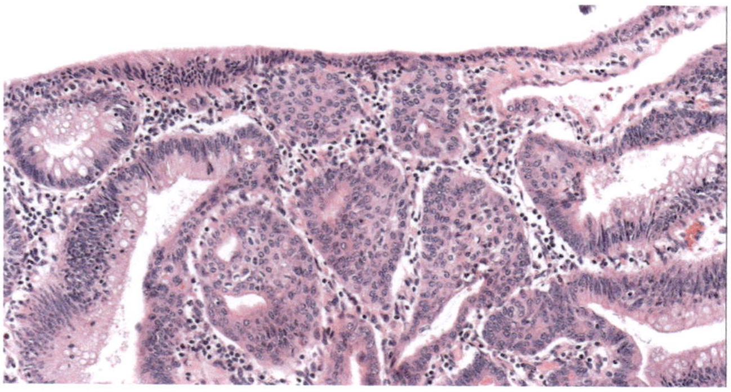

Fig. 1.44 Composite intestinal adenoma-microcarcinoid

1.9.4 Eroded Adenomas

Trauma in large adenomas may result in a superficial increase in lamina propria inflammation, granulation tissue formation, and smooth muscle proliferation in the lamina propria, as in Fig. 1.45. These may be associated with architectural

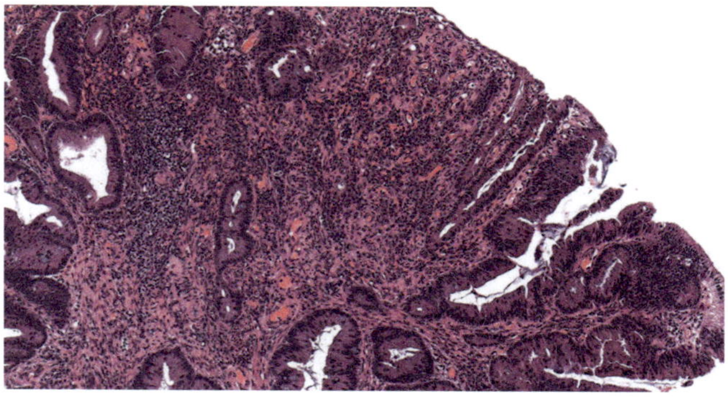

Fig. 1.45 Adenoma variant with erosions

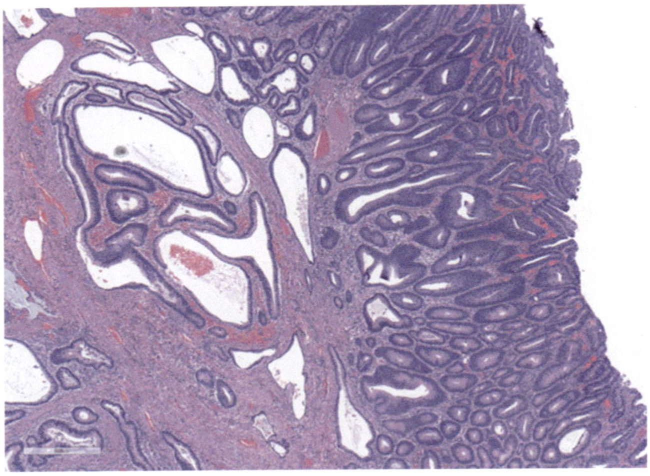

Fig. 1.46 Adenoma with epithelial misplacement (low-power view)

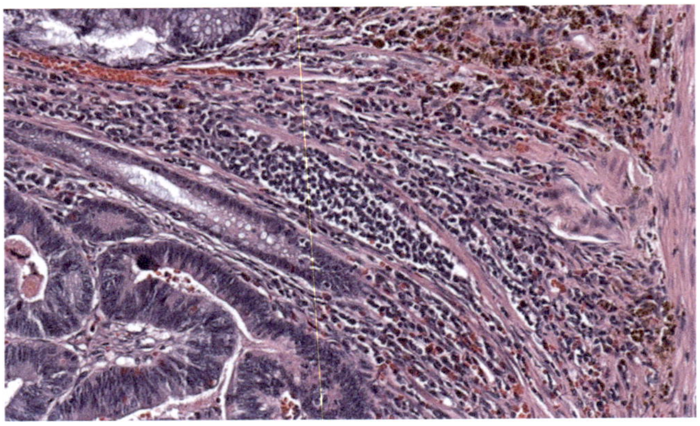

Fig. 1.47 Adenoma with epithelial misplacement (higher magnification)

distortion and increased cytologic atypia, which may mimic high-grade dysplasia or even invasive carcinoma [32]. A careful assessment of the polyp base is required in such cases to assess for the presence of an infiltrative edge and presence of a desmoplastic reaction.

1.9.5 Epithelial Misplacement

Epithelial misplacement in adenomas is a common phenomenon in the left colon, particularly the sigmoid; it results from repeated episodes of trauma, hemorrhage, and ischemia to the base of the polyp, or from previous biopsy. As a result, adenomatous epithelium and its associated lamina propria herniate below the mucosa into the underlying submucosa. The characteristic finding of low power is that of dilated, round to diamond-shaped crypts associated with surrounding hemorrhage and hemosiderin, distortion of the associated muscularis mucosae, and variable mucin pools (Fig. 1.46). It is important to recognize these features of epithelial misplacement, as the phenomenon can mimic the morphologic findings of invasive adenocarcinoma. The terms *mucosal herniation* and *pseudoinvasion* are also used to describe this phenomenon, although the latter term is discouraged, as it may create confusion.

On higher magnification (Fig. 1.47), the misplaced glands are seen to be associated with their corresponding lamina propria, which is characterized by a chronic inflammatory infiltrate of plasma cells, lymphocytes and eosinophils. The surrounding lamina propria hence has a characteristic red-white-blue appearance, which contrasts with the pale, desmoplastic response typically associated with invasive carcinomas. Hemorrhage, in the form of either red blood cells or hemosiderin-laden macrophages (*top right*), is also a helpful finding and should suggest the possibility of epithelial displacement whenever it is present.

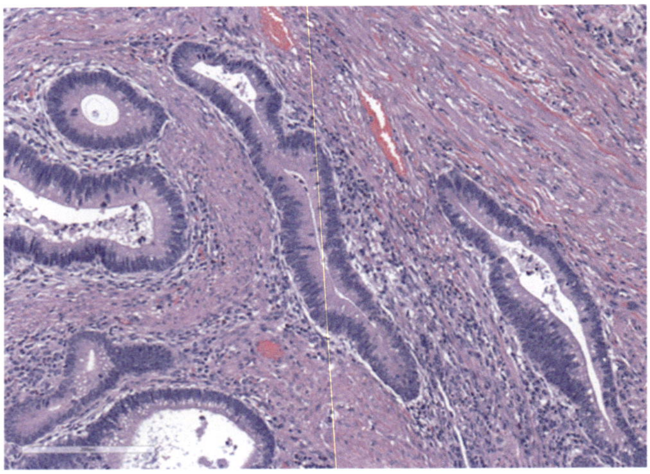

Fig. 1.48 Adenoma with epithelial misplacement

The misplaced glands may not always have readily identifiable lamina propria around their entire periphery, nor are they always of the characteristic round shape. In Fig. 1.48, the gland on the right lacks lamina propria around a large portion of its periphery, but it is morphologically identical otherwise to its neighboring glands with benign features. It is also similar to the overlying adenoma (*not shown*).

Mucin pools are frequently seen in cases with epithelial displacement, and may raise the possibility of an associated mucinous carcinoma. In contrast to malignant mucin pools, mucin pools in benign epithelial displacement are either acellular or are associated with a single layer of adenomatous epithelium in long strips within the mucin or lining the periphery of the pool, as in Fig. 1.49. In contrast, mucinous carcinoma contains either single cells (often signet ring–like) or irregular clusters of malignant cells within the mucin pools.

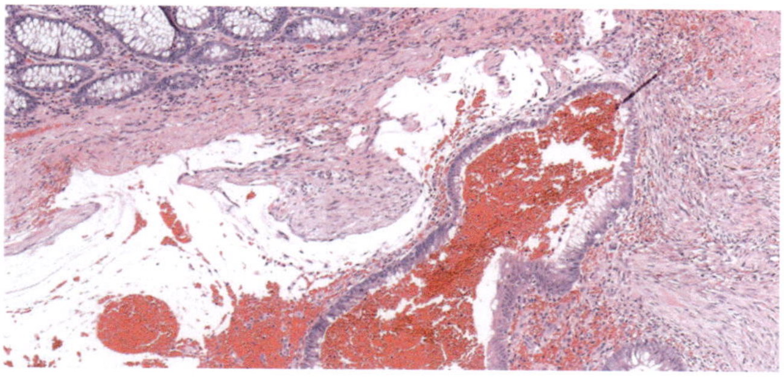

Fig. 1.49 Adenoma with epithelial misplacement and mucin pool

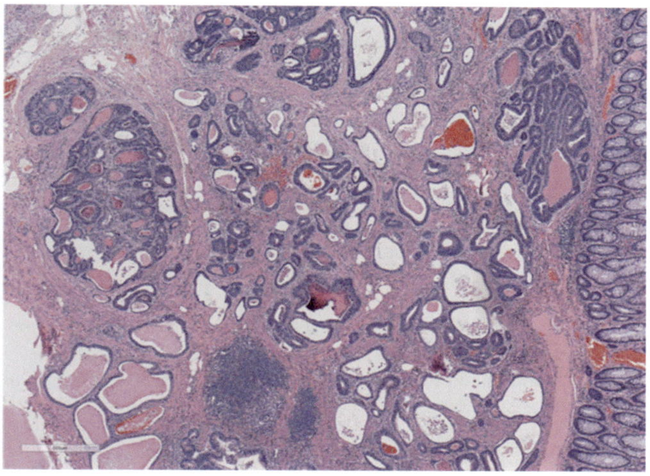

Fig. 1.50 Adenoma with epithelial misplacement and high-grade dysplasia

The constellation of aforementioned findings usually result in the correct identification of misplaced epithelium. It is typically not necessary to include this feature in a diagnostic line, as it has no clinical significance other than being necessary for pathologists to identify. Problematic situations include the aforementioned absence of lamina propria, *bona fide* very well-differentiated adenocarcinomas, and high-grade dysplasia that involves misplaced epithelium, as in Fig. 1.50, where two foci of crowded, cytologically distinct adenomatous epithelium are present in the left-side of the image.

Higher magnification (Fig. 1.51) shows that these foci show increased gland crowding, and are cytologically more high-grade than the remainder of the adenoma. The presence of adjacent glands with low-grade dysplasia surrounded by lamina propria, as well as focal hemosiderin amidst the high-grade dysplasia, are most compatible with an interpretation of high-grade dysplasia within misplaced mucosa, rather than invasive carcinoma. Although invasive carcinoma cannot be excluded in rare cases, such cases rarely warrant further management, as the equivocal foci typically lack features associated with nodal metastases and are distant from the margins. Polypectomy usually suffices as treatment, regardless of whether an equivocal focus is diagnosed as carcinoma

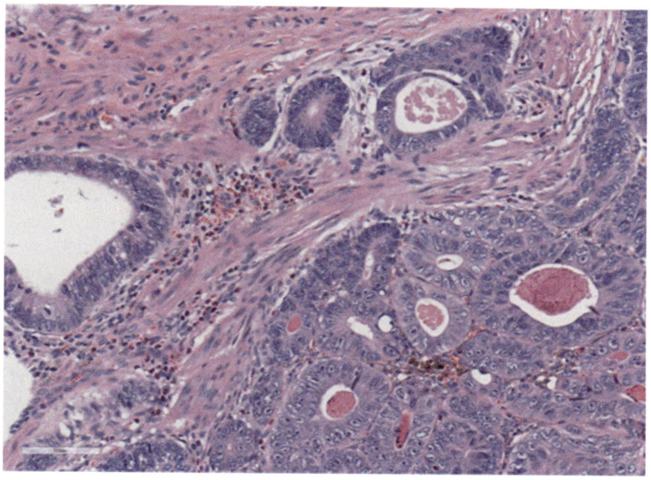

Fig. 1.51 Adenoma with epithelial misplacement and high-grade dysplasia (high-power view)

or misplaced epithelium. Immunohistochemistry (p53, E-cadherin) has been suggested as an adjunctive test in challenging cases [33, 34].

References

1. Jepsen JM, Persson M, Jakobsen NO, Christiansen T, Skoubo-Kristensen E, Funch-Jensen P, et al. Prospective study of prevalence and endoscopic and histopathologic characteristics of duodenal polyps in patients submitted to upper endoscopy. Scand J Gastroenterol. 1994;29:483–7.
2. Kelly JK, Langevin JM, Price LM, Hershfield NB, Share S, Blustein P. Giant and symptomatic inflammatory polyps of the colon in idiopathic inflammatory bowel disease. Am J Surg Pathol. 1986;10:420–8.
3. Chetty R, Bhathal PS, Slavin JL. Prolapse-induced inflammatory polyps of the colorectum and anal transitional zone. Histopathology. 1993;23:63–7.
4. Meniconi RL, Caronna R, Benedetti M, Fanello G, Ciardi A, Schiratti M, et al. Inflammatory myoglandular polyp of the cecum: case report and review of literature. BMC Gastroenterol. 2010;10:10.
5. Shaco-Levy R, Jasperson KW, Martin K, Samadder NJ, Burt RW, Ying J, Bronner MP. Morphologic characterization of hamartomatous gastrointestinal polyps in Cowden syndrome, Peutz-Jeghers syndrome, and juvenile polyposis syndrome. Hum Pathol. 2016;49:39–48.
6. Iqbal U, Chaudhary A, Karim MA, Anwar H, Merrell N. Cronkhite-Canada syndrome: a rare cause of chronic diarrhea. Gastroenterology Res. 2017;10:196–8.
7. Jansen M. Mucosal prolapse in the pathogenesis of Peutz-Jeghers polyposis. Gut. 2006;55:1–5.
8. Sethi A, Anspach-Hanson J. A morphologic reappraisal of endoscopically but not histologically apparent polyps and the emergence of the overlooked goblet cell--rich hyperplastic polyp. Hum Pathol. 2015;46:1147–52.
9. Choi EY, Appelman HD. A historical perspective and exposé on serrated polyps of the colorectum. Arch Pathol Lab Med. 2016;140:1079–84.

10. Huang CC, Frankel WL, Doukides T, Zhou XP, Zhao W, Yearsley MM. Prolapse-related changes are a confounding factor in misdiagnosis of sessile serrated adenomas in the rectum. Hum Pathol. 2013;44:480–6.
11. Torlakovic E, Skovlund E, Snover DC, Torlakovic G, Nesland JM. Morphologic reappraisal of serrated colorectal polyps. Am J Surg Pathol. 2003;27:65–81.
12. Quirke P, Risio M, Lambert R, von Karsa L, Vieth M. Quality assurance in pathology in colorectal cancer screening and diagnosis—European recommendations. Virchows Arch. 2011;458:1–19.
13. Huang CS, Farraye FA, Yang S, O'Brien MJ. The clinical significance of serrated polyps. Am J Gastroenterol. 2011;106:229–40.
14. Snover DC. Update on the serrated pathway to colorectal carcinoma. Hum Pathol. 2011;42:1–10.
15. Winawer SJ, Zauber AG, Fletcher RH, Stillman JS, O'Brien MJ, Levin B, US Multi-Society Task Force on Colorectal Cancer, American Cancer Society, et al. Guidelines for colonoscopy surveillance after polypectomy: a consensus update by the US Multi-Society Task Force on Colorectal Cancer and the American Cancer Society. Gastroenterology. 2006;130:1872–85.
16. Lieberman DA, Rex DK, Winawer SJ, Giardiello FM, Johnson DA, Levin TR. Guidelines for colonoscopy surveillance after screening and polypectomy: a consensus update by the US Multi-Society Task Force on Colorectal Cancer. Gastroenterology. 2012;143:844–57.
17. Higuchi T, Sugihara K, Jass JR. Demographic and pathological characteristics of serrated polyps of colorectum. Histopathology. 2005;47:32–40.
18. Oka S, Tanaka S, Hiyama T, Ito M, Kitadai Y, Yoshihara M, et al. Clinicopathologic and endoscopic features of colorectal serrated adenoma: differences between polypoid and superficial types. Gastrointest Endosc. 2004;59:213–9.
19. Snover DC, Jass JR, Fenoglio-Preiser C, Batts KP. Serrated polyps of the large intestine: a morphologic and molecular review of an evolving concept. Am J Clin Pathol. 2005;124:380–91.
20. Lash RH, Genta RM, Schuler CM. Sessile serrated adenomas: prevalence of dysplasia and carcinoma in 2139 patients. J Clin Pathol. 2010;63:681–6.
21. Jass JR. Serrated route to colorectal cancer: back street or super highway? J Pathol. 2001;193:283–5.
22. Torlakovic EE, Gomez JD, Driman DK, Parfitt JR, Wang C, Benerjee T, Snover DC. Sessile serrated adenoma (SSA) vs. traditional serrated adenoma (TSA). Am J Surg Pathol. 2008;32:21–9.. Erratum in: Am J Surg Pathol. 2008;32:491
23. Levin B, Lieberman DA, McFarland B, Andrews KS, Brooks D, Bond J, American Cancer Society Colorectal Cancer Advisory Group, US Multi-Society Task Force, American College of Radiology Colon Cancer Committee, et al. Screening and surveillance for the early detection of colorectal cancer and adenomatous polyps, 2008: a joint guideline from the American Cancer Society, the US Multi-Society Task Force on Colorectal Cancer, and the American College of Radiology. Gastroenterology. 2008;134:1570–95.
24. East JE, Saunders BP, Jass JP. Sporadic and syndromic hyperplastic polyps and serrated adenomas of the colon: classification, molecular genetics, natural history and clinical management. Gastroenterol Clin N Am. 2008;37:25–46.
25. Groff RJ, Nash R, Ahnen DJ. Significance of serrated polyps of the colon. Curr Gastroenterol Rep. 2008;10:490–8.
26. Schick BA, McLean CA, Driman DK. Negative colorectal polyp biopsies: the utility of cutting deeper levels. Virchows Arch. 2015;467:635–40.
27. Wu ML, Dry SM, Lassman CR. Deeper examination of negative colorectal biopsies. Am J Clin Pathol. 2002;117:424–8.
28. Nash JW, Niemann T, Marsh WL, Frankel WL. To step or not to step: an approach to clinically diagnosed polyps with no initial pathologic finding. Am J Clin Pathol. 2002;117:419–23.
29. Shi C, Scudiere JR, Cornish TC, Lam-Himlin D, Park JY, Fox MR, Montgomery EA. Clear cell change in colonic tubular adenoma and corresponding colonic clear cell adenocarcinoma is associated with an altered mucin core protein profile. Am J Surg Pathol. 2010;34:1344–50.
30. Mahon M, Xu J, Yi X, Liu X, Gao N, Zhang L. Paneth cell in adenomas of the distal colorectum is inversely associated with synchronous advanced adenoma and carcinoma. Sci Rep. 2016;6:26129.
31. Lin J, Goldblum JR, Bennett AE, Bronner MP, Liu X. Composite intestinal adenoma-microcarcinoid. Am J Surg Pathol. 2012;36:292–5.
32. Tanizawa T, Seki T, Nakano M, Kamiyama R. Pseudoinvasion of the colorectal polypoid tumors: serial section study of problematic cases. Pathol Int. 2003;53:584–90.
33. Yantiss RK, Bosenberg MW, Antonioli DA, Odze RD. Utility of MMP-1, p53, E-cadherin, and collagen IV immunohistochemical stains in the differential diagnosis of adenomas with misplaced epithelium versus adenomas with invasive adenocarcinoma. Am J Surg Pathol. 2002;26:206–15.
34. Panarelli NC, Somarathna T, Samowitz WS, Kornacki S, Sanders SA, Novelli MR, et al. Diagnostic challenges caused by endoscopic biopsy of colonic polyps: a systematic evaluation of epithelial misplacement with review of problematic polyps from the Bowel Cancer Screening Program, United Kingdom. Am J Surg Pathol. 2016;40:1075–83.

2 Colorectal Carcinoma

Aaron Pollett

Colorectal carcinoma is the most common cancer of the digestive tract. It is the third most common cancer in men and women and the third leading cause of cancer death worldwide. Colorectal cancers are divided into three main anatomic areas: the right colon, left colon, and rectum. While the definition of the rectum varies, anatomically it is marked by the fusion of the tenia coli of the sigmoid to form a circumferential longitudinal muscle. As opposed to the sigmoid, which is intraperitoneal with a mesentery, the rectum has a partial or no peritoneal covering and no mesentery. The colon on the right side of the splenic flexure is considered the right colon and the colon on the left side of the splenic flexure is considered the left colon. The underlying molecular biology appears to be different between cancers of the right and left colon; right-sided colonic cancers are more likely to have high-frequency microsatellite instability (MSI-H) and harbor BRAF mutations. The clear majority (> 95%) of colorectal carcinomas are of glandular origin; rare types of carcinoma include adenosquamous, squamous, spindle cell, and undifferentiated carcinoma. The World Health Organization (WHO) classification of colorectal carcinomas includes six histologic subtypes of invasive adenocarcinoma, cribriform comedo-type adenocarcinoma, medullary carcinoma, micropapillary carcinoma, colloid carcinoma, serrated carcinoma, and signet ring cell carcinoma. Adenocarcinoma NOS is the most common type of colorectal adenocarcinoma, accounting for 80% of colorectal adenocarcinomas. The histologic subtype of the carcinoma gives prognostic information and different morphologies are associated with different underlying molecular changes. While immunohistochemistry is rarely needed for the diagnosis, colorectal carcinomas are typically positive for cytokeratin 20 (CK20), CDX2, special AT-rich sequence-binding protein 2 (SATB2), and villin, and are negative for cytokeratin 7 (CK7). CDX2 can be lost in high-grade colorectal adenocarcinoma and is associated with a worse prognosis. MSI-H colorectal carcinomas can have aberrant immunohistochemical expression, including loss of CK20 expression and CK7 positivity. The possibility of an MSI-H colorectal carcinoma should be considered with colorectal tumors with unusual morphologies and atypical immunohistochemical expression.

Low-grade tubuloglandular carcinoma is a subtype found in approximately 10% of adenocarcinomas arising in inflammatory bowel disease (IBD). While typically associated with dysplastic changes, the dysplasia in IBD can be subtle, and tubuloglandular carcinoma can be associated with low-grade dysplastic changes, making it difficult to detect on biopsies (Figs. 2.1, 2.2, 2.3, 2.4, 2.5, 2.6, 2.7, 2.8, 2.9, 2.10, 2.11, 2.12, 2.13, 2.14, 2.15, 2.16, 2.17, 2.18, 2.19, 2.20, 2.21, 2.22, 2.23, 2.24, 2.25, 2.26, 2.27, 2.28, 2.29, 2.30, 2.31, 2.32, 2.33, 2.34, 2.35, 2.36, and 2.37).

H. H. Li-Chang et al., *Atlas of Intestinal Pathology*, Atlas of Anatomic Pathology,
https://doi.org/10.1007/978-3-030-12379-6_2

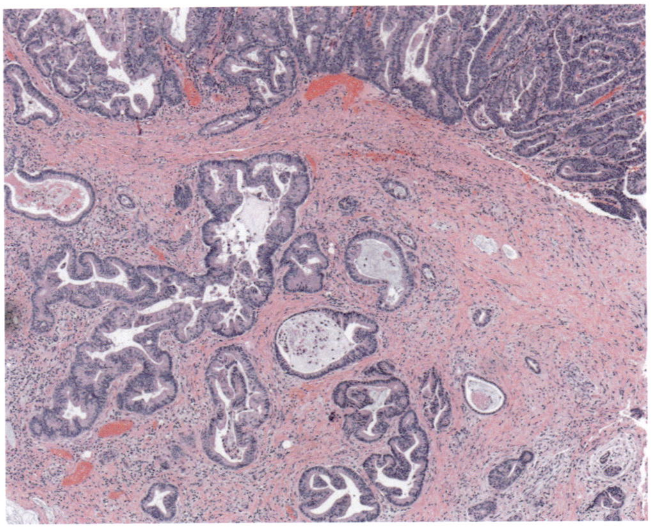

Fig. 2.1 Well-differentiated adenocarcinoma. The grading of colorectal adenocarcinomas is based on the extent of glandular formation. Excluding the leading front edge, the tumor grade is based on the region with the highest grade. Well-differentiated adenocarcinomas are >95% gland-forming and account for 15–20% of colorectal adenocarcinomas. The glands tend to be well formed; while a desmoplastic stromal reaction is typically present, it is not required for diagnosis. Some well-differentiated adenocarcinomas may have a lamina propria, so the presence of lamina propria does not exclude invasion

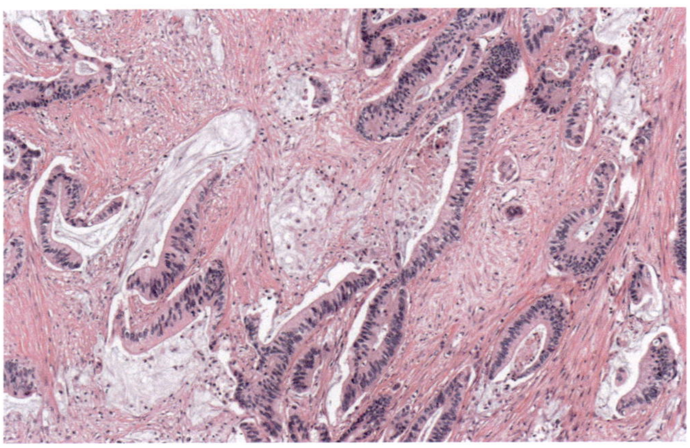

Fig. 2.2 Moderately-differentiated adenocarcinoma. Moderately differentiated adenocarcinoma is the most common colorectal adenocarcinoma, accounting for 60–70% of cases. The tumors are 50–95% gland forming. The glands tend to be more disorganized than the glands of well-differentiated adenocarcinomas and are often filled with necrotic debris ("dirty necrosis"). In some grading systems, well-differentiated and moderately differentiated tumors are combined as low-grade adenocarcinomas, but currently a 3– (or 4–) grade system is preferred for describing colorectal adenocarcinomas

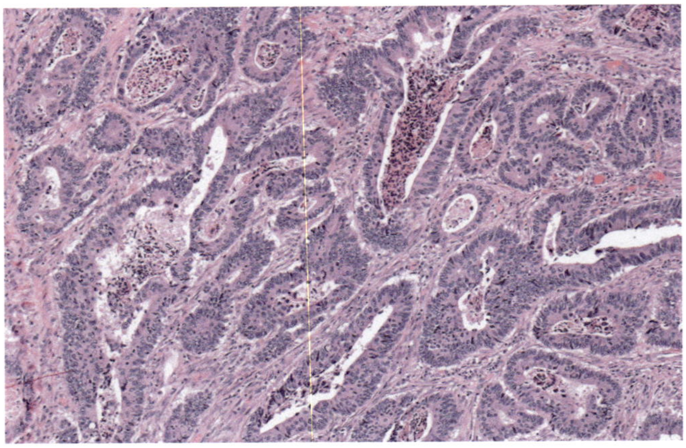

Fig. 2.3 Moderately differentiated adenocarcinoma with dirty necrosis. Intraluminal necrosis (as seen in this case) is common in colorectal carcinomas. The degree of glandular differentiation and cellular atypia is typical for a moderately differentiated colorectal adenocarcinoma

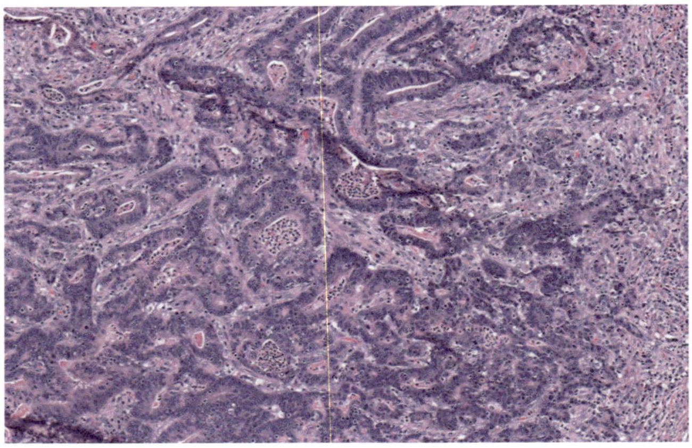

Fig. 2.4 Moderately differentiated colonic adenocarcinoma. Most invasive colorectal adenocarcinomas are associated with a desmoplastic stromal reaction (as seen in this case). There are exceptions with some low-grade colorectal adenocarcinomas, in particular the low-grade tubuloglandular adenocarcinomas associated with inflammatory bowel disease (*see* Figs. 2.20, 2.21, and 2.22)

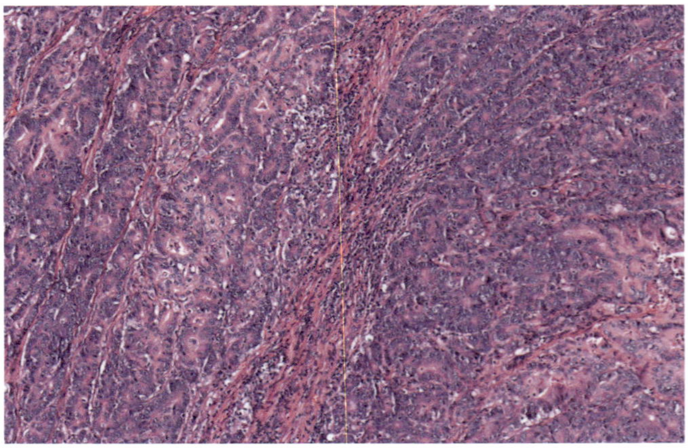

Fig. 2.5 Moderately differentiated adenocarcinoma. In this case the glands of the tumor are tightly packed together, but the tumor is still more than 50% gland-forming and should be considered moderately differentiated

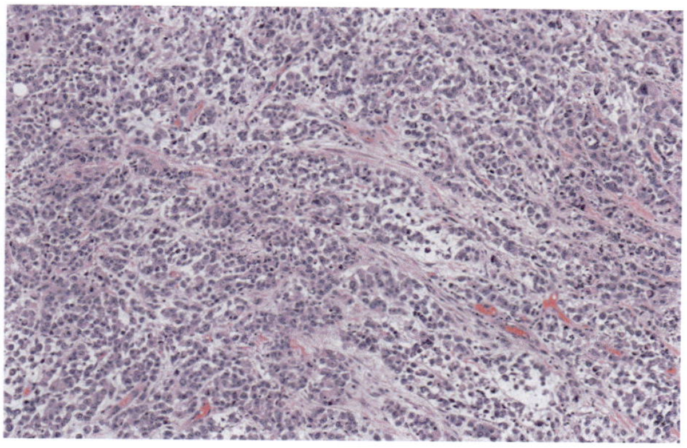

Fig. 2.6 Poorly differentiated adenocarcinoma. Poorly differentiated adenocarcinomas are <50% gland-forming. Approximately 15–20% of colorectal adenocarcinomas are poorly differentiated. The tumor can be composed of sheets of tumor cells, infiltrating nests, or individual infiltrating cells. Tumors with no glandular or mucinous differentiation can be further classified as undifferentiated adenocarcinomas (when a 4-point grading system is used). Poorly differentiated adenocarcinomas have a worse prognosis. In this case the tumor is infiltrating predominately as individual cells

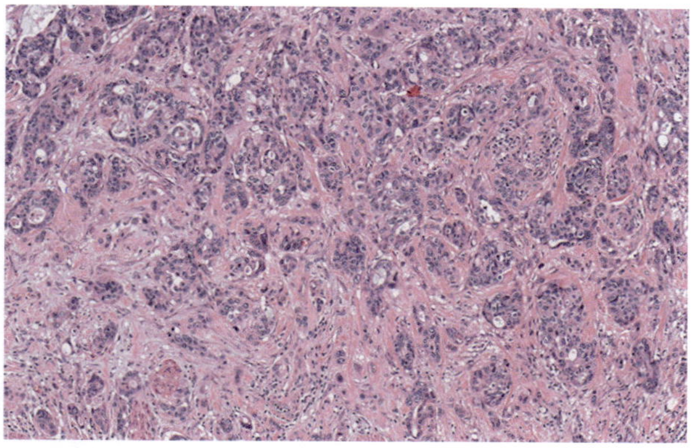

Fig. 2.7 Poorly differentiated adenocarcinoma. Poorly differentiated adenocarcinomas can also infiltrate as irregular islands. In this case the tumor islands are embedded in a desmoplastic stroma with only focal gland formation

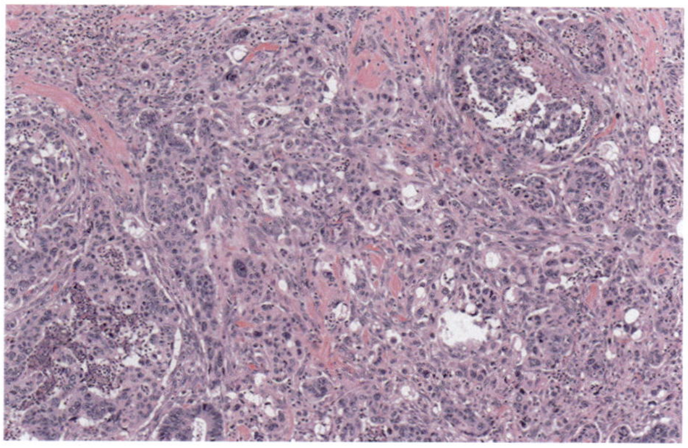

Fig. 2.8 Poorly differentiated adenocarcinoma. Poorly differentiated adenocarcinoma can also form solid areas of tumor growth. In this case the tumor also demonstrates marked cellular atypia with enlarged tumor cells. The degree of cellular atypia in this case is more than would typically be seen in moderately differentiated adenocarcinoma and supports a poorly differentiated adenocarcinoma

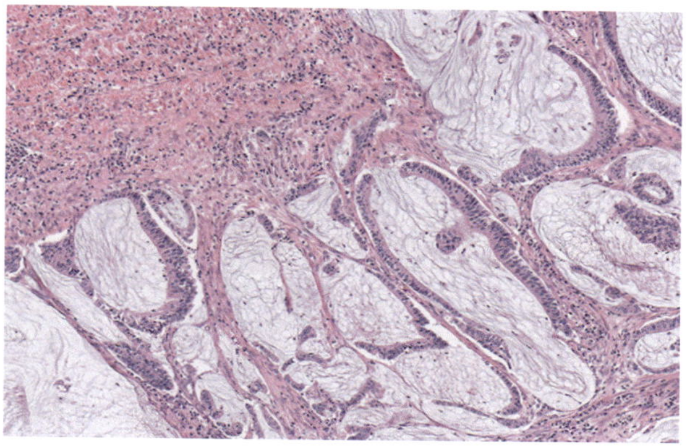

Fig. 2.9 Colloid (mucinous) adenocarcinoma. Mucinous adenocarcinomas account for approximately 10% of colorectal adenocarcinomas. They consist of pools of mucin with malignant epithelium; >50% of the tumor must have a mucinous morphology to be considered a mucinous adenocarcinoma. Most mucinous adenocarcinomas are microsatellite stable (MSS) but mucinous adenocarcinomas are more likely to have high-frequency microsatellite instability (MSI-H) than conventional adenocarcinomas. KRAS mutations are also more common in mucinous adenocarcinomas compared to conventional adenocarcinomas. The prognosis of mucinous adenocarcinomas compared to conventional (moderately differentiated) colorectal adenocarcinomas is debatable, with mucinous carcinomas having a similar or slightly worse prognosis. In this case the tumor is composed of mucin lakes lined by malignant epithelium

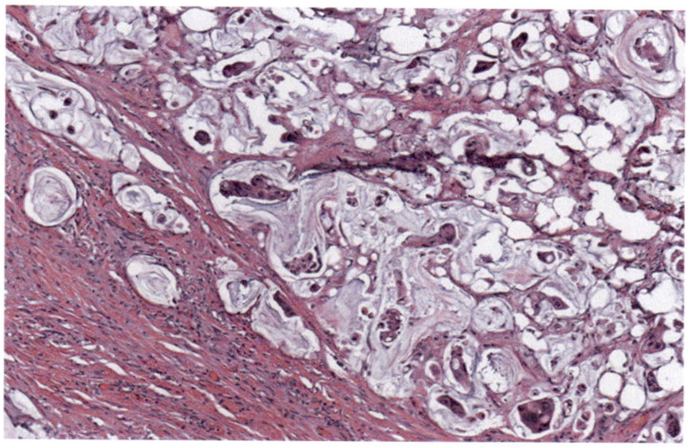

Fig. 2.10 Colloid (mucinous) adenocarcinoma. Mucinous adenocarcinoma can also be composed of tumor islands floating in mucin. The nuclear atypia seen in the floating tumor islands can vary. This case shows poorly differentiated tumor cells but the nuclei may show clusters of well-differentiated or moderately differentiated tumor cells

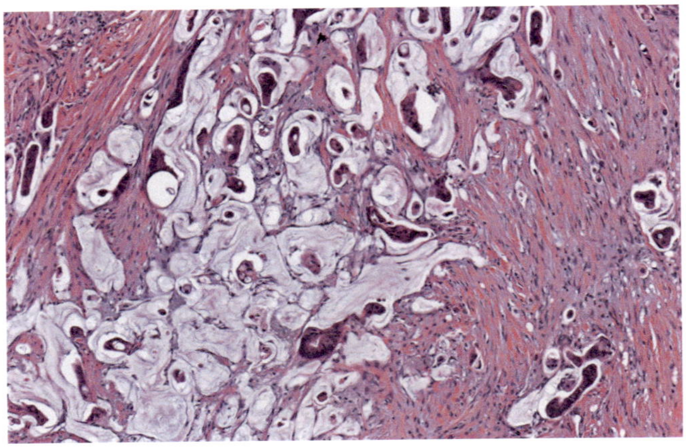

Fig. 2.11 Colloid carcinoma with scattered signet ring tumor cells. Scattered signet ring tumor cells can be seen in colloid (mucinous) adenocarcinomas. For a tumor to be classified as a signet ring carcinoma, >50% of the tumor cells have to be signet ring cells. The presence of signet ring tumor cells in any adenocarcinoma is a poor prognostic figure, and this tumor will behave more aggressively than colloid carcinomas without signet ring cells

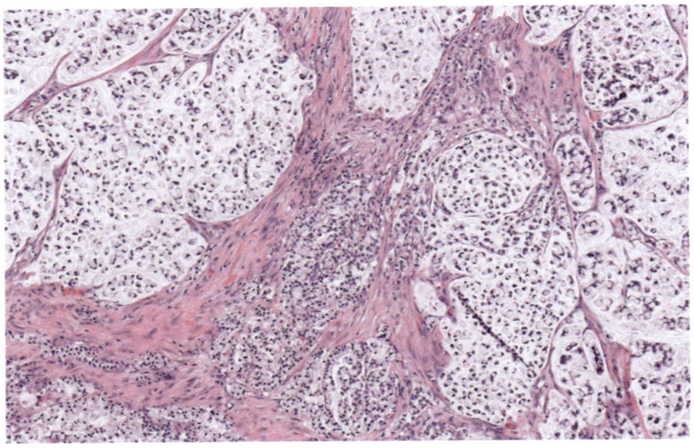

Fig. 2.12 Signet ring carcinoma. True signet ring cell colorectal adenocarcinomas are rare (<1% of colorectal adenocarcinomas). Signet ring cells are composed of tumor cells with a prominent intracytoplasmic mucin vacuole, while classic signet rings have a displaced, hyperchromatic nucleus. Signet ring carcinomas are composed of >50% signet ring cells. The tumor cells may be associated with mucin pools or may diffusely invade the colonic wall. Signet ring carcinomas have a worse prognosis than conventional colorectal adenocarcinoma. In cases where signet ring cells are <50% of tumor cells, the presence of signet ring tumor cells is a poor prognostic feature

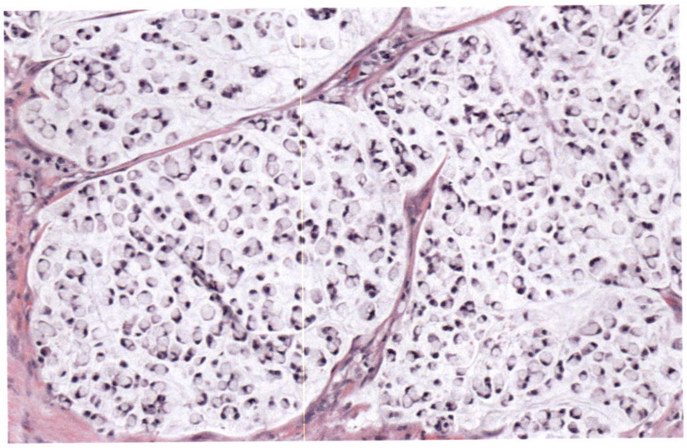

Fig. 2.13 Signet ring carcinoma. A medium-power view of a signet ring carcinoma. Individual malignant cells are seen floating in mucin. While occasionally colonic signet ring carcinomas can infiltrate the wall of the colon, similar to the way gastric signet ring carcinoma extends into the gastric wall, signet ring carcinomas of the colon are more often associated with extracellular mucin

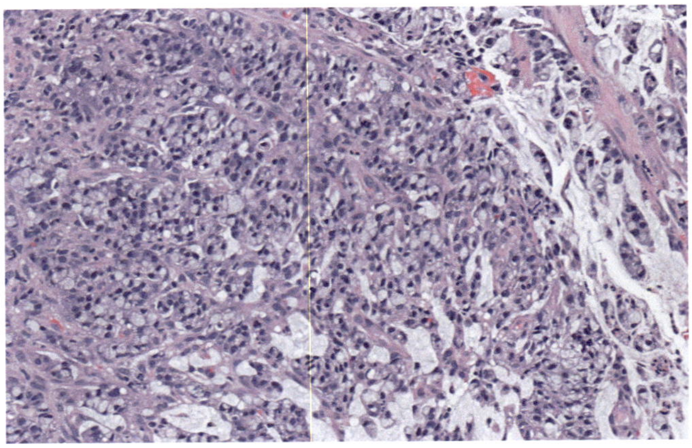

Fig. 2.14 Signet ring carcinoma. Signet ring carcinomas can have variable cellularity, including areas of individual cell infiltration into the wall of the colon or areas of solid tumor growth. In order to be classified as a signet ring carcinoma, >50% of the tumor cells need to have a signet ring morphology

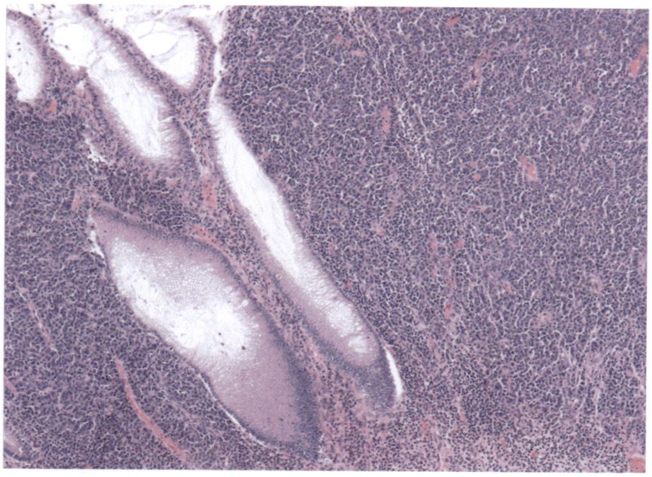

Fig. 2.15 Medullary carcinoma. A rare adenocarcinoma (<1% of cases), medullary carcinoma is composed of sheets of malignant cells with vesicular nuclei, prominent nucleoli, and abundant pink cytoplasm associated with a prominent infiltration by intraepithelial lymphocytes. Medullary carcinomas are strongly associated with high-frequency microsatellite instability (MSI-H), and despite the poorly differentiated epithelium, have a favorable prognosis

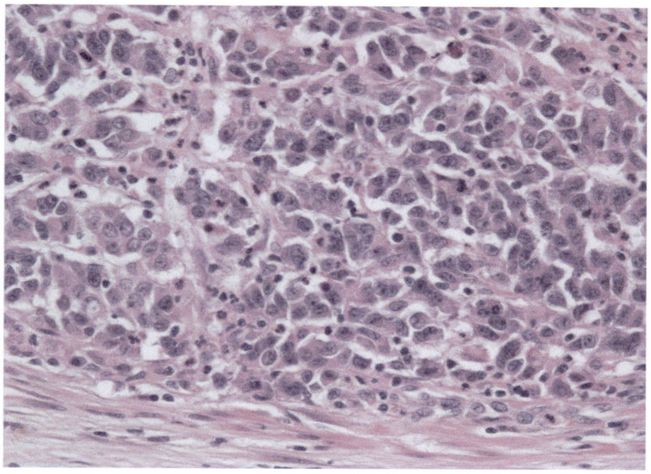

Fig. 2.16 Medullary carcinoma. The higher-power view of the medullary carcinoma highlights the poorly differentiated tumor cells, marked lymphoid infiltrate and rounded ("pushing") nature of the invasive tumor front

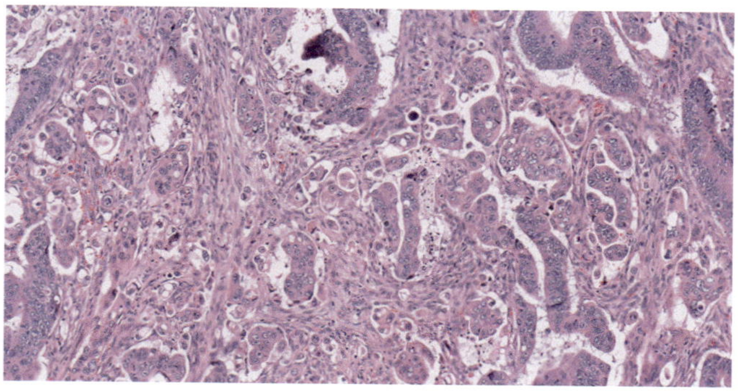

Fig. 2.17 Micropapillary carcinoma. Micropapillary adenocarcinomas are identified by small clusters of malignant cells with abundant eosinophilic cytoplasm and pleomorphic nuclei. The tumor nests have the apical surface towards the periphery rather than the center, giving it a micropapillary appearance similar to that seen in other tumor types. Micropapillary features can be found in 9–20% of colorectal adenocarcinoma and are commonly seen in association with conventional colorectal adenocarcinoma. The presence of a micropapillary component is a poor prognostic feature; lymphovascular and lymph node metastasis are common even with T1 or T2 tumors

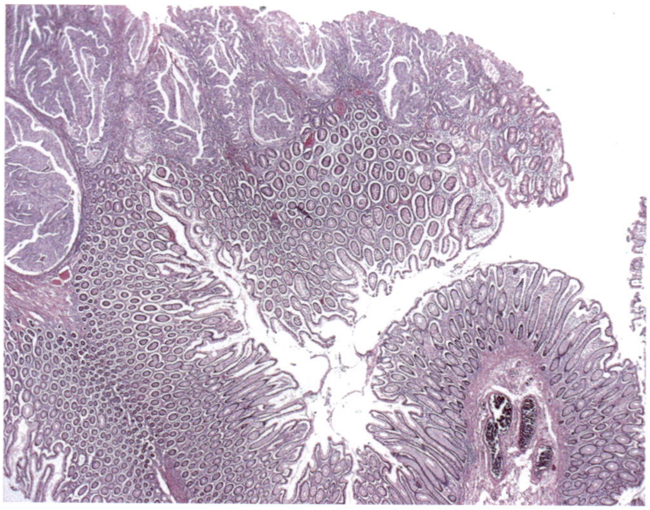

Fig. 2.18 Serrated adenocarcinomas. Serrated adenocarcinomas account for approximately 10% of all colorectal adenocarcinomas. The epithelium has serrations with epithelial tufts and lack true papillary projects. There is abundant clear or eosinophilic cytoplasm. Necrosis is absent or only focally present. Serrated adenocarcinomas are more aggressive than conventional adenocarcinomas. They are associated with a more rapid appearance and growth pattern. BRAF mutations are commonly found in serrated adenocarcinomas

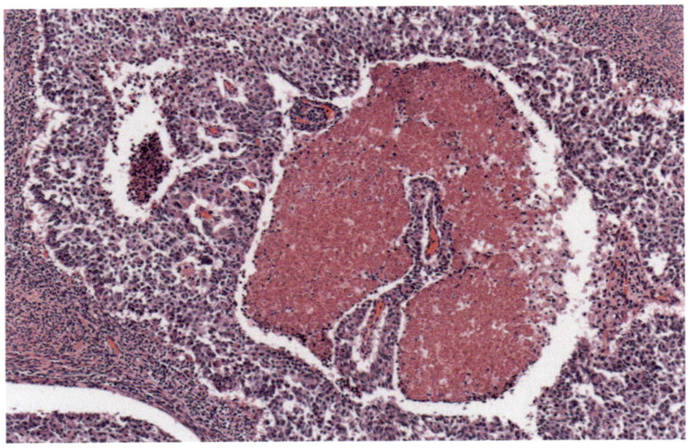

Fig. 2.19 Cribriform carcinoma with comedo necrosis. Colonic cribriform carcinoma represents 5–10% of all colonic adenocarcinomas. It tends to present as a late stage tumor and the majority show extensive invasion and lymphovascular space invasion. The tumor cells have abundant basophilic cytoplasm and form solid nests with "punched-out" spaces, resembling cribriform adenocarcinoma of the salivary glands or comedo-type ductal carcinoma in situ (DCIS) of the breast. These tumors behave in an aggressive manner and are associated with a worse prognosis (stage for stage) than conventional colonic adenocarcinomas

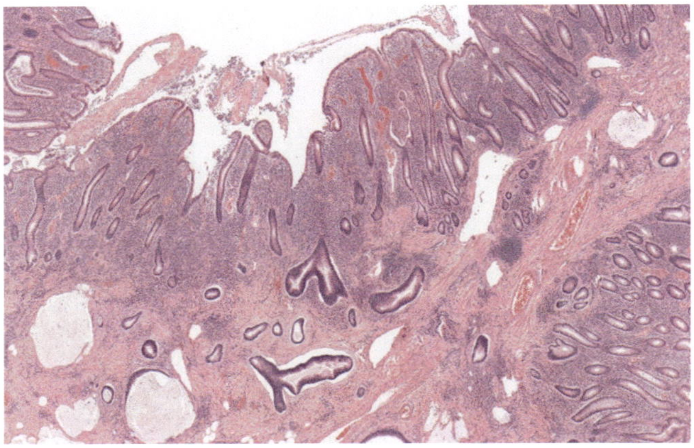

Fig. 2.20 Low-grade tubuloglandular adenocarcinoma. Tubuloglandular adenocarcinoma is a very low-grade adenocarcinoma seen in approximately 10% of adenocarcinomas associated with inflammatory bowel disease (both ulcerative colitis and Crohn's). The glands show minimal atypia but are seen extending through the wall of the colon and into pericolonic adipose tissue. The overlying mucosa may show only low-grade dysplastic changes (see Fig. 2.21). This tumor shows very mild cytologic or architectural features of malignancy, and parts of the tumor can be seen with a lamina propria

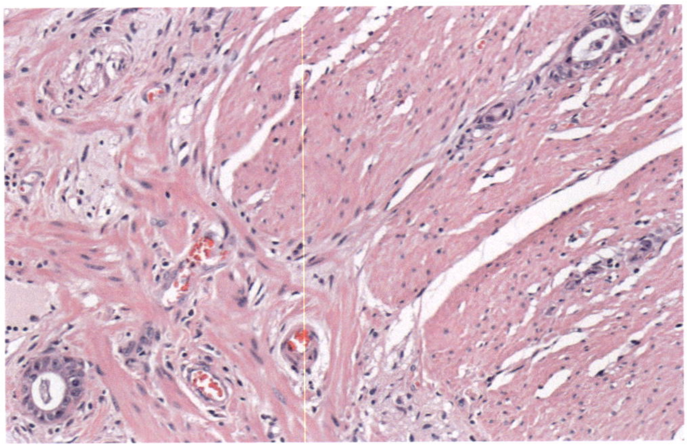

Fig. 2.21 Low-grade tubuloglandular adenocarcinoma. A high-power view of the tubuloglandular adenocarcinoma shows very bland glands haphazardly infiltrating the wall of the bowel. There is no desmoplastic reaction, and the tumor cells show minimal atypia. It is only by the architecture that the malignant growth pattern can be identified

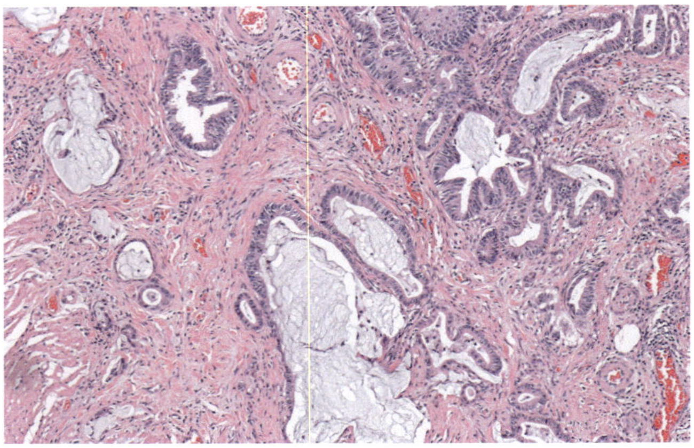

Fig. 2.22 Tubuloglandular carcinoma associated with conventional colorectal adenocarcinoma. At medium power, a component of the tumor with conventional, moderately differentiated adenocarcinoma is evident. When present, the associated conventional adenocarcinoma makes it easier to identify the tumor as an invasive colorectal adenocarcinoma

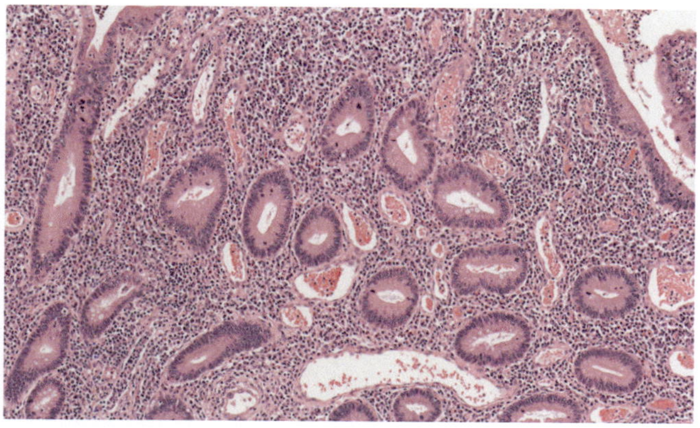

Fig. 2.23 Dysplasia overlying tubuloglandular adenocarcinoma. Low-grade dysplastic changes overlying an invasive tubuloglandular carcinoma. The lack of conventional or high-grade dysplastic changes overlying tubuloglandular carcinomas can make them hard to detect on biopsy. A high level of suspicion is need when glands in the biopsy are low-grade but with a meandering, infiltrative pattern. Given the difficulty and inconsistency of recognizing dysplasia in inflammatory bowel disease (IBD), a new classification is being proposed for dysplasia in IBD. This classification system was presented at USCAP in 2017 [1] and includes seven categories for dysplasia: conventional adenoma-like, hypermucinous, sessile serrated polyp-like, traditional serrated adenoma-like, "Terminal epithelial differentiation," goblet cell deficient, serrated NOS, and unclassified

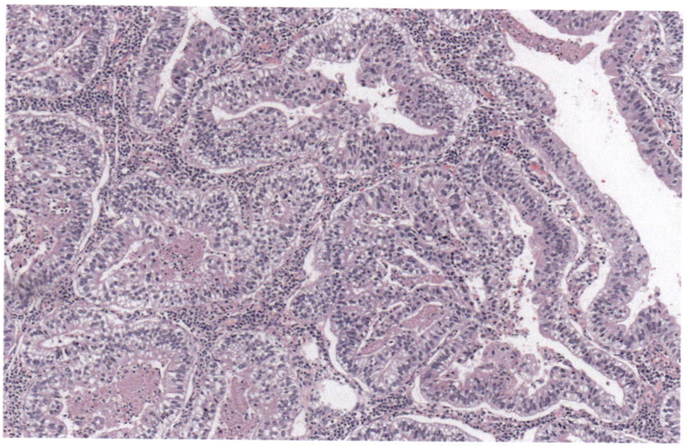

Fig. 2.25 Clear cell (enteroblastic) adenocarcinoma. Clear cell adenocarcinoma of the colon is very rare (<0.1% of colorectal adenocarcinomas). Immunohistochemical staining can be used to separate primary colorectal clear cell adenocarcinoma from metastatic disease. Given its rare nature it is difficult to determine the prognosis of this histologic finding. The enteroblastic component of the tumor can be highlighted by staining for glypican 3 or SALL4. AFP staining can be seen in approximately 45% of tumors with enteroblastic differentiation

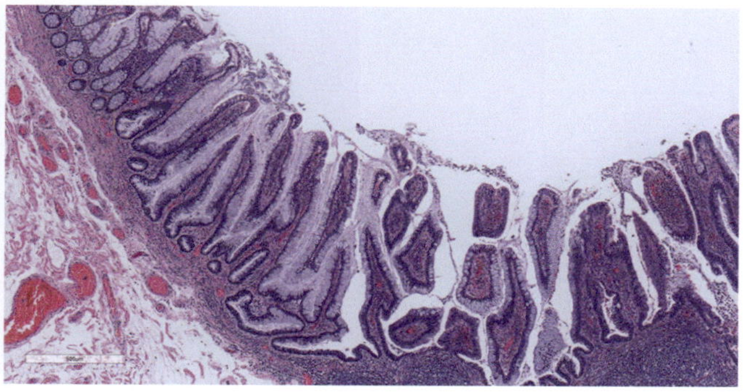

Fig. 2.24 Low-grade dysplasia in inflammatory bowel disease (hypermucinous subtype). Hypermucinous dysplasia is one of the subtypes of dysplasia put forward by Harpaz et al. at the 2017 USCAP meeting. The hypermucinous subtype of dysplasia associated with inflammatory bowel disease (IBD) includes epithelium with prominent cytoplasmic mucin, but without the serrated appearance of a serrated adenoma. The expanded classification of dysplasia will hopefully identify patients who are at risk for developing IBD associated adenocarcinoma and prevent the development of carcinomas in this population

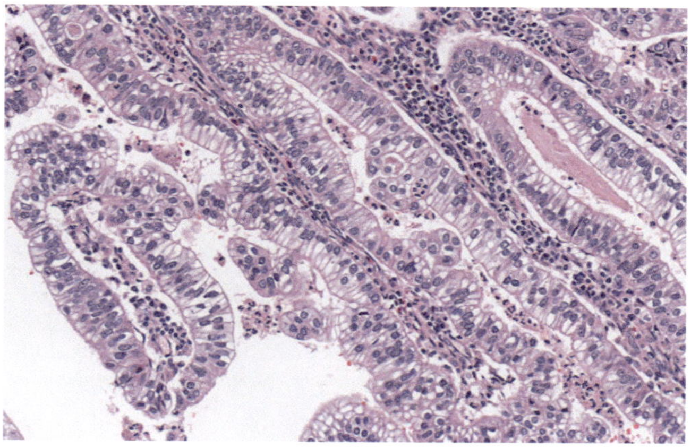

Fig. 2.26 Clear cell carcinoma. At a higher power the more columnar nature of the tumor cells and the nuclear characteristics make it possible to separate colonic clear cell carcinoma from clear cell renal carcinoma

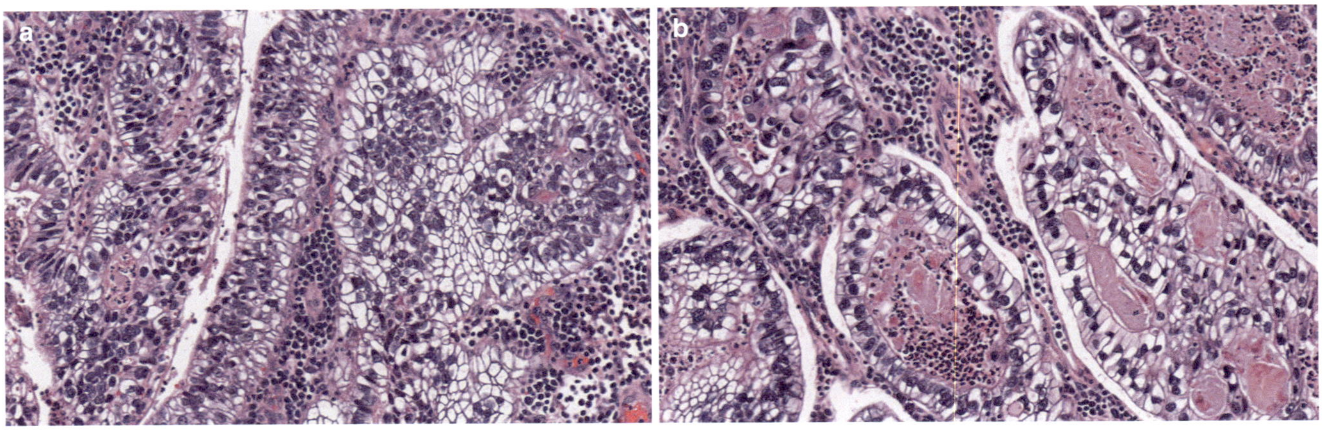

Fig. 2.27 (**a**, **b**), Clear cell carcinomas of the colon can be associated with areas showing a more primitive histologic appearance. The term *enteroblastic carcinoma* is used for these clear cell carcinomas with primitive appearing areas. Given the rare nature, it is difficult to determine the significance of this histologic appearance, but it appears that these tumors have a worse prognosis compared to conventional colorectal adenocarcinomas

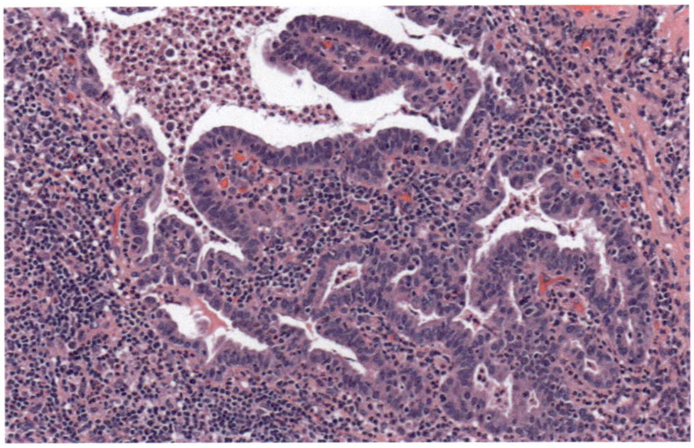

Fig. 2.28 Tumor infiltrating lymphocytes (TIL). Tumor infiltrating lymphocytes consists of T-lymphocytes extending into the stroma or epithelium of the infiltrating tumor. A marked TIL (>2 / hpf) is associated with tumors having high-frequency microsatellite instability (MSI-H) and are associated with a better prognosis, independent of microsatellite status

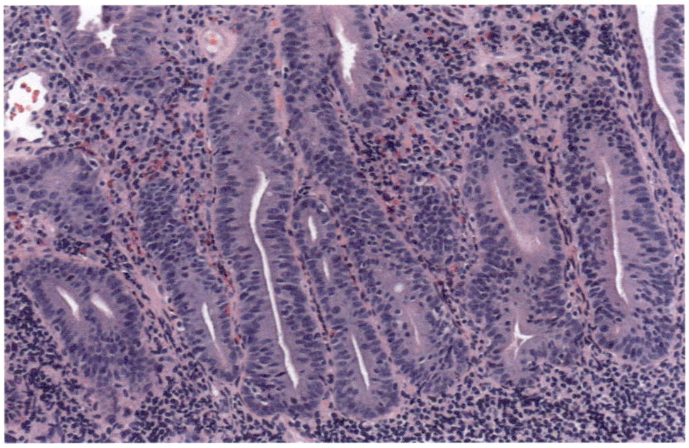

Fig. 2.29 Tumor infiltrating lymphocytes (TIL) with associated increased inflammatory infiltrate. Tumors with a high degree of tumor infiltrating lymphocytes may have increased eosinophils in the adjacent stroma and increased lymphocytes at the infiltrative tumor edge

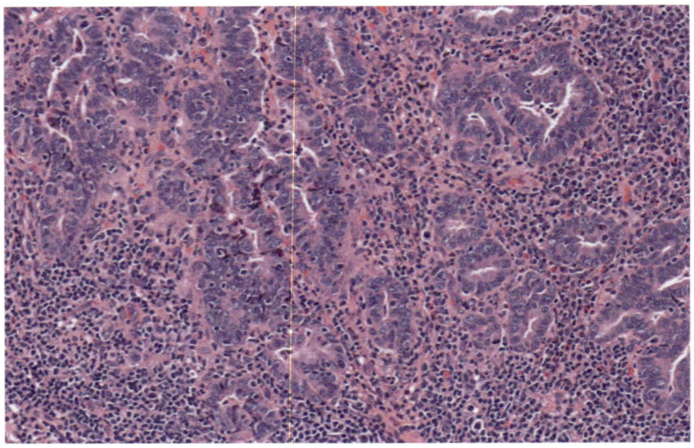

Fig. 2.30 Tumor infiltrating lymphocytes (TIL) with gland disruption. Extensive TILs can lead to glandular disruption, making it difficult to make out the tumor architecture. It is important to separate out tumors that are disrupted because of TILs (a good prognostic feature) from tumor budding (a poor prognostic feature). Thankfully adenocarcinomas with tumor budding tend not to be associated with TILs. If necessary, immunohistochemistry (pan-cytokeratin or cytokeratin 20) can be used to help outline the tumor architecture

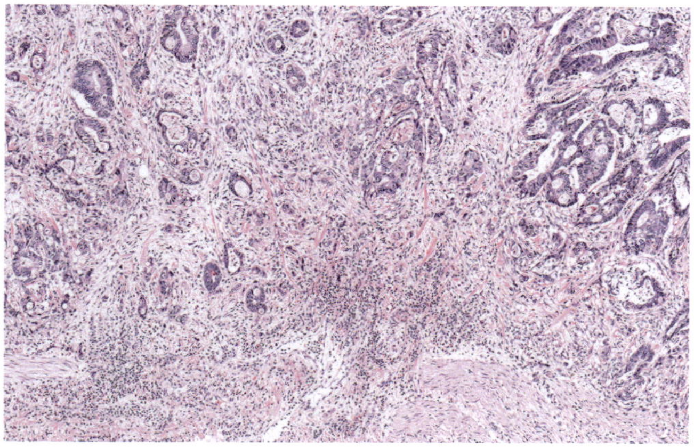

Fig. 2.31 High-grade tumor budding (low magnification). Tumor buds are single cells or small clusters (<5 cells) of infiltrating tumor cells at the advancing front of the tumor. Tumors with 10 or more buds at 200× magnification (0.785 mm^2) are considered to have high-grade tumor budding. High-grade tumor budding is associated with a worse prognosis and is considered a high-risk factor for patients with stage II colorectal adenocarcinoma. At low power the aggressive infiltrating edge of the tumor is evident

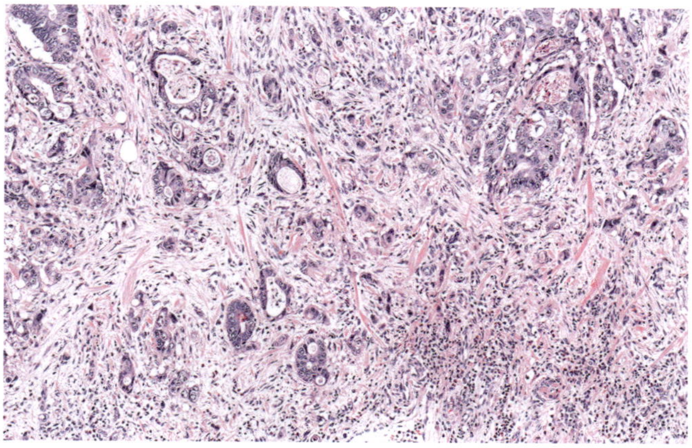

Fig. 2.32 Medium-power view of tumor budding. At medium power the tumor budding is more evident. The small nests (<5 cells) and single cell infiltration can be seen

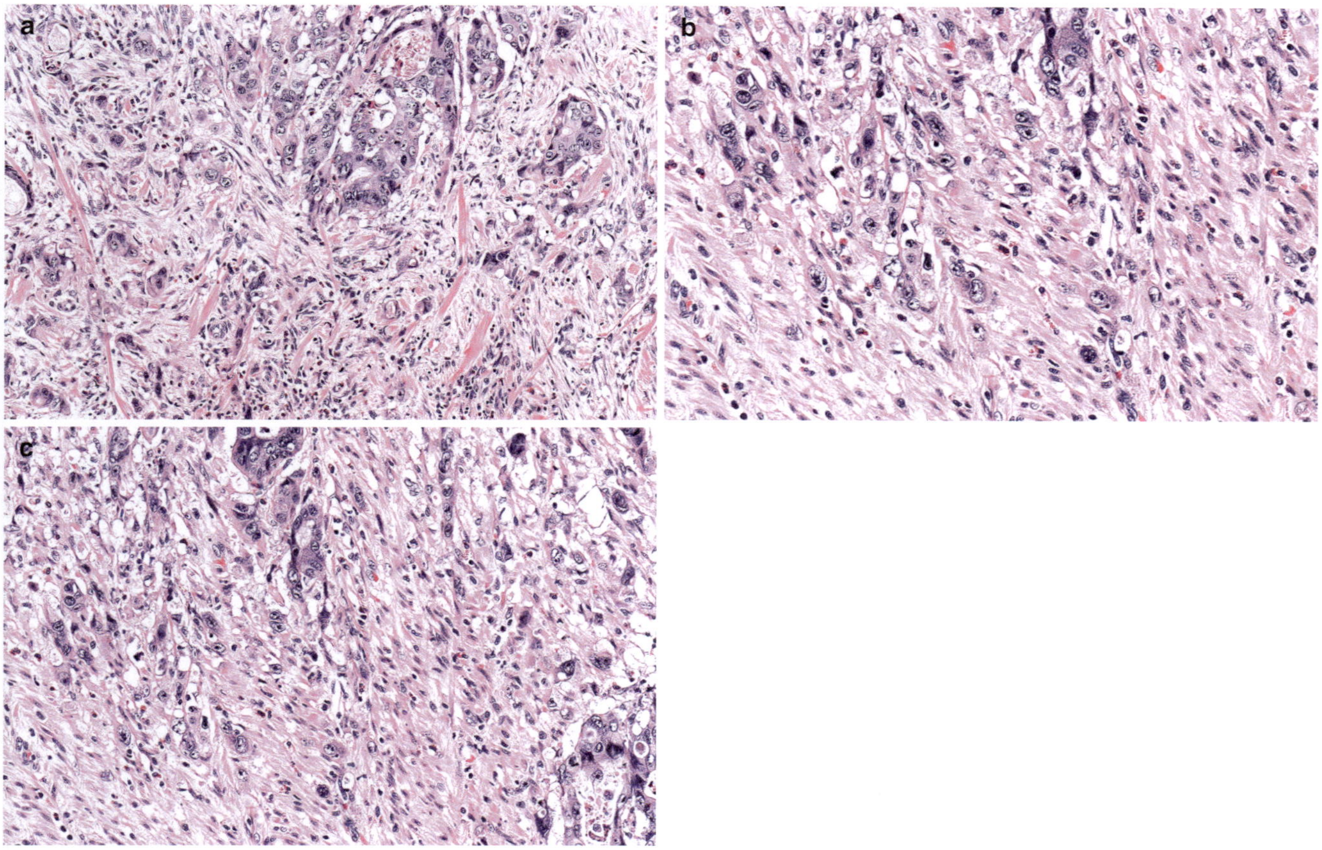

Fig. 2.33 (**a**–**c**) High-power view of tumor budding. The tumor buds are evidence on H&E at high power. A total of 10 buds need to be identified on H&E to classify the tumor as having high-grade tumor budding

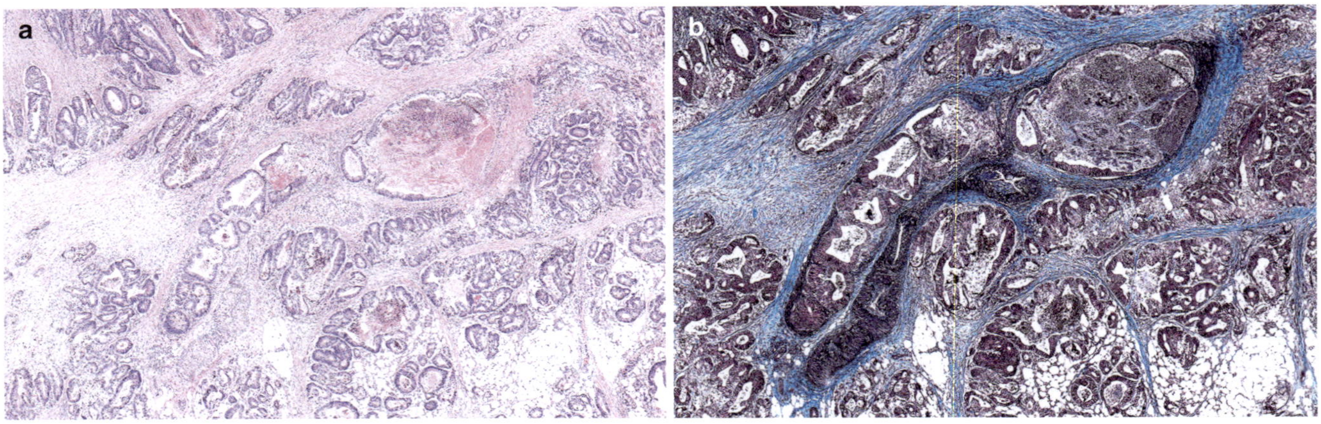

Fig. 2.34 Extramural venous invasion, H&E (**a**) and elastic trichrome (**b**) staining. Extramural venous invasion is a poor prognostic factor and is a recognized risk factor for liver metastasis. Given its significance, it is recommended that small vessel (capillary) vascular invasion be reported separately from venous (large vessel) invasion. The presence of tumor deposits adjacent to arterioles with an identified vein ("orphan arteriole" sign) or elongated tumor nodules extending into adipose tissue ("protruding tongue" sign) are highly suspicious for venous invasion. The use of elastic stains can improve the detection of venous invasion. The orphan arteriole is evident in this section; the vascular spaces are highlighted by the elastic-trichrome stain

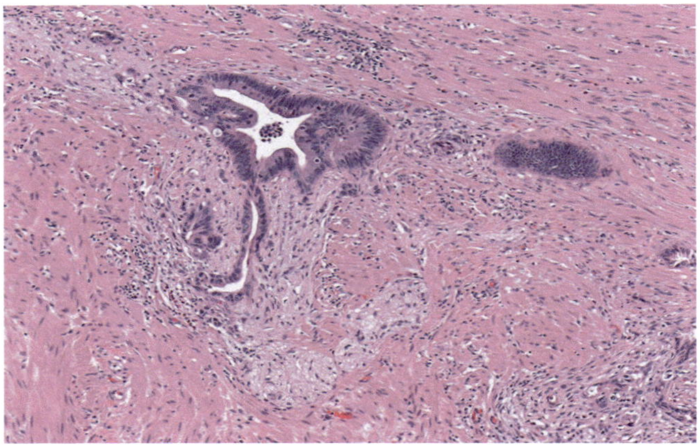

Fig. 2.35 Perineural invasion. While there is some controversy over the significance, most studies have found perineural invasion to be a poor prognostic indicator. As in this case, perineural invasion can be seen with low-grade adenocarcinomas (including low-grade tubuloglandular carcinomas). Extramural perineural invasion may have a worse prognosis than intramural invasion, but the significance of the location of perineural invasion has not been established

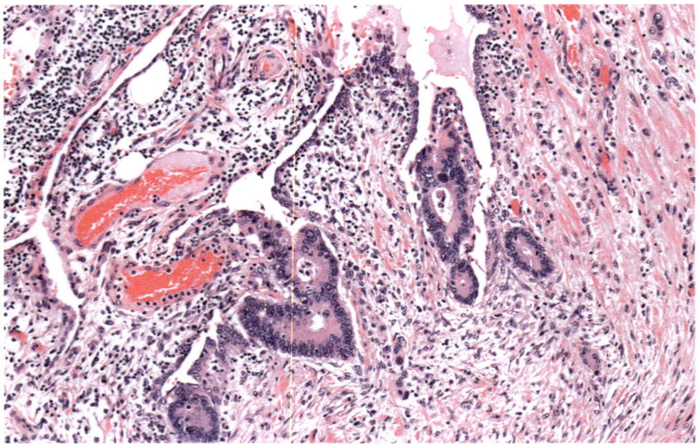

Fig. 2.36 Serosal invasion. Tumor infiltration of the serosa is a poor prognostic factor. Visceral serosal involvement can be missed and thorough sampling of the serosa in the regions of deep tumor infiltration is warranted. Serosal invasion can be assumed if there is tumor extension to the serosal surface, tumor cells at the serosal surface associated with inflammation and reactive mesothelial changes, or tumor perforation with tumor at the serosal surface. Elastic stains can be helpful in some situations, demonstrating involvement of the subperitoneal elastic lamina. In this case the tumor at the serosal surface is seen in association with inflammation at the serosal surface

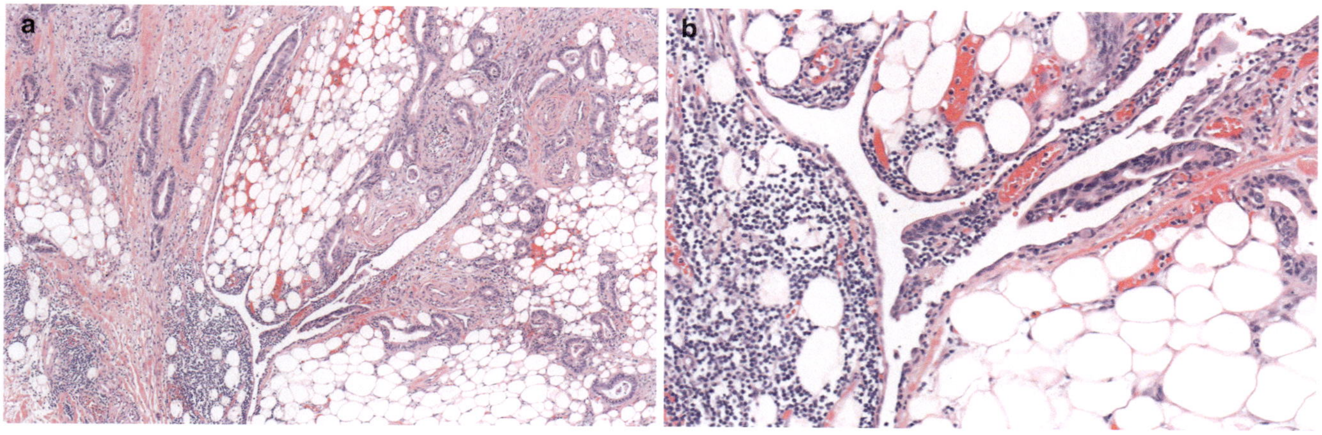

Fig. 2.37 Serosal invasion in a cleft low power (**a**) and high power (**b**). Serosal involvement can be difficult to pick up when involving clefts along the colonic surface (as in this case). At low power (**a**), tumor can be seen extending out into the lobules of adipose tissue. At high power (**b**), tumor is evident involving the mesothelium lining the adipose tissue lobule

Reference

1. Riddell R. Dysplasia (and serrated lesions) in IBD. Robert Haggitt Memorial Lecture. USCAP 2017. Augusta: United States and Canadian Academy of Pathology; 2017. Available at https://handouts.uscap.org/AN2017/2017_CM16_Ridde_0501_post.pdf.

Suggested Reading

Bosman FT, Carneiro F, Hruban RH, Theise ND, WHO Classification of Tumours of the Digestive System, editors. WHO Classification of Tumours, vol. 3. 4th ed. Lyon: IARC; 2010.

Dawson H, Kirsch R, Driman DK, Messenger DE, Assarzadegan N, Riddell RH. Optimizing the Detection of Venous Invasion in Colorectal Cancer: The Ontario, Canada, Experience and Beyond. Front Oncol. 2015;4:354.

Lee HJ, Eom DW, Kang GH, Han SH, Cheon GJ, Hs O, et al. Colorectal micropapillary carcinomas are associated with poor prognosis and enriched in markers of stem cells. Mod Pathol. 2013;26(8):1123–31.

Lino-Silva LS, Salcedo-Hernández RA, Herrera-Gómez A, Padilla-Rosciano A, Ramírez-Jaramillo M, Herrera-Goepfert RE, et al. Colonic Cribriform Carcinoma, a Morphologic Pattern Associated with Low Survival. Int J Surg Pathol. 2015;23(1):13–9.

Levi GS, Harpaz N. Intestinal Low-Grade Tubuloglandular Adenocarcinoma in Inflammatory Bowel Disease. Am J Surg Pathol. 2006;30(8):1022–9.

Lugli A, Kirsch R, Aijoka Y, Bosman F, Cathomas G, Dawson H, et al. Recommendations for reporting tumor budding in colorectal cancer based on the International Tumor Budding Consensus Conference (ITBCC) 2016. Mod Pathol. 2017;30(9):1299–311.

Mäkinen MJ. Colorectal serrated adenocarcinoma. Histopathology. 2007;50(1):131–50.

3 Mesenchymal Neoplasms

Aysegul Sari, Richard Kirsch, and James Conner

As in the stomach, gastrointestinal stromal tumors (GIST) comprise the majority of malignant mesenchymal neoplasms in the small and large intestine. In addition, there is a diverse array of other nonepithelial tumors, both benign and malignant. Many benign mucosal and submucosal mesenchymal neoplasms may present as colorectal polyps, and recognition of these entities can be useful in some situations to explain the endoscopic impression of a polyp in the absence of typical adenomatous or hyperplastic epithelial changes. Some mesenchymal lesions are entirely harmless in isolation but may indicate the presence of an underlying hereditary cancer syndrome. Recognizing these associations and flagging appropriate patients may prompt clinical genetic evaluation and modification of cancer surveillance protocols. This chapter reviews key histologic features of the most common mesenchymal neoplasms in the small and large intestine.

3.1 Gastrointestinal Stromal Tumors

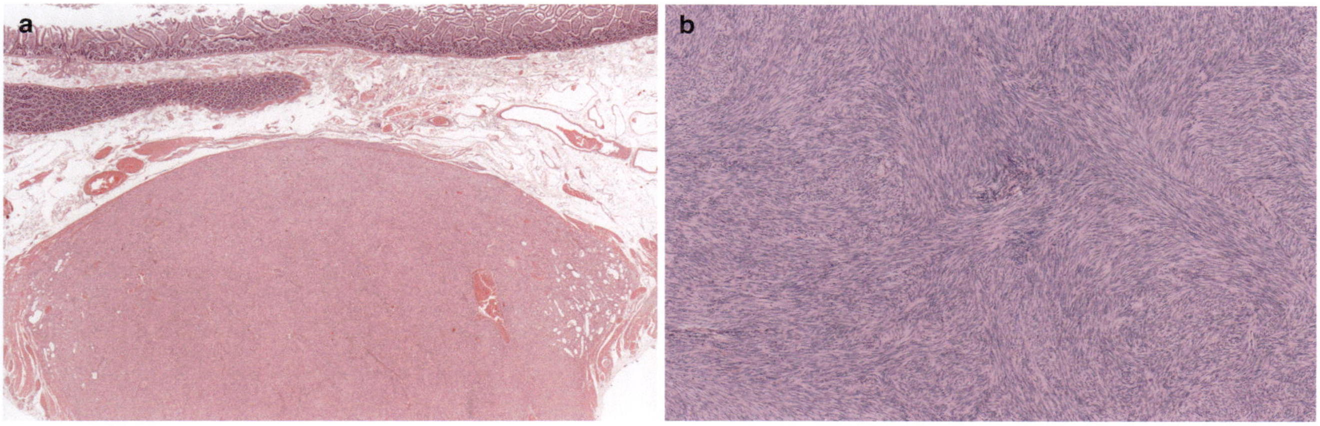

Spindle cell gastrointestinal stromal tumor (GIST). Over 90% of intestinal GISTs have a spindle cell morphology. The primary lesions are centered in the muscularis propria (**a**), where they arise from native interstitial cells of Cajal (ICC). Most cases are relatively well circumscribed but unencapsulated. The architecture may vary, but most cases have a fascicular growth pattern (**b**). The cell density can also be variable (especially after treatment), but moderately to highly cellular lesions are most common (**c**). Some cases may have a prominent myxoid stroma in which tumor cells can exhibit a striking palisading architecture (**d**). Tumor cell nuclei are generally uniform, with mostly blunt (but occasionally pointed) ends, evenly distributed and finely textured chromatin, and small nucleoli (**e**). Perinuclear cytoplasmic vacuoles are common and can be a prominent feature, but these are not entirely specific for GIST and can be seen in other spindle cell tumors (e.g., leiomyoma) (**f**). Skeinoid fibers are strands of dense, eosinophilic collagen bundles in the extracellular matrix. This feature is almost entirely limited to GISTs arising in the small intestine (**g**). Some data suggest that their presence is associated with a favorable prognosis

H. H. Li-Chang et al., *Atlas of Intestinal Pathology*, Atlas of Anatomic Pathology,
https://doi.org/10.1007/978-3-030-12379-6_3

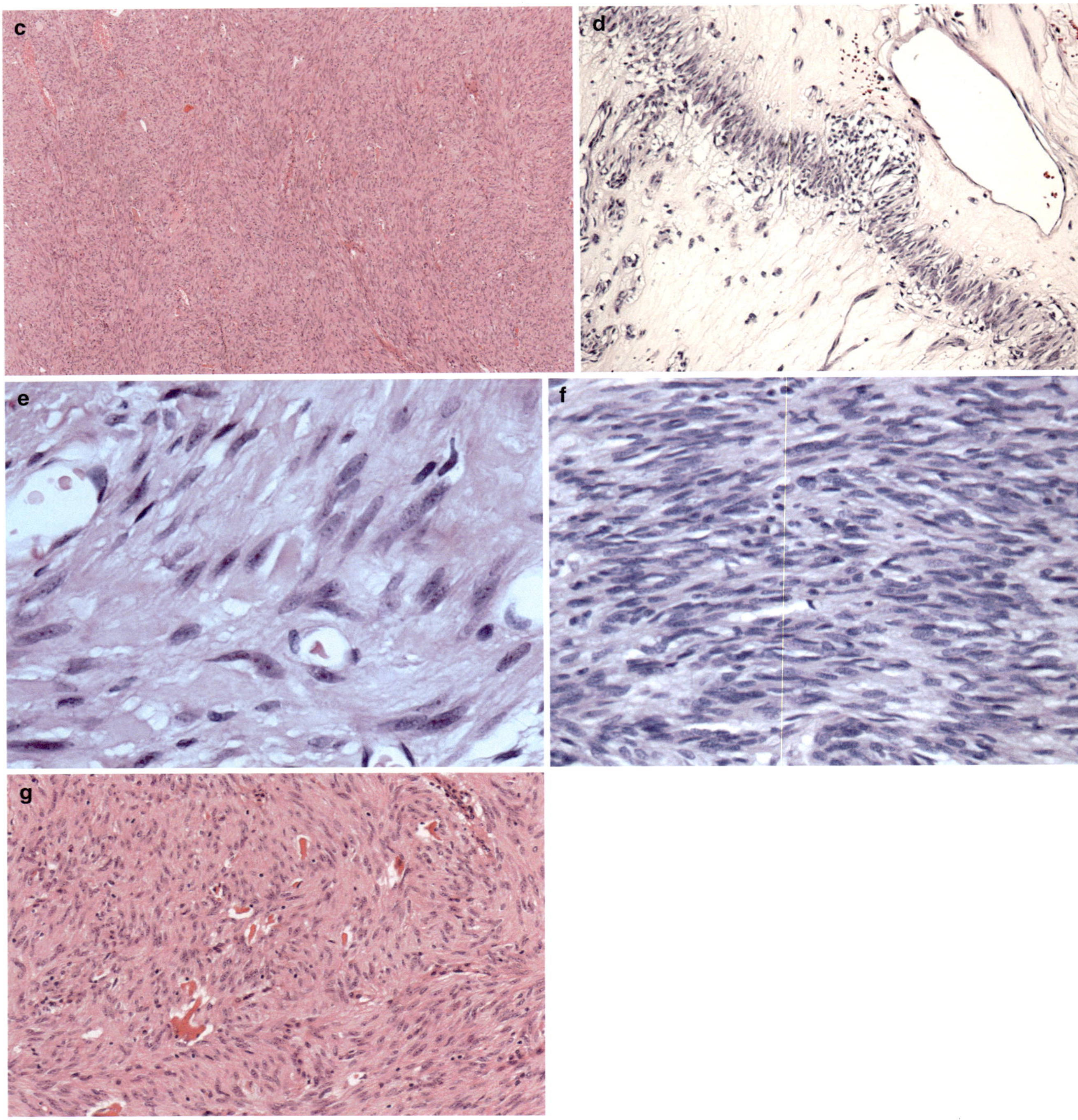

(continued)

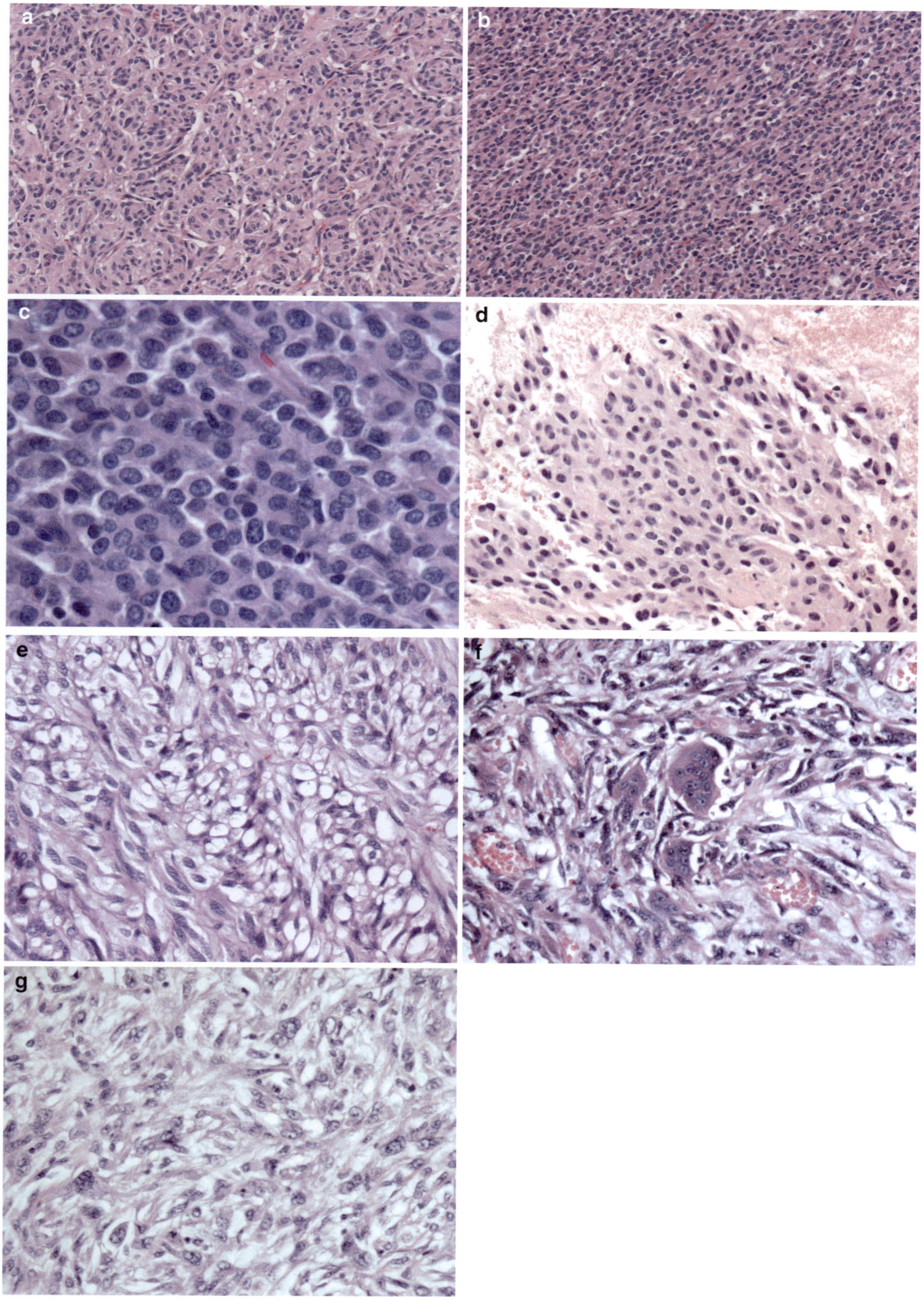

Epithelioid GIST. Epithelioid morphology is seen rarely in intestinal GISTs, occurring much less frequently than in the stomach. At low power, these lesions may have a nested growth pattern (**a**) or a solid growth pattern (**b**). The typical cytomorphology consists of centrally placed round nuclei with moderate to copious amounts of cytoplasm (**c**), which may be eosinophilic (**d**) or clear (**e**). Some cases may have multinucleated giant cells (**f**). Although most epithelioid GISTs have a relatively uniform cytomorphology, some cases may show a greater degree of nuclear pleomorphism (**g**). The morphologic differential diagnosis in these cases includes other malignant mesenchymal and epithelial neoplasms, and in more pleomorphic variants, metastatic melanoma [1, 2]. In these cases, immunohistochemistry may be required for definitive diagnosis (Table 3.1)

Table 3.1 Morphologic and Immunohistochemical Features of the Most Commonly Encountered GIST Mimics

Tumor	Typical morphology	Most Common Anatomic Site	Immunohistochemistry
Spindle Cell Tumors			
Leiomyoma	Well-circumscribed, fascicular architecture; bland, elongated, cigar-shaped nuclei and abundant eosinophilic cytoplasm	Esophagus (larger tumors of the muscularis propria) Colon and rectum (small tumors of the muscularis mucosa)	CD117 negative DOG1 negative SMA positive Desmin positive
Schwannoma	Well-circumscribed with a peripheral lymphoid cuff; elongated nuclei with tapered ends	Stomach (muscularis propria)	CD117 negative DOG1 negative S100 positive
Fibromatosis	Infiltrative lesion with long fascicles of spindle cells embedded in collagenous and myxoid matrix; bland cytology	Mesentery (may infiltrate into the wall of the tubal gut)	CD117 negative DOG1 negative Nuclear B-catenin positive SMA patchy positive
Inflammatory myofibroblastic tumor	Myofibroblastic cells embedded in myxoid or collagenous matrix with abundant inflammatory cells (three subtypes: myxoid vascular, compact spindle cell, and hypocellular sclerotic)	Mesentery	CD117 negative DOG1 negative ALK-1 positive (40–60%) SMA patchy positive
Inflammatory fibroid polyp	Loose proliferation of bland spindle cells in myxoid or collagenous matrix, often concentric around blood vessels; inflammatory infiltrate with numerous eosinophils	Gastric submucosa Small intestine (may involve full thickness of the intestinal wall)	CD117 negative DOG1 negative CD34 positive
Epithelioid Cell Tumors			
Neuroendocrine tumor	Nested, trabecular, acinar, rosette-like, or solid growth of monotonous cells with characteristic coarse granular chromatin	Gastric (mucosa, may extend into submucosa and muscularis propria) Small intestine (may present as metastasis) Pancreas (may present as metastasis)	CD117 negative DOG1 negative Cytokeratin positive Chromogranin positive Synaptophysin positive
Spindle or Epithelioid			
Melanoma	Variable; commonly dyscohesive epithelioid cells with prominent nucleoli and variable amounts of cytoplasm; may be amelanotic	Any site	CD117 positive (up to 50% of cases; usually focal) DOG1 occasionally positive S100 positive MART-1 positive HMB-45 positive
Carcinoma	Variable; poorly cohesive tumors without gland formation may be particularly difficult to distinguish from GIST	Any site; may be associated with a precursor lesion in the overlying mucosa	CD117 negative DOG1 negative AE1/AE3 Pan-cytokeratin positive (may be focal)

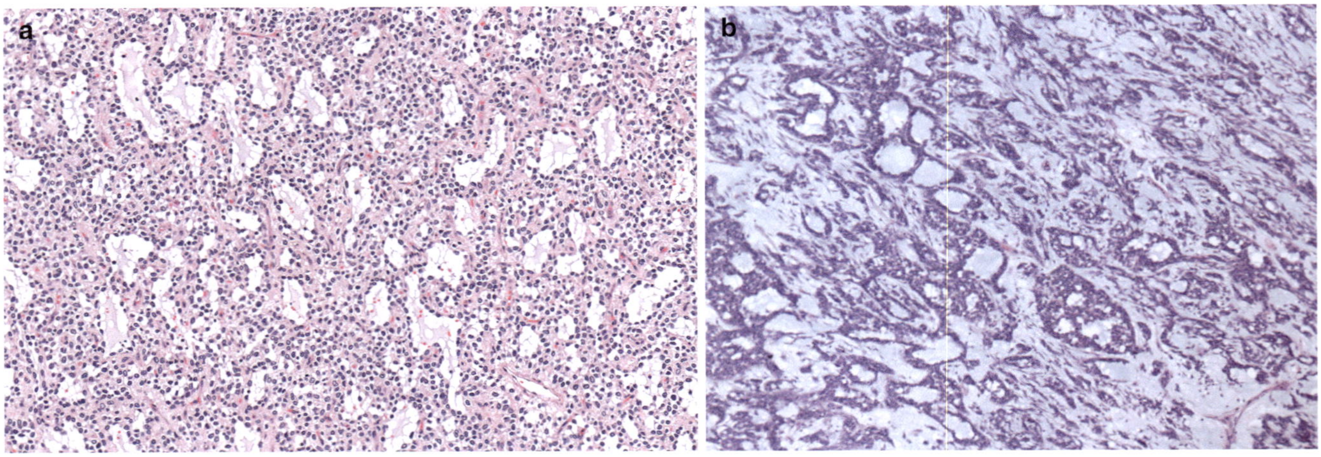

Unusual morphologic patterns. Unusual morphologic patterns may be seen in some GISTs, including pseudoglandular architecture (**a**, **b**), rhabdoid cytomorphology (**c**), signet ring–cell cytomorphology (**d**), and osteoid matrix (**e**)

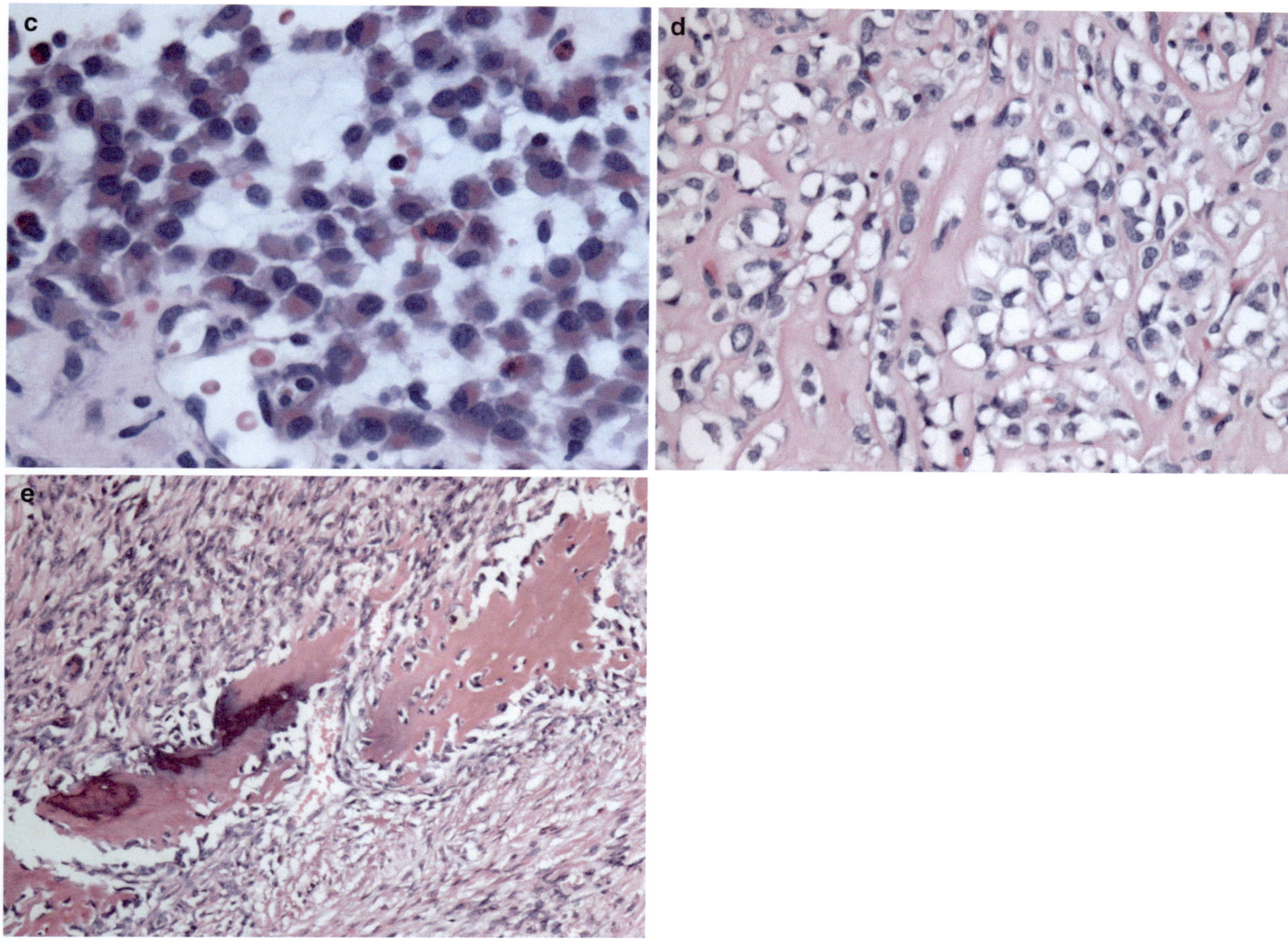

(continued)

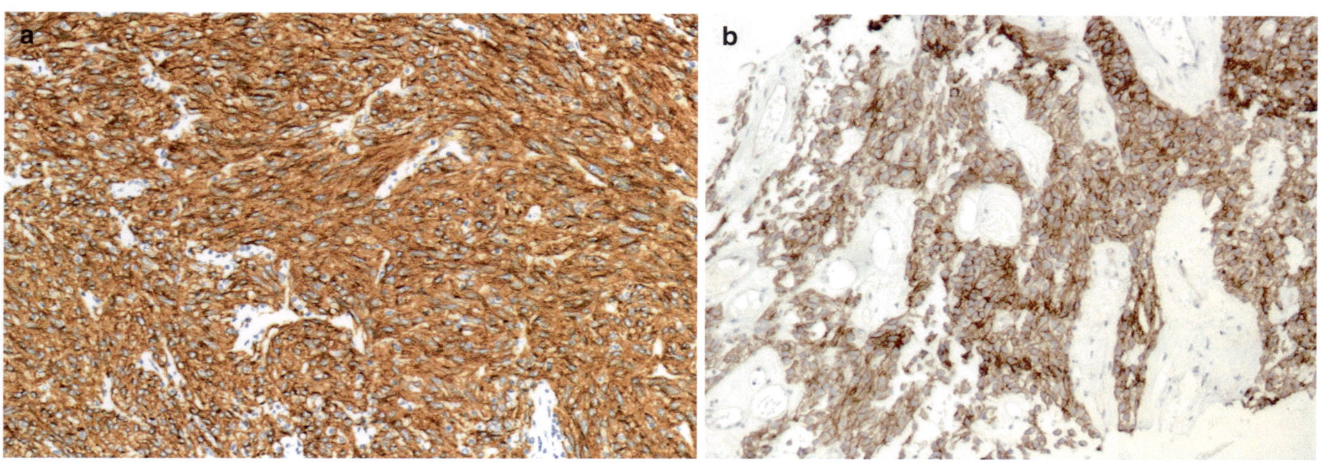

Immunohistochemical features of GIST. (**a**), CD117 (c-KIT) immunohistochemistry most often shows diffuse cytoplasmic positivity. (**b**), Occasional tumors may have a membranous pattern of expression. (**c**), Others may show perinuclear "dot-like" staining, as in this example of a GIST with more limited/focal CD117 staining. Epithelioid GISTs may show only weakly positive or even negative staining with CD117. (**d**), DOG-1 (discovered on GIST 1) is another highly sensitive and specific GIST marker, which stains 95% of GISTs. This GIST shows diffuse cytoplasmic staining and patchy membranous staining for DOG-1. Other commonly expressed but nonspecific markers include CD34 (~70%), h-Caldesmon (~80%), SMA (~40%) (**e**), and S100 (~5–10%)

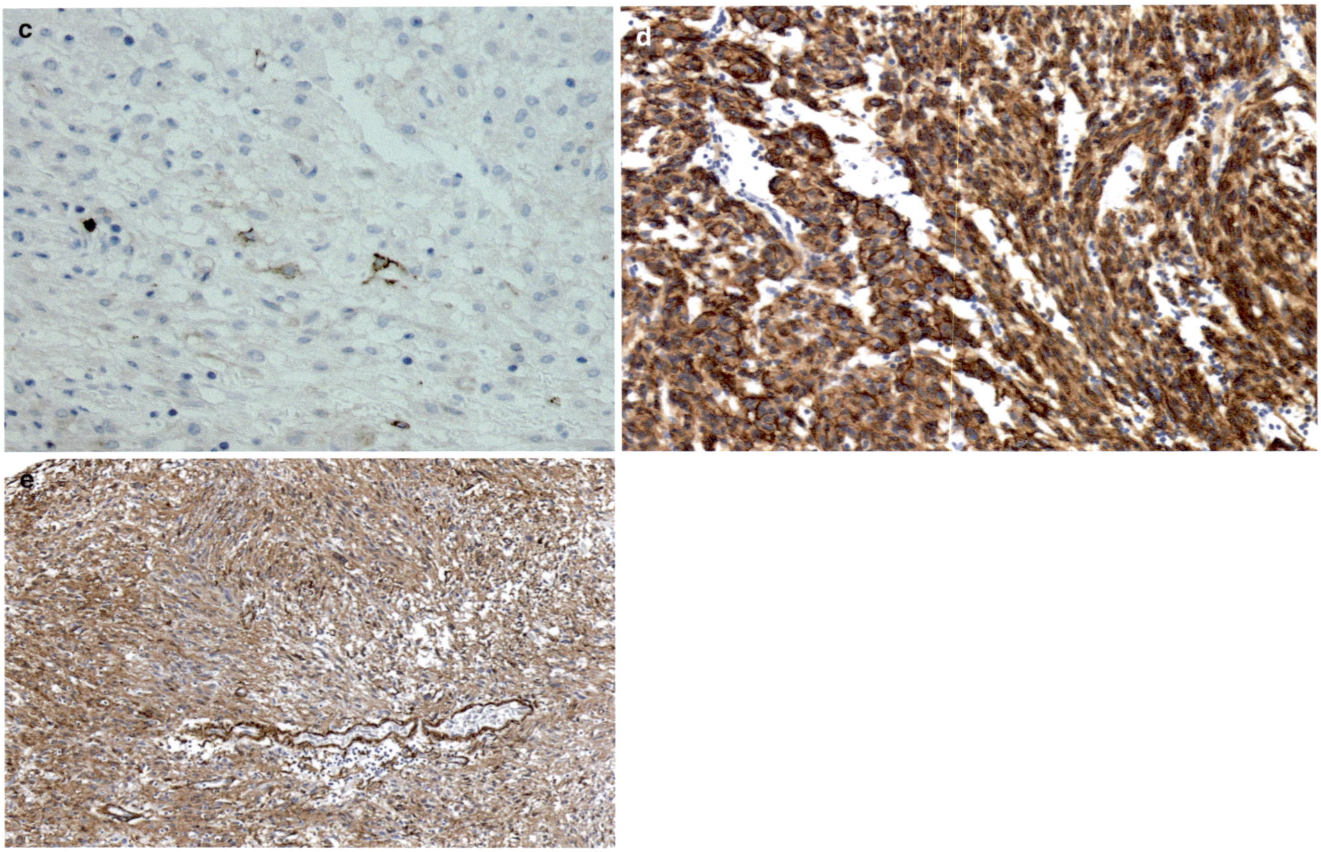

(continued)

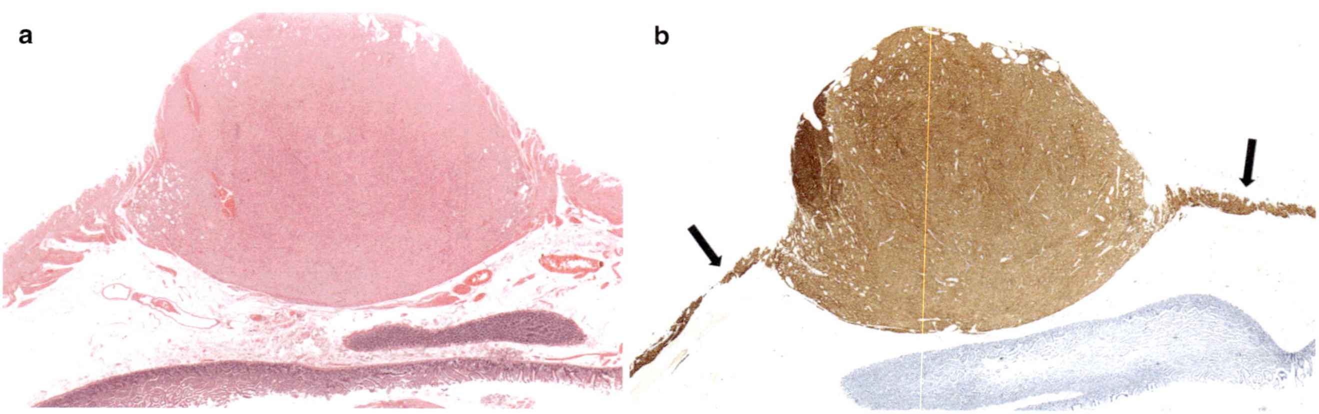

Diffuse hyperplasia of interstitial cells of Cajal (ICC). Diffuse ICC hyperplasia is seen mostly in GISTs associated with familial GIST syndrome and neurofibromatosis (NF) type 1, although it may occasionally occur sporadically [3, 4]. (**a** and **b**), CD117 immunohistochemistry performed on a GIST from a patient with familial GIST syndrome (due to a germline *KIT* mutation). Note the adjacent diffuse ICC hyperplasia (**b**, *arrows*). (**c**), A higher-power view also shows this diffuse ICC hyperplasia. (**d**), Another example of multifocal GISTs and ICC hyperplasia associated with familial GIST syndrome (CD117). Because GISTs may be the first presentation in patients with NF1, it is important to recognize ICC hyperplasia and its potential association with NF-1. NF-1–related GISTs occur mainly in the small intestine (usually jejunum) and are typically wild-type for *KIT* and *PDGFRA*. *See* Table 3.2. Rare examples of sporadic ICC hyperplasia have been reported under various terms, including *sporadic segmental ICC hyperplasia* (microscopic GIST), *long segmental hyperplasia of ICC*, *diffuse infiltrating GIST,* and *gut wall replacing type of GIST*. All have shown exon 11 *KIT* mutations, and almost all were associated with diverticular disease. (**e**, **f**), This rectosigmoid resection shows diffuse longitudinal and micronodular ICC hyperplasia on a background of diverticular disease, highlighted by CD117 immunohistochemistry (an exon 11 *KIT* mutation was identified). (**g**), Diffuse ICC proliferation in sporadic forms tends to replace the full thickness of the muscularis propria, whereas in familial forms, ICC hyperplasia occurs in Aurbach's plexus within intermuscular space (**c**).

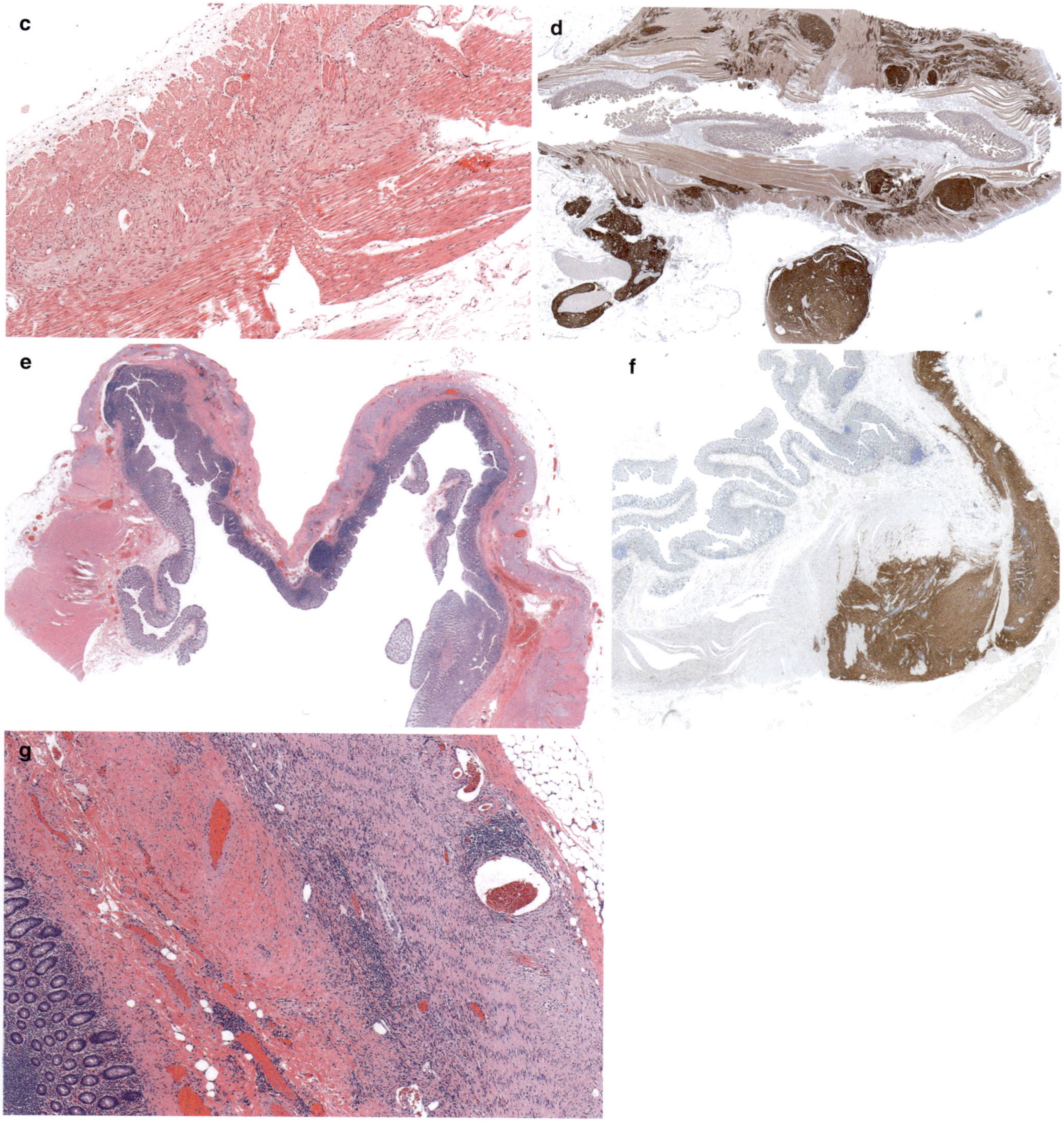

(continued)

Table 3.2 Syndromes Associated with Gastrointestinal Stromal Tumors (GIST)

Syndrome	Germline Alterations	Inheritance	Characteristic Features of GIST	Other Associated Neoplasms
Familial GIST syndrome	*KIT* or *PDGFRA* mutations	Autosomal dominant	Multiple primary GISTs Background ICC hyperplasia	Cutaneous lesions Hematologic neoplasms
Carney's triad	Unknown	Most cases sporadic Predominantly female patients	Epithelioid cytomorphology Multinodular, plexiform growth Loss of *SDHB* expression	Pulmonary chondromas Paragangliomas
Carney-Stratakis syndrome	*SDHB*, *SDHC*, *SDHD* mutations	Autosomal dominant (incomplete penetrance) Equal female: male ratio	Epithelioid cytomorphology Multinodular, plexiform growth Loss of *SDHB* expression	Paragangliomas
Neurofibromatosis type 1.	*NF1*	Autosomal dominant	Multiple primary GISTs Background ICC hyperplasia Predominantly small intestinal May be S100 reactive (40–60%)	Skin lesions ("café-au-lait" spots) Neural tumors

ICC interstitial cells of Cajal

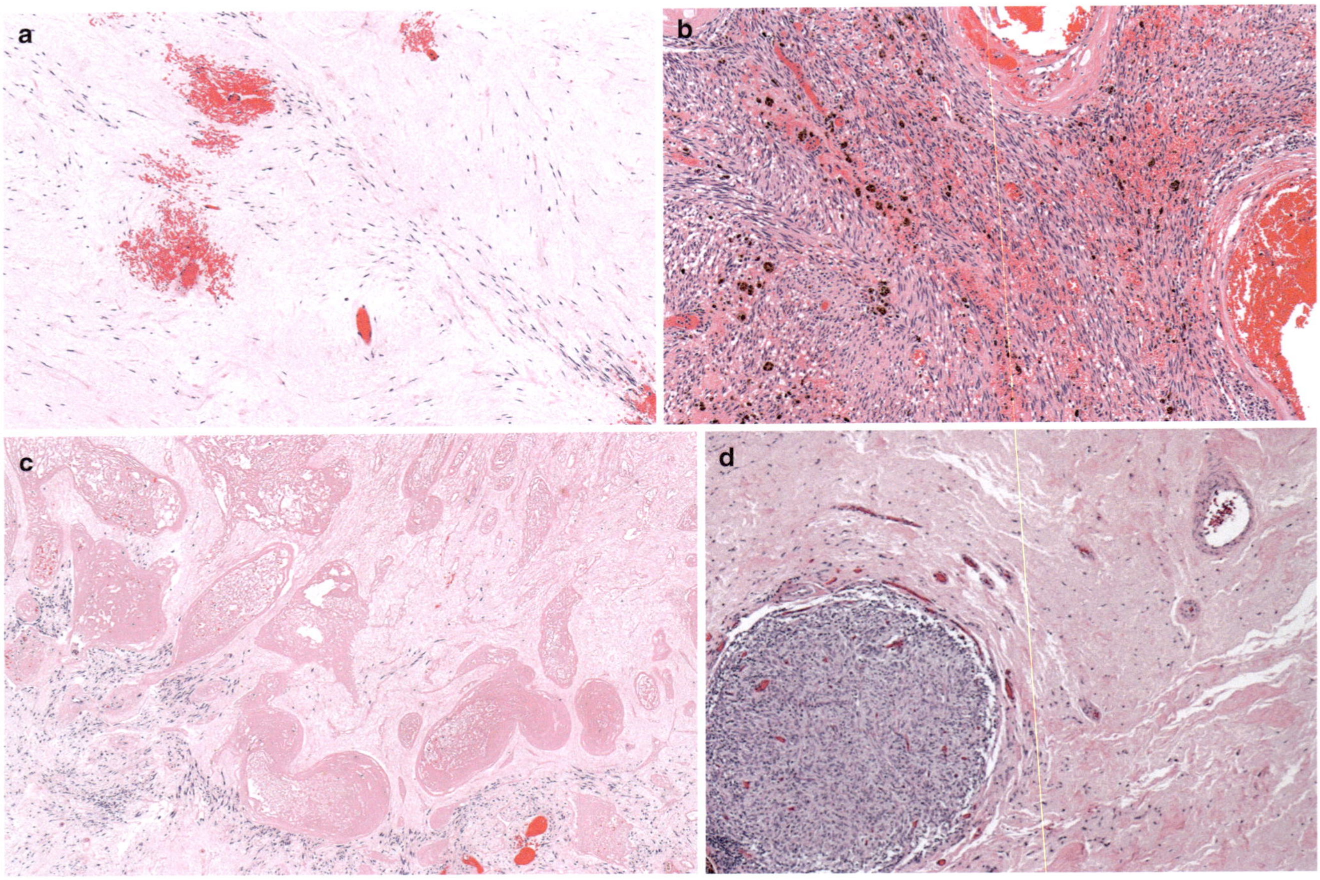

Posttreatment changes in GIST. Histological features following imatinib treatment are usually heterogeneous [5]. The most frequent changes include hyalinization, sometimes with no viable tumor cells or only scattered residual spindled tumor cells (**a**). Other posttreatment changes include hemorrhage and hemosiderin deposition (**b**), myxoid degeneration, foamy histiocytes, cystic change, or rarely tumor necrosis. Areas of coagulative necrosis can be seen (**c**). Even in tumors with a very good treatment response, focal residual viable tumor nodules can be found (**d**). Occasionally, phenotypic alterations, such as a switch from a spindled to an epithelioid phenotype can occur. CD117 immunoreactivity may be lost, but DOG1 immunoreactivity is usually retained

Risk Stratification in GIST

Mitoses per 5 mm^2	Size, *cm*	Risk of Progression or Mortality: Stomach	Jejunum/Ileum
≤5	≤2	None (0%)	None (0%)
	>2–≤5	Very low (1.9%)	Low (4.3%)
	>5–≤10	Low (3.6%)	Moderate (24%)
	>10	Moderate (12%)	High (52%)
>5	≤2	None (0%)[a]	High (50%)[a]
	>2–≤5	Moderate (16%)	High (73%)
	>5–≤10	High (55%)	High (85%)
	>10	High (86%)	High (90%)

[a]Very few cases of tumors ≤2 cm with >5 mitoses/5mm^2 were identified [2].

Molecular Classification of GIST

Gene	Exon/ Allele	Frequency	Response to Imatinib
KIT	Exon 11	60–70%	85%
	Exon 9	10–15%	45% (higher dose)
	Exon 13	1–4%	Few cases
	Exon 17	<1%	Few cases
PDGFRA	Exon 18	4–5%	Poor
	Exon 12	<1%	Few cases
	Exon 14	<1%	Few cases
SDHB deficient (mutation or epigenetic alterations in any SDH subunit gene)		8–10%	Poor
BRAF	V600E	1–2%	Limited data

3.2 Tumors of Neural Origin

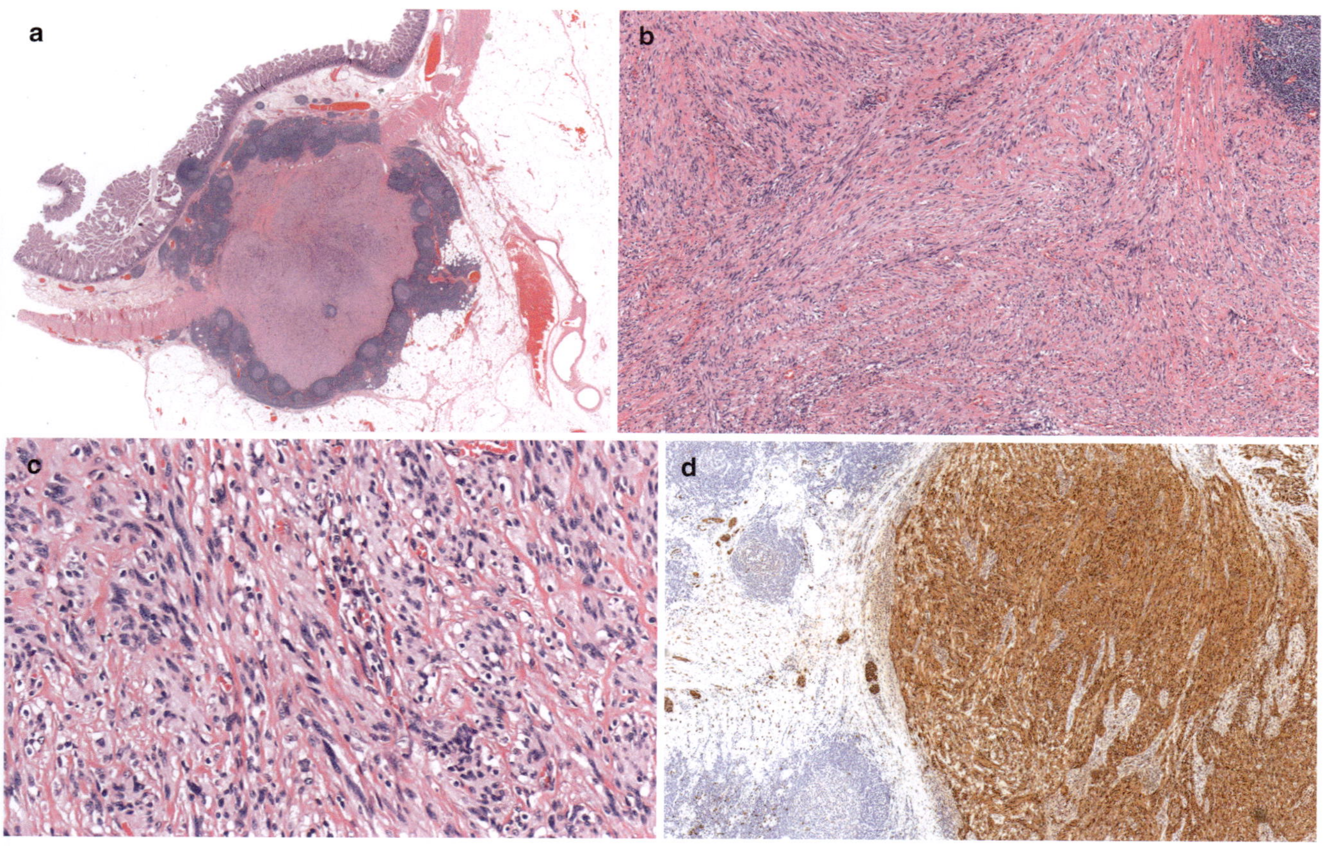

Schwannoma. Schwannomas are benign peripheral nerve sheath tumors that are relatively rare in the GI tract. The stomach is the most common site, followed by the colon and rectum [6, 7]. (**a**), At low power, these tumors are typically well circumscribed and have a characteristic peripheral lymphoid cuff, often with germinal centers. (**b**), GI schwannomas are composed of spindle cells, often arranged in short fascicles or a micro-trabecular pattern in a variably collagenous stroma. A myxoid stroma may be observed. (**c**), Nuclei are elongated, wavy, and have tapered ends, they may have small, inconspicuous nucleoli. Focal cytologic atypia and occasional mitoses can be seen, but are usually <5 per 10 HPF. Of note, classic features of soft tissue schwannomas, such as Verocay bodies, hyalinized vessels, and prominent nuclear palisading are not typical of GI schwannomas. (**d**), GI schwannomas are diffusely immunoreactive with S100. CD117 and DOG1 are negative

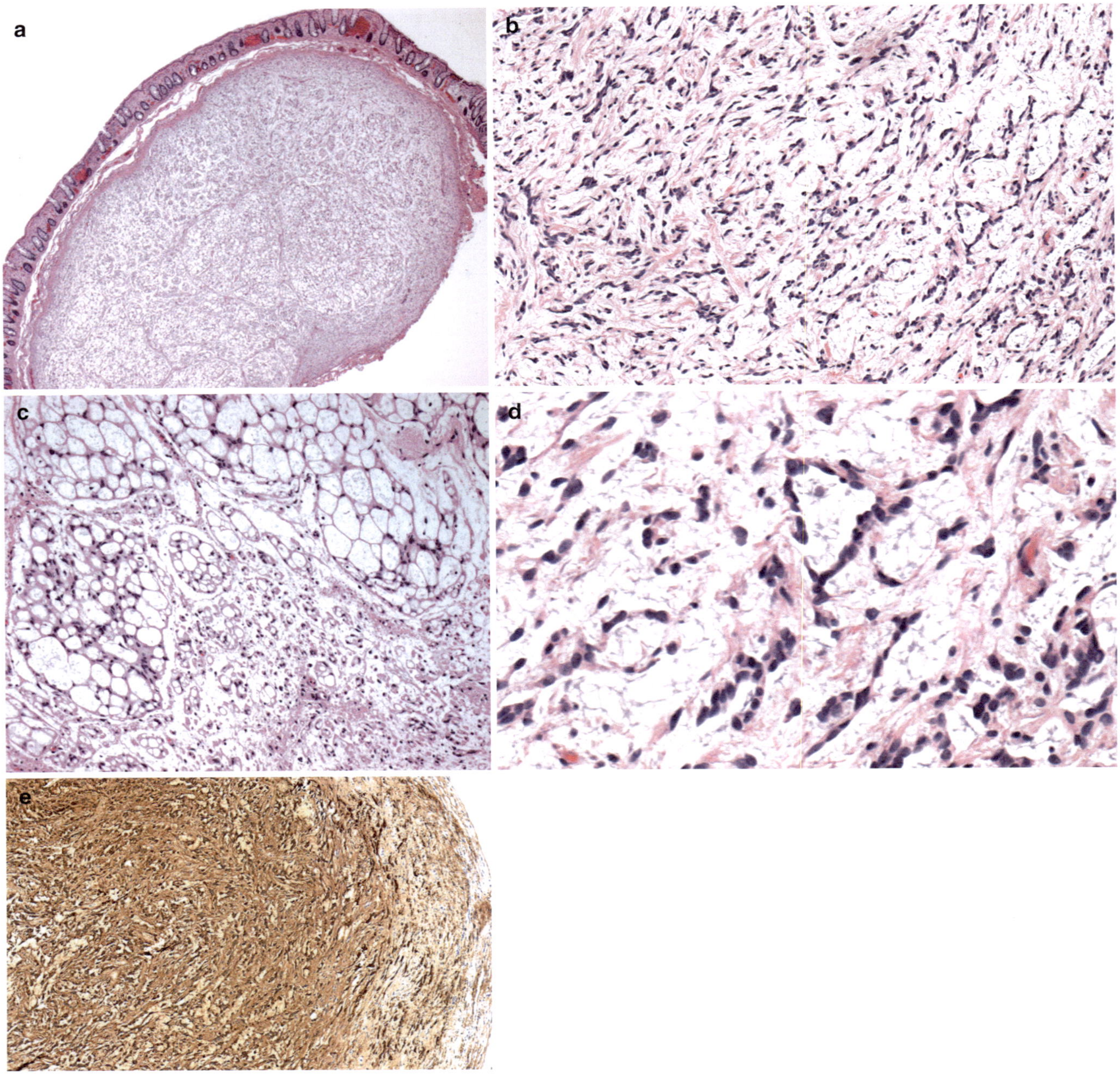

Microcystic schwannoma (MCS). MCS is a rare variant of schwannoma most commonly seen in the colon and rectum [8–10]. It commonly presents as a submucosal polyp (**a**). Tumor cells are often arranged around a loose, myxoid stroma, imparting a microcystic or sponge-like reticular architecture (**b**); it can mimic cribriforming glands (**c**). Tumor cells are uniform and typically round to ovoid in shape, although areas with spindle cell morphology may be seen in some lesions. There is no significant cytologic atypia (**d**). Involvement of the muscularis mucosae, with extension into the mucosa, is not uncommon. In biopsy specimens, these tumors may mimic both signet ring–cell carcinoma and GIST with prominent myxoid changes. Diffuse and strong immunoreactivity with S100 (**e**), along with negative CD117 and pankeratin stains, helps in the differential diagnosis in problematic cases

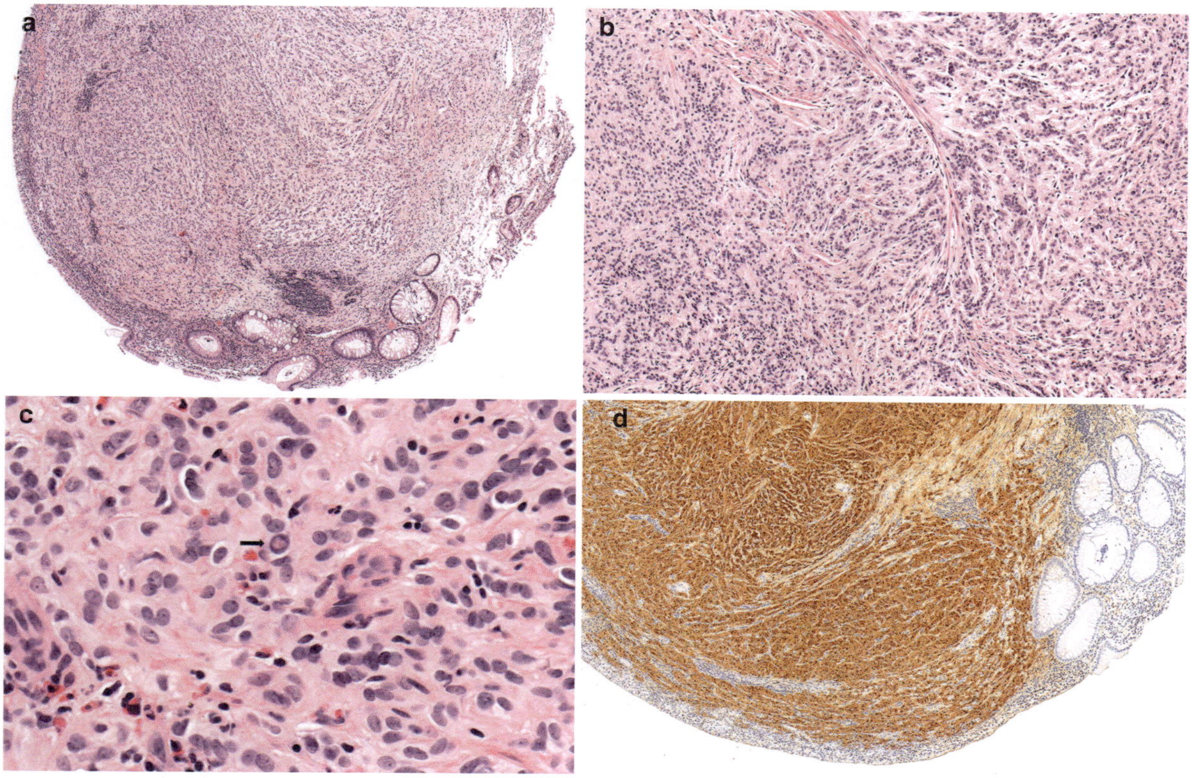

Mucosal benign epithelioid nerve sheath tumor (mBENST). This is a rare entity with similar morphology to epithelioid schwannoma of the soft tissues [11–13]. These tumors are usually identified at colonoscopy as incidental polyps. Histologically, the lesion is composed of a diffuse proliferation of small epithelioid tumor cells, which resemble nevus cells, arranged in trabecula or loosely cohesive small clusters in a collagenous stroma (**a**, **b**). Most commonly, the lesion is centered in the lamina propria and may extend into the superficial submucosa. (In the example shown, however, the epicenter of the lesion is mainly in the submucosa.) Note the associated mucosal ulceration (**a**). Higher magnification (**c**) shows uniform epithelioid cells with eosinophilic fibrillary cytoplasm and round-oval nuclei with fine chromatin and small inconspicuous nucleoli. Intranuclear pseudo-inclusions may be present (*arrow*). There is no atypia or mitotic activity. S-100 is diffusely positive (**d**). CD117 is negative and helps in the differential diagnosis with GISTs. The clinical course of mBENST is benign

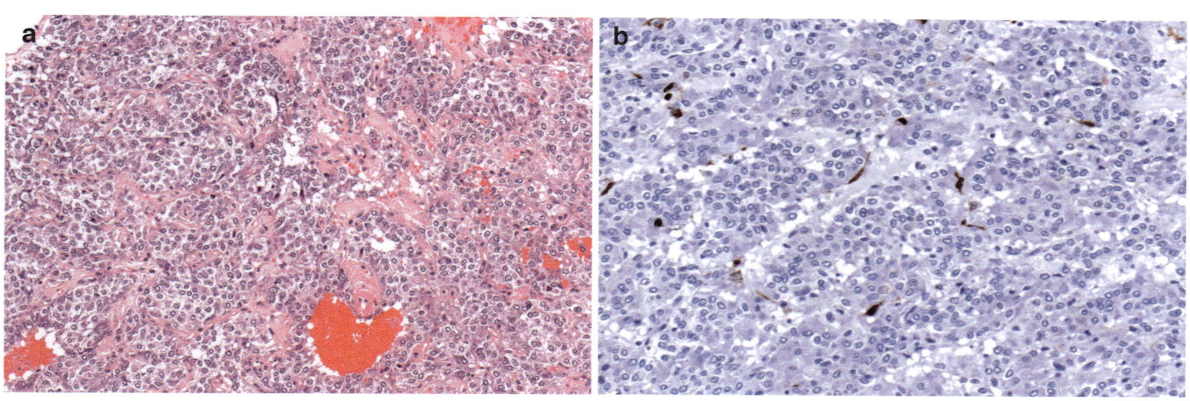

Paraganglioma and gangliocytic paraganglioma. GI paragangliomas are rare and mostly affect the duodenum. They originate from the external surface of the bowel and grow inwards. Although mostly sporadic, familial forms associated with germline loss of function mutations in SDH (succinate dehydrogenase) genes may occur. They may also be part of a tumor syndrome such as NF-1, MEN 2, VHL disease, Carney's triad, or a variant of GIST paraganglioma syndrome. (**a**), Example of a paraduodenal paraganglioma composed predominantly of nests of epithelioid cells (zellballen) with centrally placed round nuclei and granular, amphophilic cytoplasm. (**b**), Some of the nests are partially surrounded by spindle cells that are S100 positive and interpreted as sustentacular cells. Abundant small and medium-size blood vessels are seen throughout the tumor. (**c**), Tumor cells are diffusely immunoreactive for GATA3 [14]. (**d**), They can show variable, often heterogeneous, expression with neuroendocrine markers such as chromogranin. Epithelioid GIST (including the paragangliomalike variant) is in the differential diagnosis. Expression of GATA3 and neuroendocrine markers and lack of CD117 expression helps differentiate paragangliomas from GIST. (**e**), Gangliocytic paragangliomas are located almost exclusively in the duodenum and affect the submucosa. (**f**, **g**), They are composed of three cell types in varying proportions: spindle cells with a neural phenotype (**f**), ganglion cells, and epithelioid cells with neuroendocrine features forming a carcinoidlike pattern (**f**, **g**). The prognosis is excellent after surgical resection

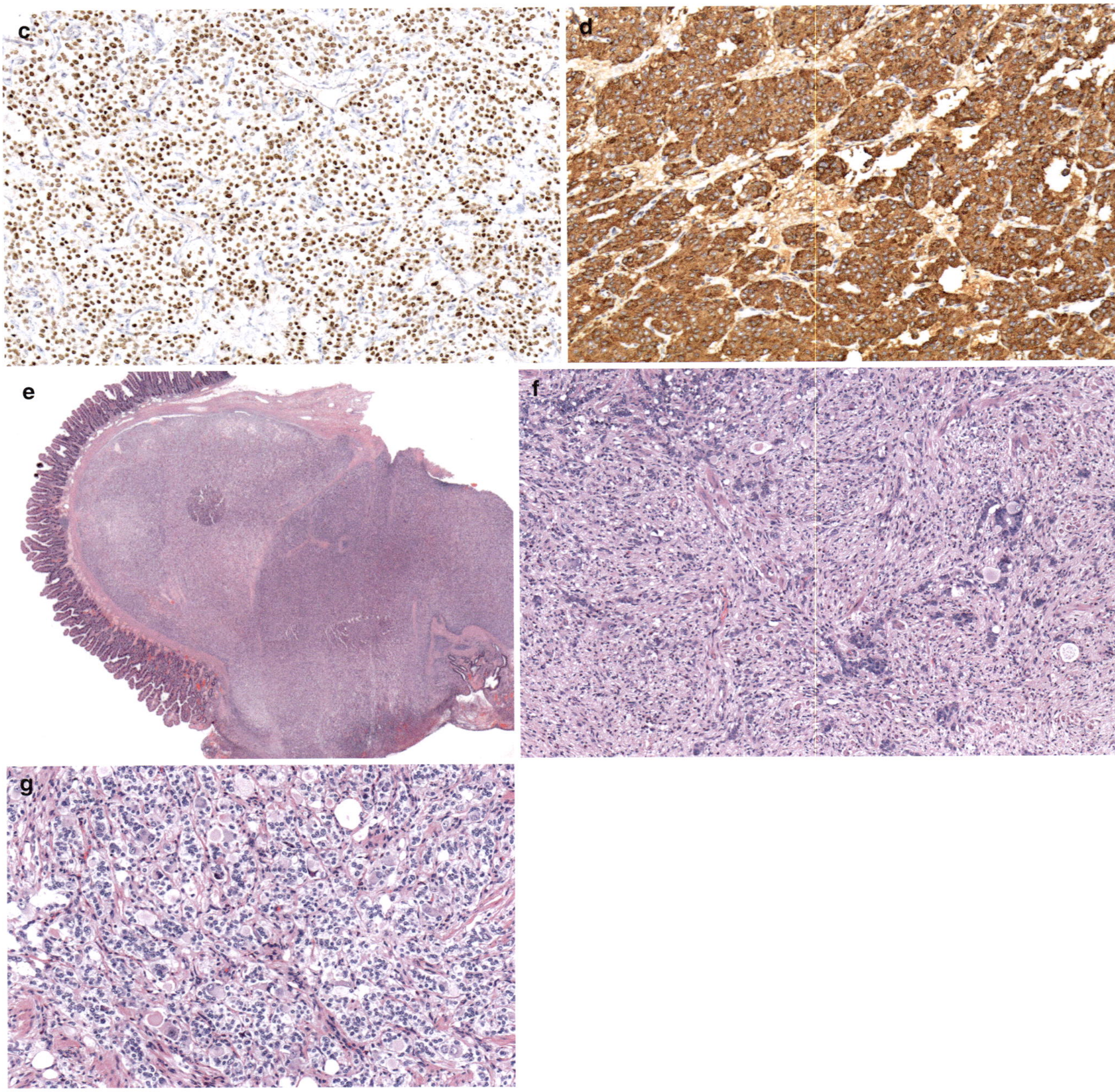

(continued)

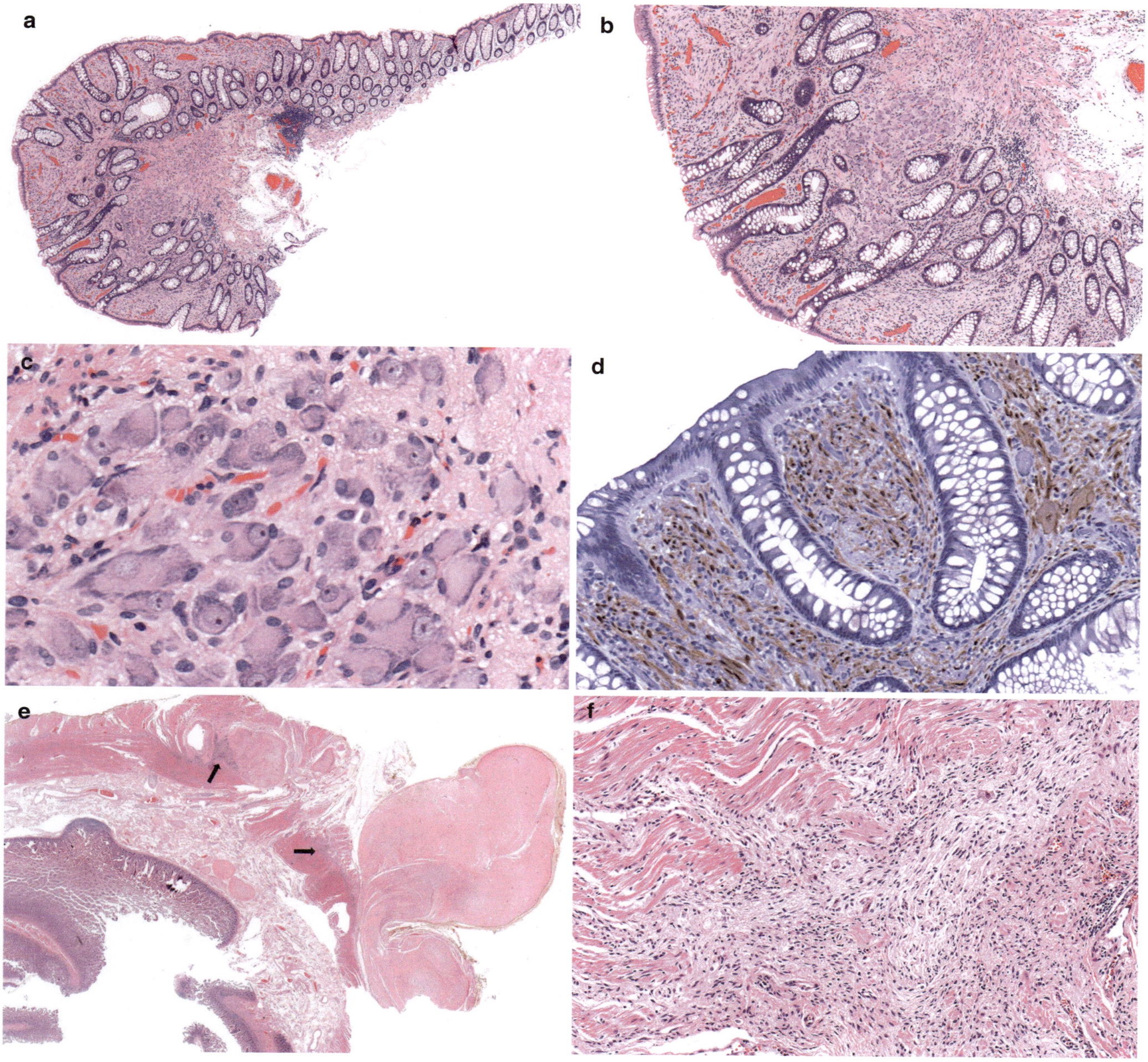

Ganglioneuromas. Polypoid ganglioneuromas are small mucosal or submucosal sessile polyps, usually discovered incidentally at colonoscopy. They may be either solitary or few in number. (**a**), The lamina propria is expanded by a poorly circumscribed neuronal proliferation causing distortion of entrapped crypts, hence resembling an inflammatory/juvenile polyp at low power. Occasionally, they may have a more nodular architecture (not shown here). (**b**), Scattered large ganglion cells with unusual morphology are interspersed between a proliferation of spindle-shaped Schwann cells. The ganglion cells may occur singly or in small clusters. Entrapped native submucosal ganglion cells should not be interpreted as evidence of a ganglioneuroma in other mucosal neural proliferations. (**c**), Note the large, atypical ganglion cells present in this polypoid ganglioneuroma. (**d**), S100 is positive. There are no known syndromic associations with isolated or a few polypoid ganglioneuromas, but two other forms of GI ganglioneuromatous proliferations are associated with hereditary syndromes. Ganglioneuromatous polyposis occurs as multiple polyps (>20), usually in the colon or rectum. It is frequently associated with extraintestinal manifestations and may herald Cowden syndrome. (**e**, **f**), Diffuse ganglioneuromatosis has a strong association with MEN2b and NF1 syndromes [15]. Unlike polypoid ganglioneuromas, which are typically superficial, diffuse ganglioneuromatosis is usually centered around the myenteric plexus (*arrow* in **e**), with intramural or transmural involvement. These are sections from the jejunum of a patient with NF1 syndrome, showing multiple neurofibromas involving all layers of the bowel wall associated with diffuse ganglioneuromatosis.

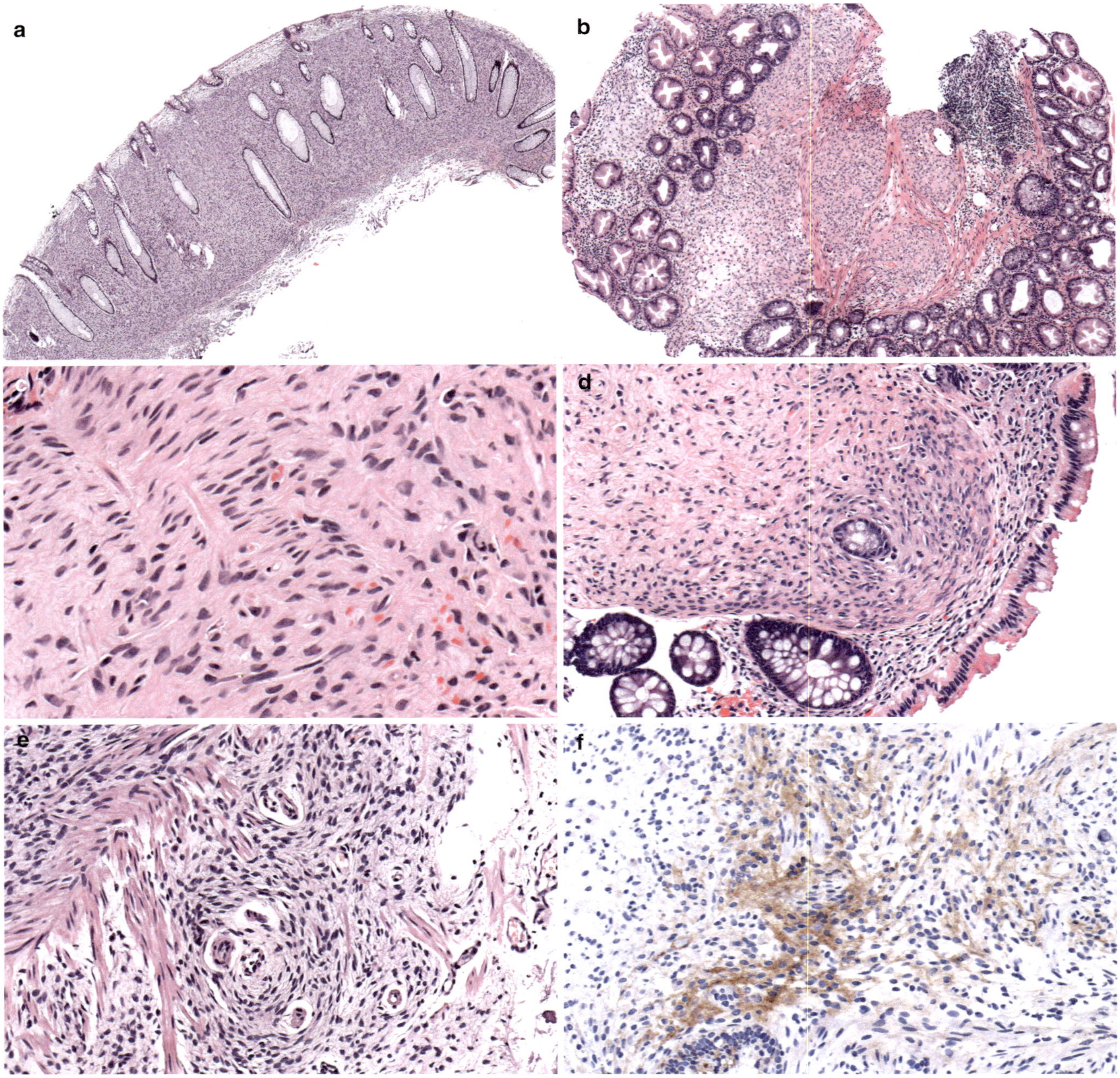

Mucosal perineurioma/benign fibroblastic polyp. Mucosal perineuriomas are benign peripheral nerve sheath tumors that are believed to represent the same entity as benign fibroblastic polyps. These small (typically 2–15 mm) mucosal colonic polyps are usually incidentally discovered during colonoscopy. The characteristic feature is expansion of the lamina propria by bland ovoid to spindle cells, often with a vague whorling pattern, which separate and entrap the crypts (**a**, **b**). Involvement of the superficial submucosa is not uncommon (**a**). Interestingly, most of these lesions are associated with either hyperplastic polyps (**b**) or sessile serrated polyps, which have been shown to harbor *BRAF* mutations. The lesional cells have pale, eosinophilic cytoplasm with indistinct cell borders and delicate, long cytoplasmic processes (**c**), which may display focal concentric arrangement around crypts and vessels (**d**, **e**). There is no atypia or mitotic activity. (Note the fairly well-demarcated lateral border in **d**.). They show variable and patchy immunoreactivity with markers of perineural differentiation such as EMA (**f**), GLUT1, and claudin-1. S100, CD117, DOG 1, SMA, SOX10, and keratin are negative. Based on their strong association with serrated polyps, some have proposed that mucosal perineuriomas may be epithelial-stromal hybrid lesions, consisting of neoplastic epithelium and a reactive perineural stromal component [16–19]

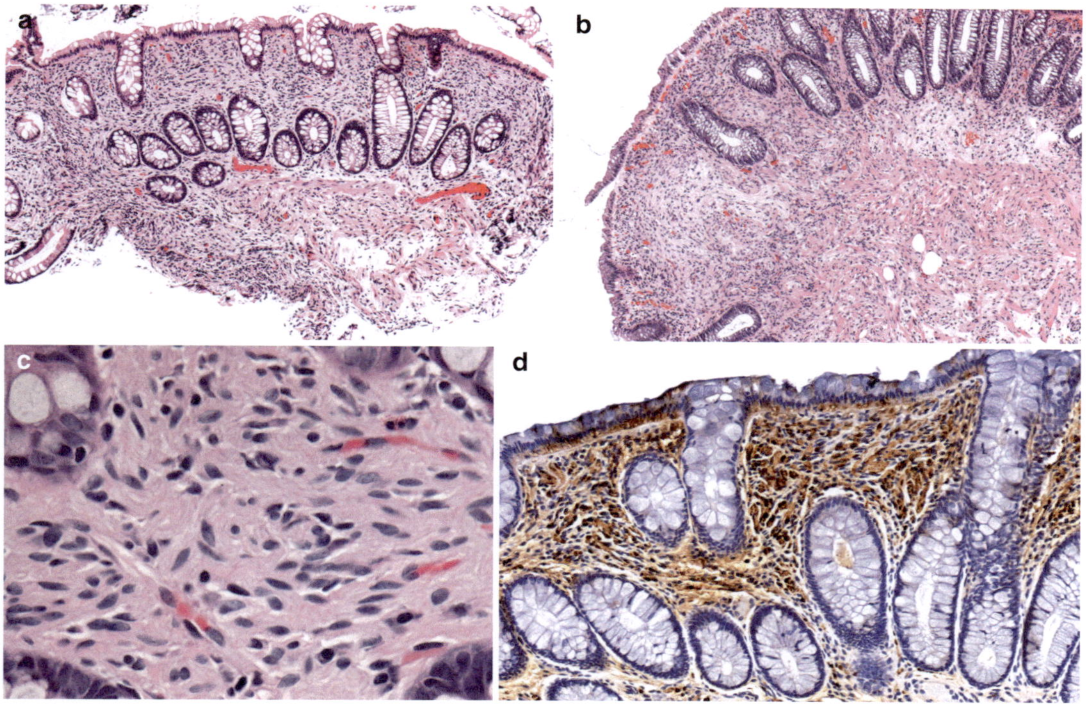

Schwann cell hamartoma (mucosal neuroma). This is a benign intramucosal Schwann cell proliferation, which is usually detected incidentally as a small sessile polypoid lesion (~1–6 mm) in the rectosigmoid region of elderly adults. The lesion consists of a diffuse, ill-defined proliferation of bland, uniform spindle cells in the lamina propria, which entraps crypts (**a**, **b**). The lesional cells have elongated or wavy tapering nuclei, inconspicuous small nucleoli, and dense eosinophilic cytoplasm with indistinct cell borders (**c**). There is no atypia or mitotic activity. No ganglion cells are present. S100 is diffusely and strongly positive (**d**). EMA, GFAP, CD34, SMA, and CD117 are negative. S100 immunoreactivity helps in the differential diagnosis with perineurioma. It is important to differentiate these tumors from neurofibromas and ganglioneuromas, because Schwann cell hamartomas are not associated with any hereditary conditions [20]

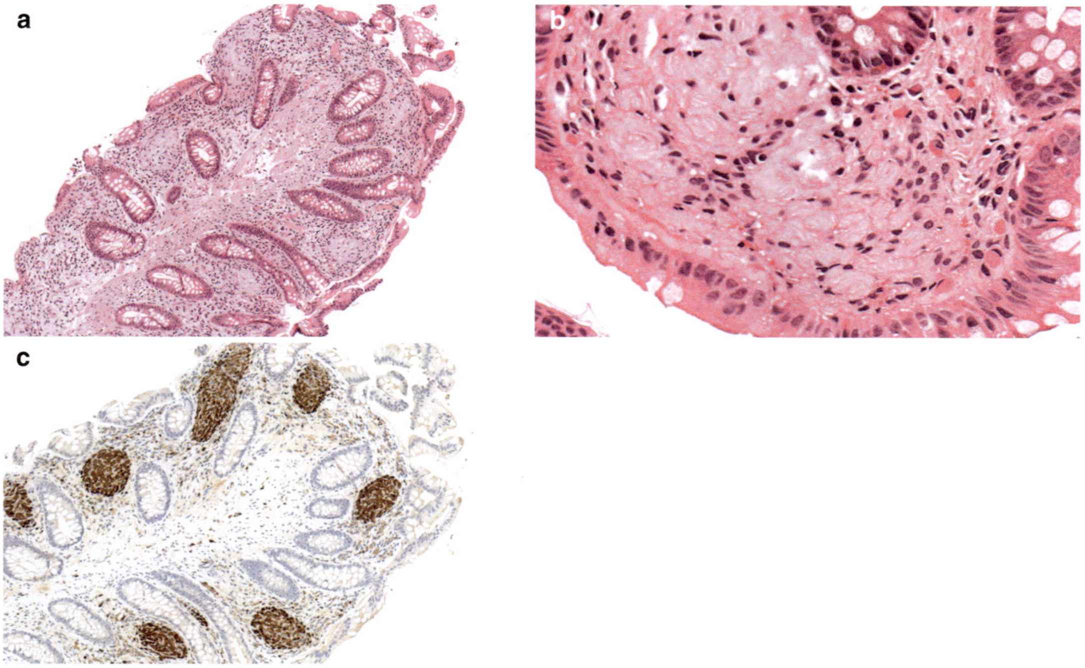

Tactile corpuscle-like bodies (Wagner-Meissner corpuscles). These are rarely seen in the GI tract and may represent part of the morphologic spectrum of Schwann cell hamartoma. They have no known syndromic associations. Like Schwann cell hamartomas, the most common location is the colon and rectum, although they may be seen throughout the GI tract [21]. (**a**, **b**), They are characterized by multiple small foci of nodular, unencapsulated clusters of lamellated, concentrically arranged spindle cells within the lamina propria between the crypts. The lesional cells have eosinophilic cytoplasm with peripherally located nuclei (**b**). (**c**), They are immunoreactive with S100

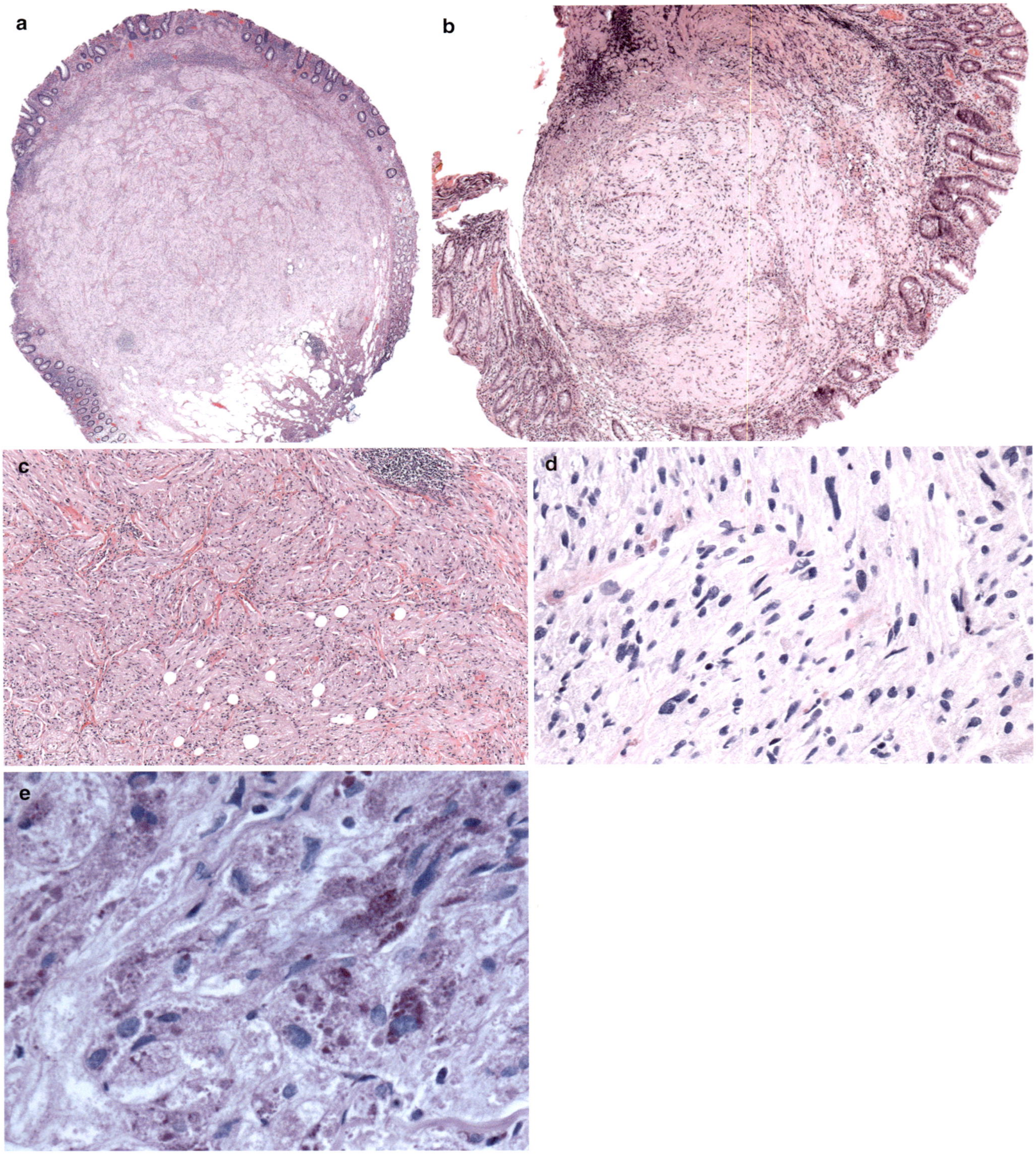

Granular cell tumor (GCT). These tumors are rare in the GI tract outside of the esophagus. Intestinal granular cell tumors are usually incidentally discovered during colonoscopy, predominantly in the right colon. They are typically centered in the submucosa and are relatively well circumscribed (**a**, **b**), although some lesions have focally infiltrative margins (**a**). Mucosal forms also exist and can have an infiltrative growth pattern. The tumor is composed of polygonal to spindled histiocyte-like cells, which are believed to be of Schwann cell origin, arranged in cohesive nests or infiltrative cords and short fascicles with intervening fibrous tissue (**c**). They have characteristic abundant granular eosinophilic cytoplasm. Nuclei are typically small and hyperchromatic, although foci of nuclear atypia, including enlargement and hyperchromasia, are occasionally present (**d**). PAS-diastase positive cytoplasmic granules, which are of lysosomal origin (**e**), and diffuse immunoreactivity for S100 and CD68 are diagnostic findings. SOX-10 is also positive. Reactive mucosal surface changes (such as crypt distortion, epithelial hyperplasia, and mucosal inflammation), a peripheral lymphoid cuff (**a**), focal dystrophic calcification, and increased amounts of peritumoral fat deposition (**a**) may be seen. Malignant GCT, though exceedingly rare, has been reported at extra-intestinal sites. To date, no distant metastasis of colorectal GCT has been reported, although occasional cases of local recurrence have been described [22–24]

Benign Polypoid Lesions of the Intestine: Typical Morphologic and Immunohistochemical Features

Tumor	Typical Morphology	Localization	Immunohistochemistry
Microcytic/reticular schwannoma	Loose myxoid stroma with a microcytic or sponge-like reticular architecture, which can mimic a cribriforming gland pattern	Submucosa	S100 positive
Benign epithelioid nerve sheath tumor	Proliferation of nevus-like epithelioid cells	Mucosa; rarely submucosa	S100 positive
Sporadic polypoid ganglioneuroma	Spindled schwannian cell proliferation admixed with atypical ganglion cells	Mucosa or submucosa	S100 positive
Perineurioma (benign fibroblastic polyp)	Expansion of lamina propria with bland slender spindle cells splaying the crypts A vague whirling pattern and foci of concentric growth around crypts and vessels Often associated with adjacent serrated polyp	Mucosa, may extend to submucosa	EMA, GLUT 1 and Claudine-1 positive (all usually focal and patchy) S100 negative
Schwann cell hamartoma	Ill-defined proliferation of bland spindle cells that entrap crypts. The cells have tapering ends and wavy nuclei	Mucosa	S100 positive EMA negative
Wagner-Meissner corpuscles (tactile corpuscle-like bodies)	Nodular arrangement of lamellated, brightly eosinophilic spindle cells with peripherally located nuclei	Mucosa	S100 positive
Granular cell tumor	Epithelioid to spindle, histiocyte-like cells with abundant granular eosinophilic cytoplasm arranged in nests or cords with intervening fibrous tissue	Mucosa or submucosa	PAS-D positive granules S100, CD 68 and SOX 10 positive
Leiomyoma of the muscularis mucosae	Well-circumscribed, fascicular growth of brightly eosinophilic, bland spindle cells with elongated, cigar-shaped nuclei merging with the muscularis mucosae	Submucosa	SMA, Desmin and Caldesmon positive
Inflammatory fibroid polyp	Proliferation of bland ovoid, spindled, and stellate cells in a loose edematous-myxoid to collagenous matrix admixed with an inflammatory infiltrate rich in eosinophils	Submucosa, may extend transmurally	Most are CD34 positive CD117, DOG 1 negative

3.3 Tumors of Smooth Muscle Origin

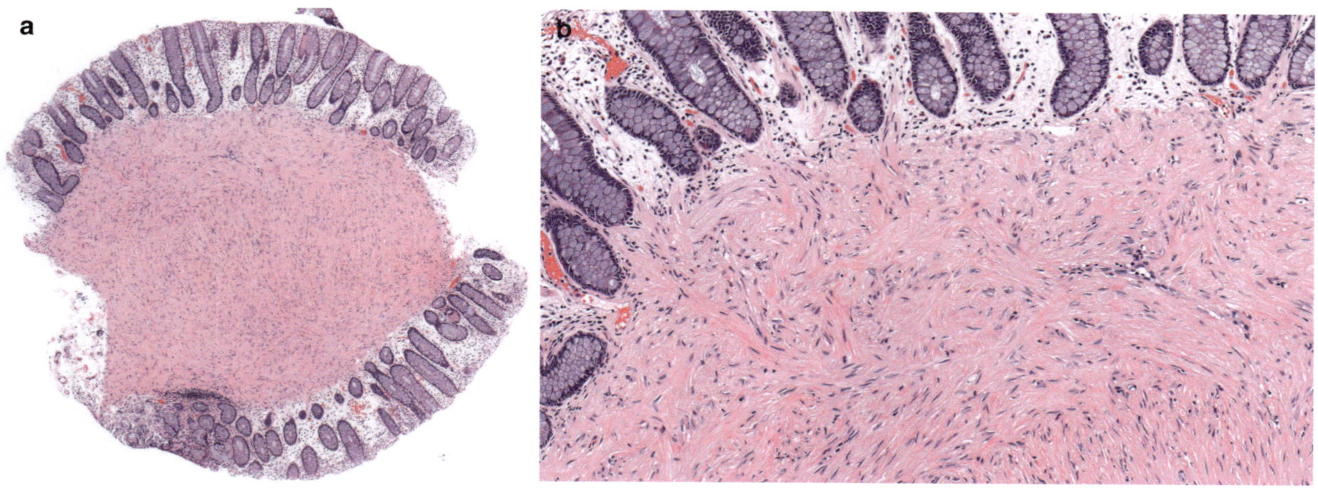

Leiomyoma of the muscularis mucosae. Leiomyomas in the GI tract can be superficial, arising from the muscularis mucosae, or deep, arising from the muscularis propria [25–28]. Leiomyoma of the muscularis mucosae is predominantly seen in the colorectum, and is the most common mesenchymal tumor of this site. These lesions are usually found incidentally as small polyps (**a**) during colonoscopy. They are typically composed of disorganized fascicles of cytologically bland smooth muscle cells with abundant eosinophilic cytoplasm. The nuclear density of the neoplastic cells is often lower than that of the native muscularis mucosae, which usually can be seen to merge with the neoplastic cells in some planes of section (**a**, **b**). Rounded, eosinophilic, desmin-positive globules may be seen in tumor cells, which can help distinguish leiomyomas from hypertrophied muscularis mucosae (**c**). Mitoses are absent or rare. Rarely, nuclear atypia analogous to uterine leiomyomas can be seen, but there are no other atypical features. Like other smooth muscle tumors, leiomyomas of the muscularis mucosae are immunoreactive with smooth muscle markers (SMA, desmin, caldesmon)

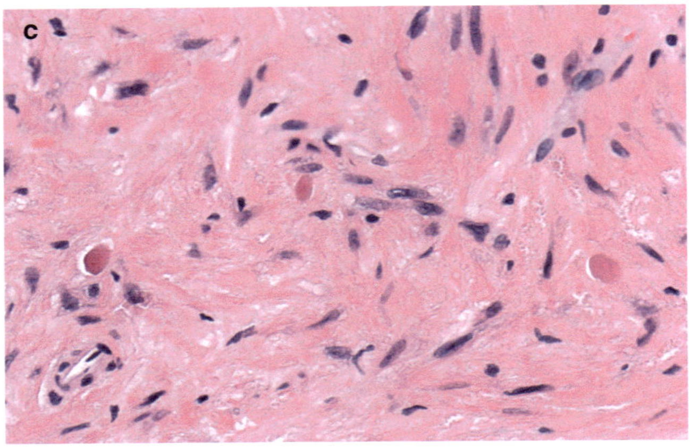

(continued)

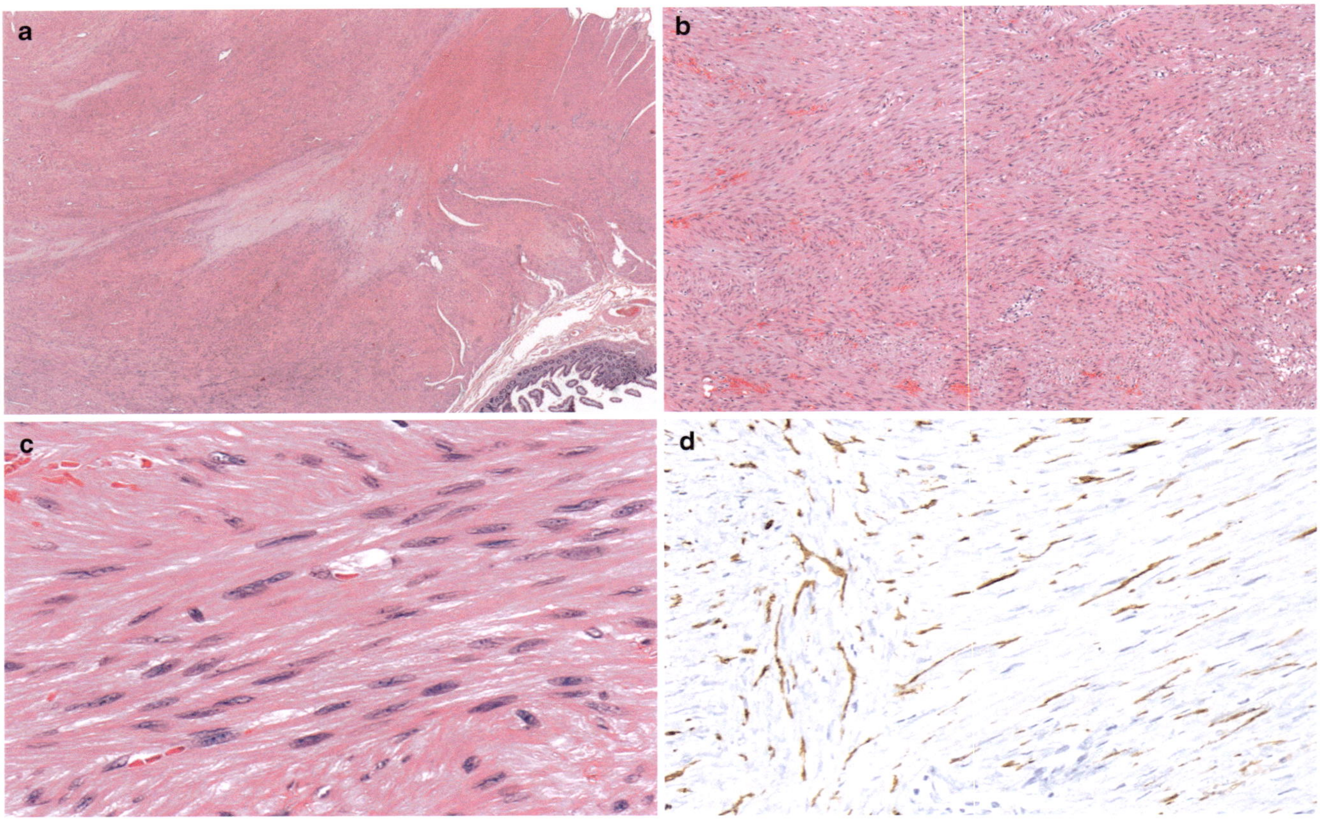

Intramural leiomyoma. (**a**), This intramural small bowel leiomyoma is originating from the muscularis propria. (**b**, **c**), These tumors are characterized by intersecting fascicles of bland, spindle-shaped cells with abundant eosinophilic cytoplasm and elongated, blunt-ended nuclei. Mitoses are absent or very scant. Tumor cells are negative for S100, C-KIT, and DOG1. Of note, mural leiomyomas in the GI tract often contain interspersed interstitial cells of Cajal, which stain positively for DOG1 (**d**) and C-KIT (**e**). Thus, the presence of admixed C-KIT and DOG1 positive cells in a lesion with typical features of leiomyoma should not on its own prompt consideration of GIST. Smooth muscle markers are diffusely positive (**f**, SMA stain). In most cases, leiomyomas are less cellular than GISTs and have plump cells with blunt-ended nuclei and dense, brightly eosinophilic cytoplasm, in contrast to the tapered nuclei and paler, fibrillary cytoplasm seen in most GISTs

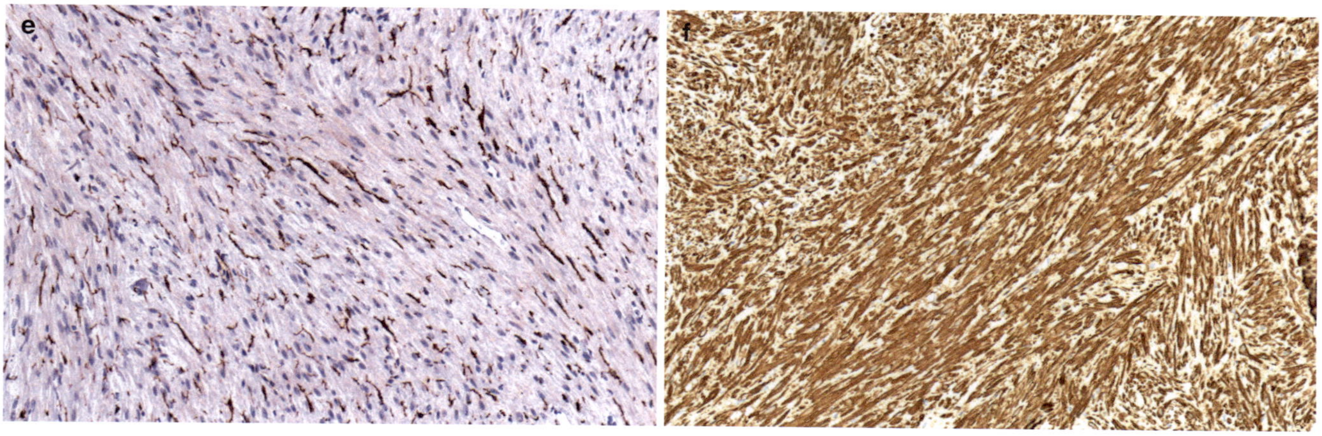

(continued)

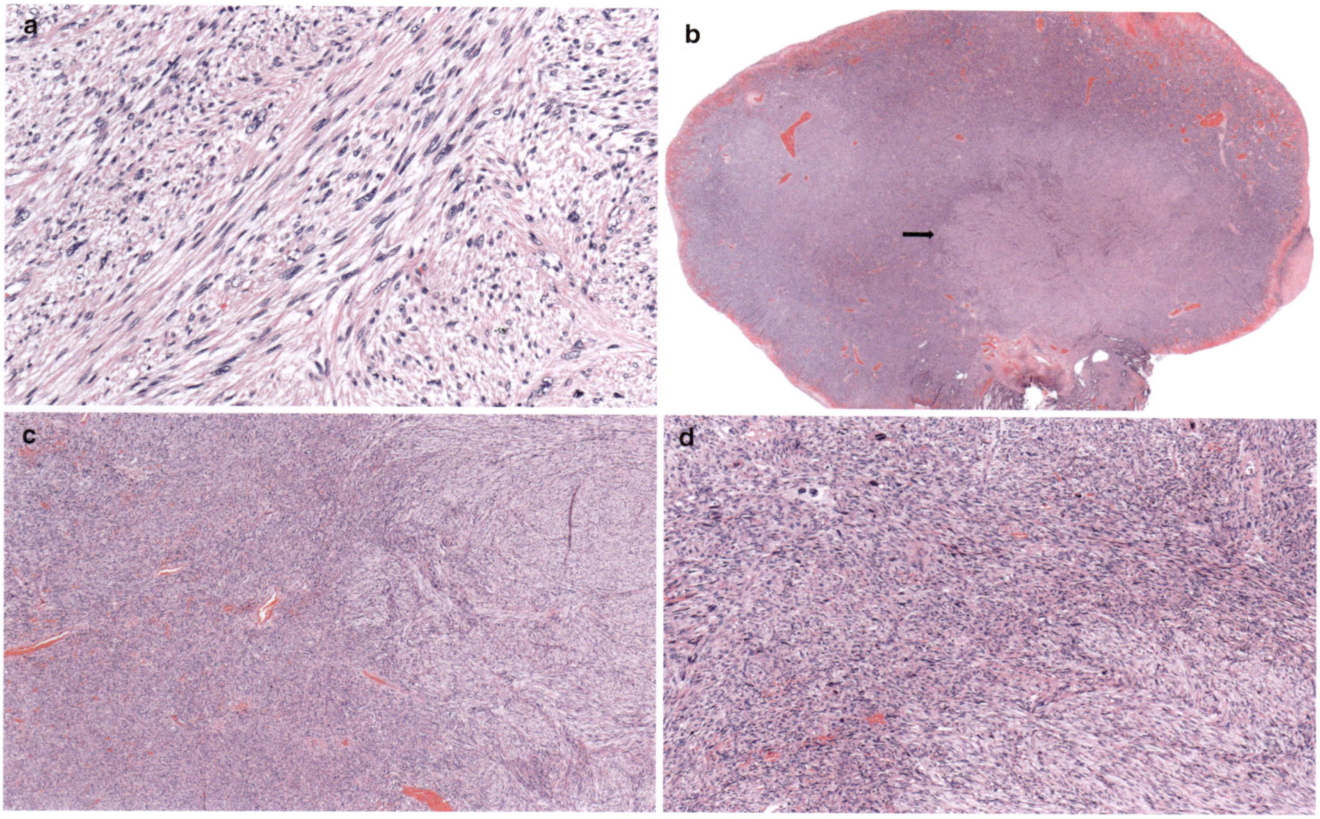

Leiomyosarcoma. Primary leiomyosarcoma in the GI tract is rare. These tumors occur mostly in the small intestine and colon. (**a**), This jejunal leiomyosarcoma shows morphologically identifiable smooth muscle differentiation. Characteristic features include right-angled, intersecting fascicles of tumor cells with blunt-ended nuclei and moderate amounts of eosinophilic cytoplasm. Distinction from leiomyoma can be made based on the presence of nuclear atypia, mitotic activity (>5 per 10 HPF in the vast majority of cases), and necrosis. Tumor cells are immunoreactive for SMA, and show variable expression of caldesmon and desmin. S100, DOG1, and CKIT are typically negative. (**b–d**), Rarely, dedifferentiation can be seen in leiomyosarcomas [29], as in this polypoid colonic mass, which shows typical smooth muscle differentiation in the center of the mass (**b**, *arrow*). (**e**), The morphologic and immunohistochemical features of smooth muscle differentiation can be lost at the periphery of the lesion (desmin stain), where there is much more marked pleomorphism. (**f**), This jejunal smooth muscle tumor of undetermined malignant potential (STUMP) appears more cellular than a typical leiomyoma, but it has mild nuclear atypia (**g**), a low mitotic rate (<5 per 10 HPF), and no necrosis. Proposed terminology for such cases, which are extremely rare in the GI tract, include *STUMP* and *low-grade leiomyosarcoma* [26, 27]. Well-defined criteria based on clinical outcomes have not been established

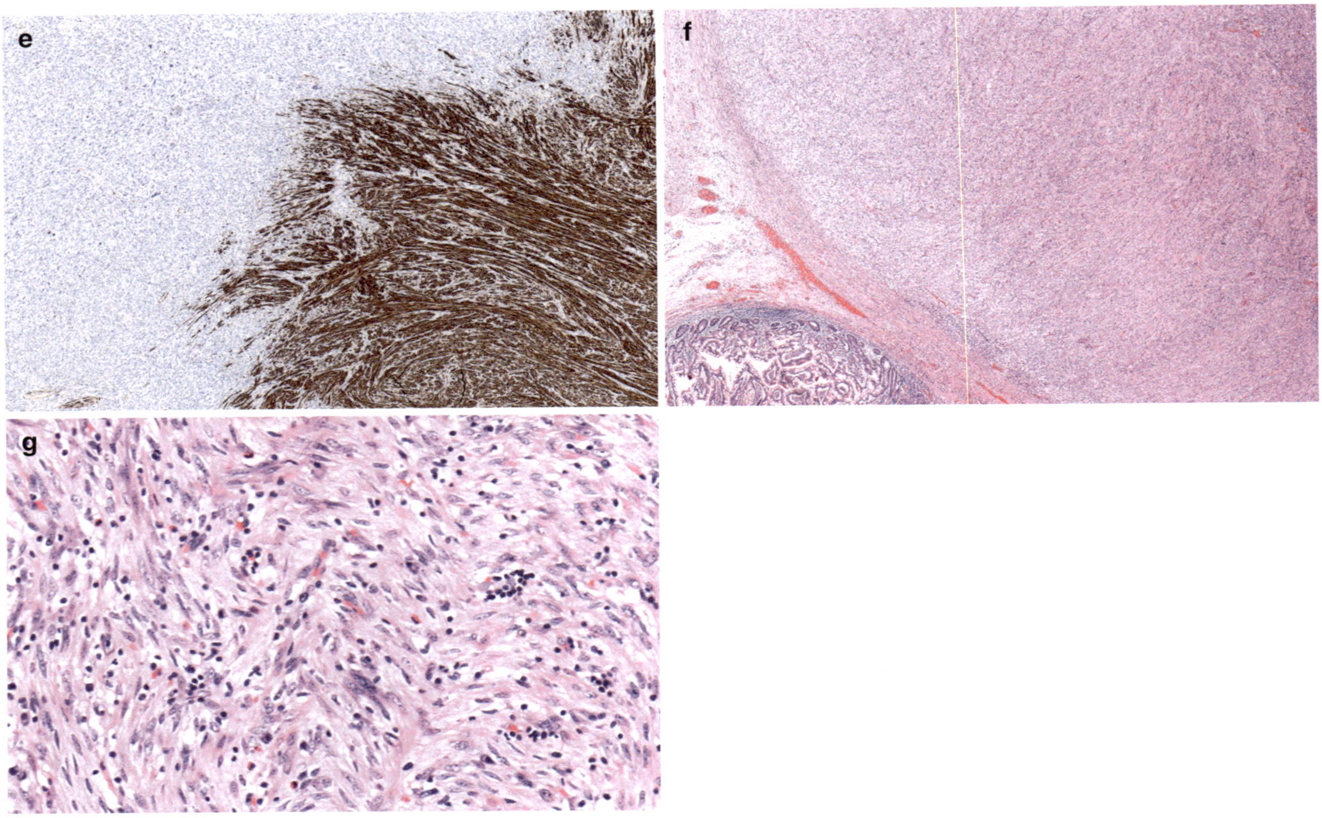

(continued)

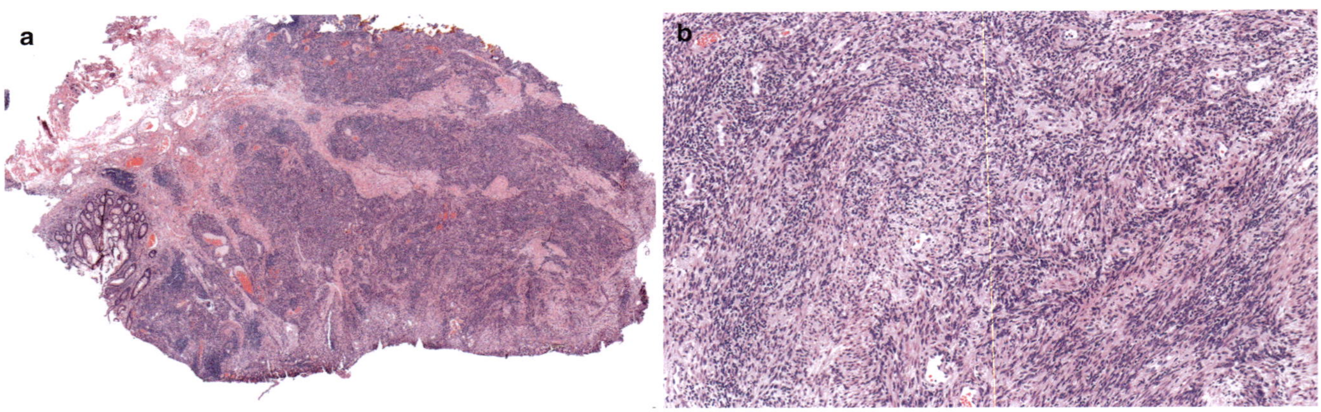

Epstein-Barr virus (EBV)–associated smooth muscle tumor (EBV-SMT). This is a rare entity, which so far has been described only in immunocompromised patients. The GI tract is one of the most common sites of involvement [30]. This colonic polyp is from a 35-year-old man with a history of renal and ureteric transplantation. He presented with melena and underwent colonoscopy, which revealed multiple polyps. At low power, the tumor is polypoid and cellular, with a somewhat lobulated appearance (**a**). A higher-power view shows spindle cells with recognizable smooth cell differentiation (**b**) admixed with more primitive ovoid-shaped cells, in which smooth muscle differentiation cannot be readily appreciated (**c**). Note the prominence of intra-tumoral lymphocytes. The tumor cells are positive for SMA (**d**) but only focally immunoreactive for desmin (**e**), as is often the case in these tumors. The diagnosis of EBV-SMT is confirmed by EBER RNA in situ hybridization (**f**). A spectrum of morphologies has been described in EBV-SMTs, ranging from appearances typical of leiomyomas to densely cellular and mitotically active tumors resembling leiomyosarcomas. There is usually a modest degree of atypia. Although most reported cases have had favorable outcomes, tumor-specific mortality has occurred in some patients. The mitotic rate does not seem to be associated with outcome

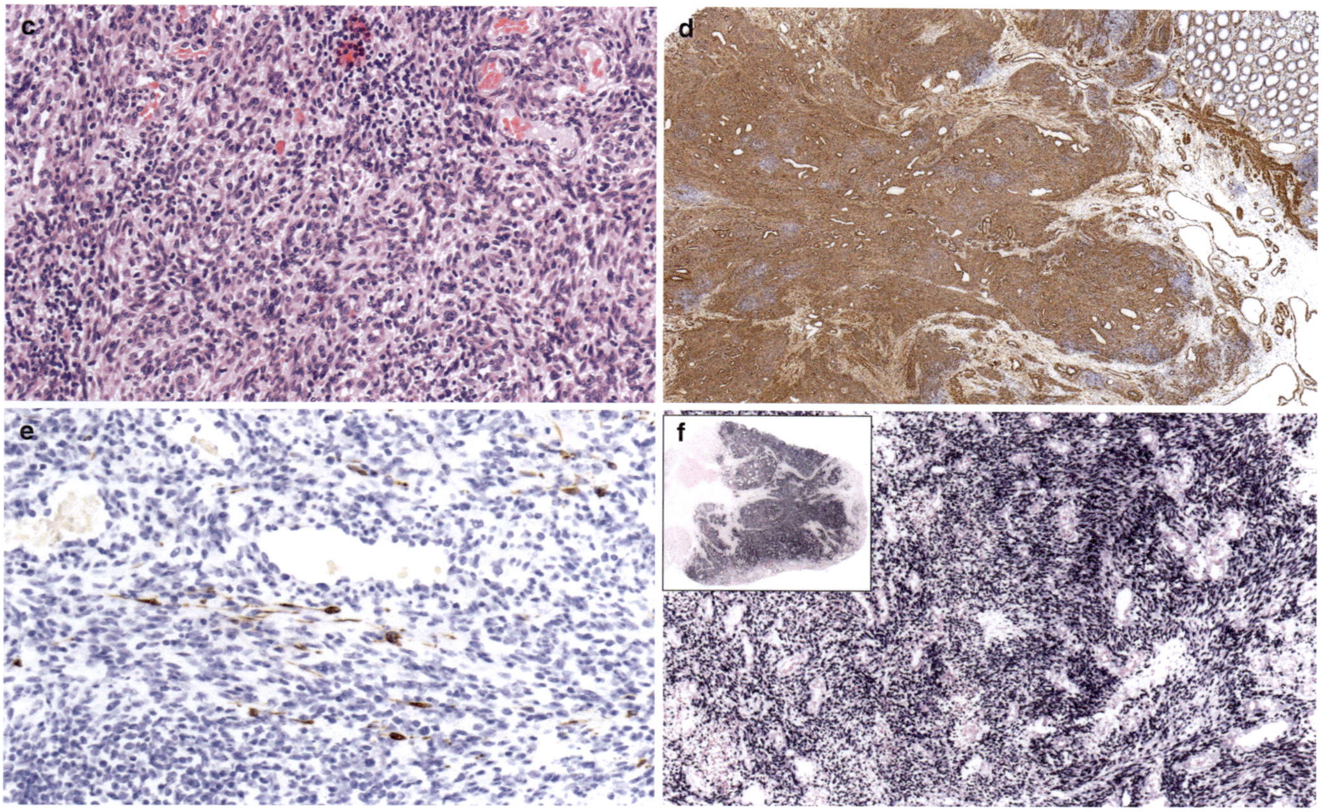

(continued)

3.4 Tumors of Fibroblastic or Myofibroblastic Origin

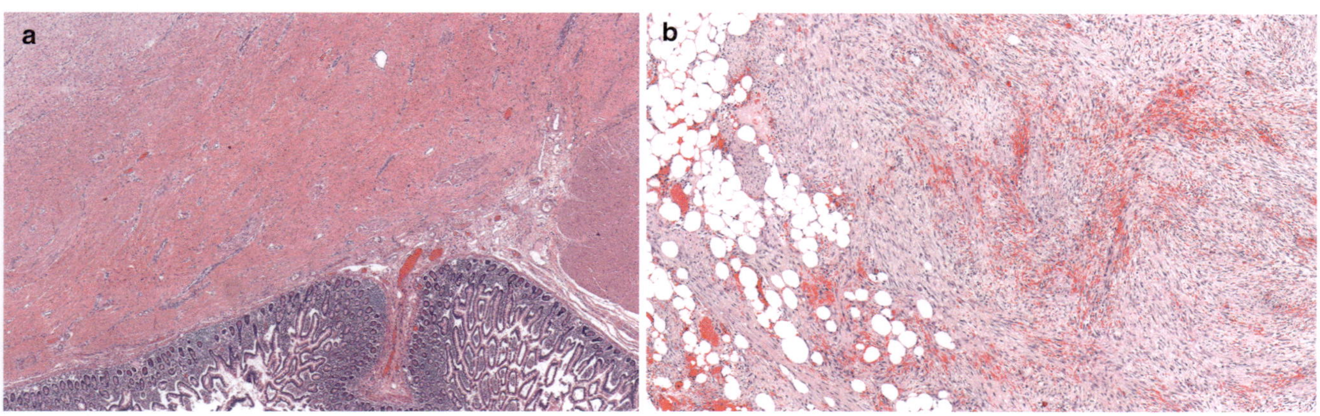

Mesenteric fibromatosis (desmoid tumor). This is the most common tumor of the mesentery [31]. It may exhibit locally aggressive behavior and can involve the wall of the bowel (**a**) or can extend into the liver and pancreas in some cases. These lesions may occur sporadically, often following trauma or abdominal surgery, or they may be associated with familial adenomatous polyposis (Gardner syndrome). They are typically paucicellular, composed of long and broad sweeping fascicles with a collagenous stroma (**b-d**), which may be dense (**a**), and have infiltrative borders (**b**, **c**). Keloid-type collagen fibers (**e**), muscular arteries, and ectatic, thin-walled veins with extravasated erythrocytes are characteristic (**d**, **e**). Storiform patterns (**f**) and myxoid stroma have also been described in some cases. At high power, bland, evenly spaced spindle to stellate cells with wavy, tapering pale eosinophilic cytoplasm and spindle-shaped nuclei with pinpoint nucleoli are characteristic, as are plumper, "tissue culture–like" stellate cells with larger nuclei and more abundant cytoplasm (**g**). Mitotic activity is generally low and atypical mitoses are not present. Immunohistochemistry for beta-catenin often shows nuclear positivity in tumor cells (**h**), although approximately 20% of cases are negative. Patchy SMA expression may be seen

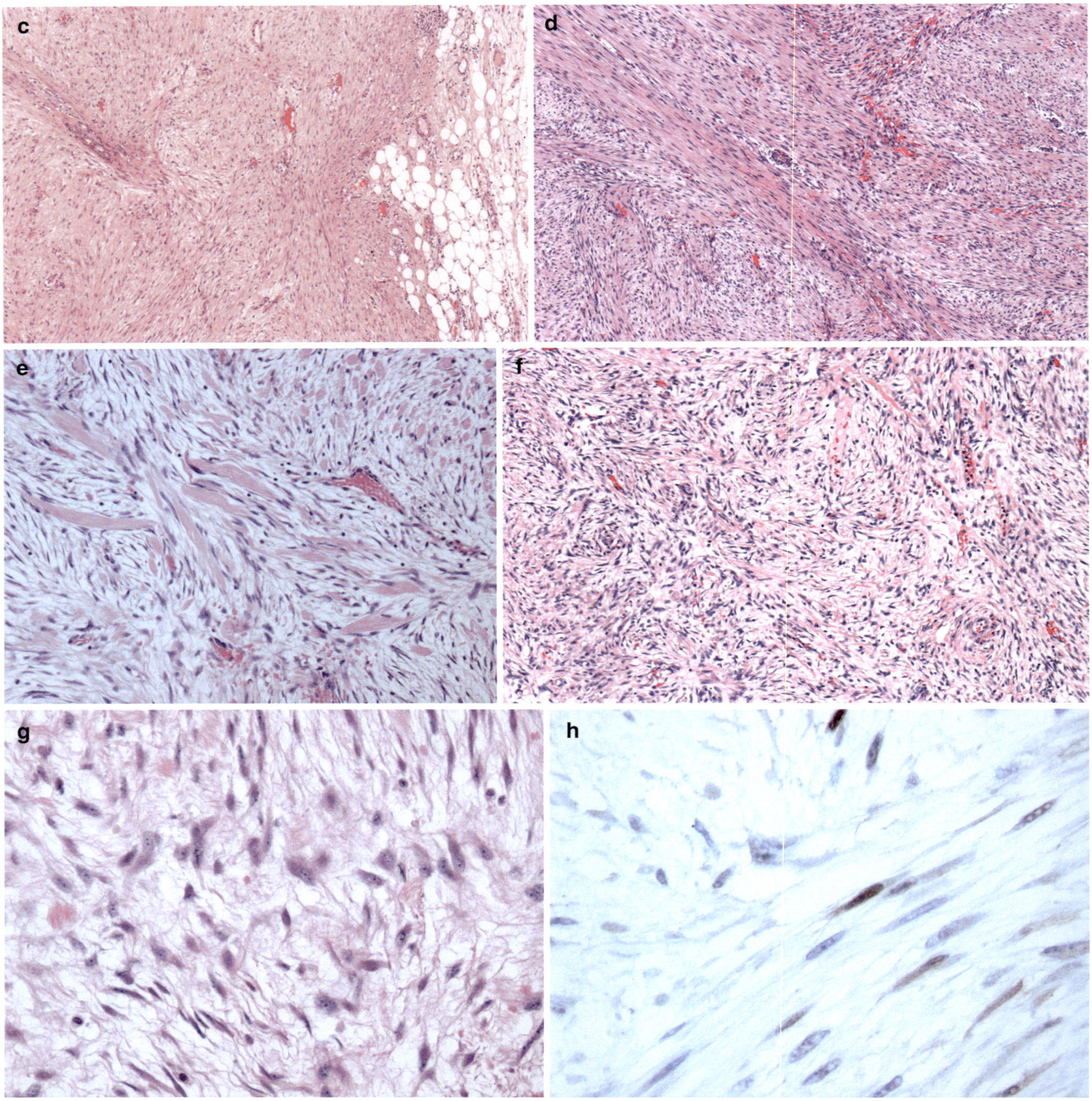

(continued)

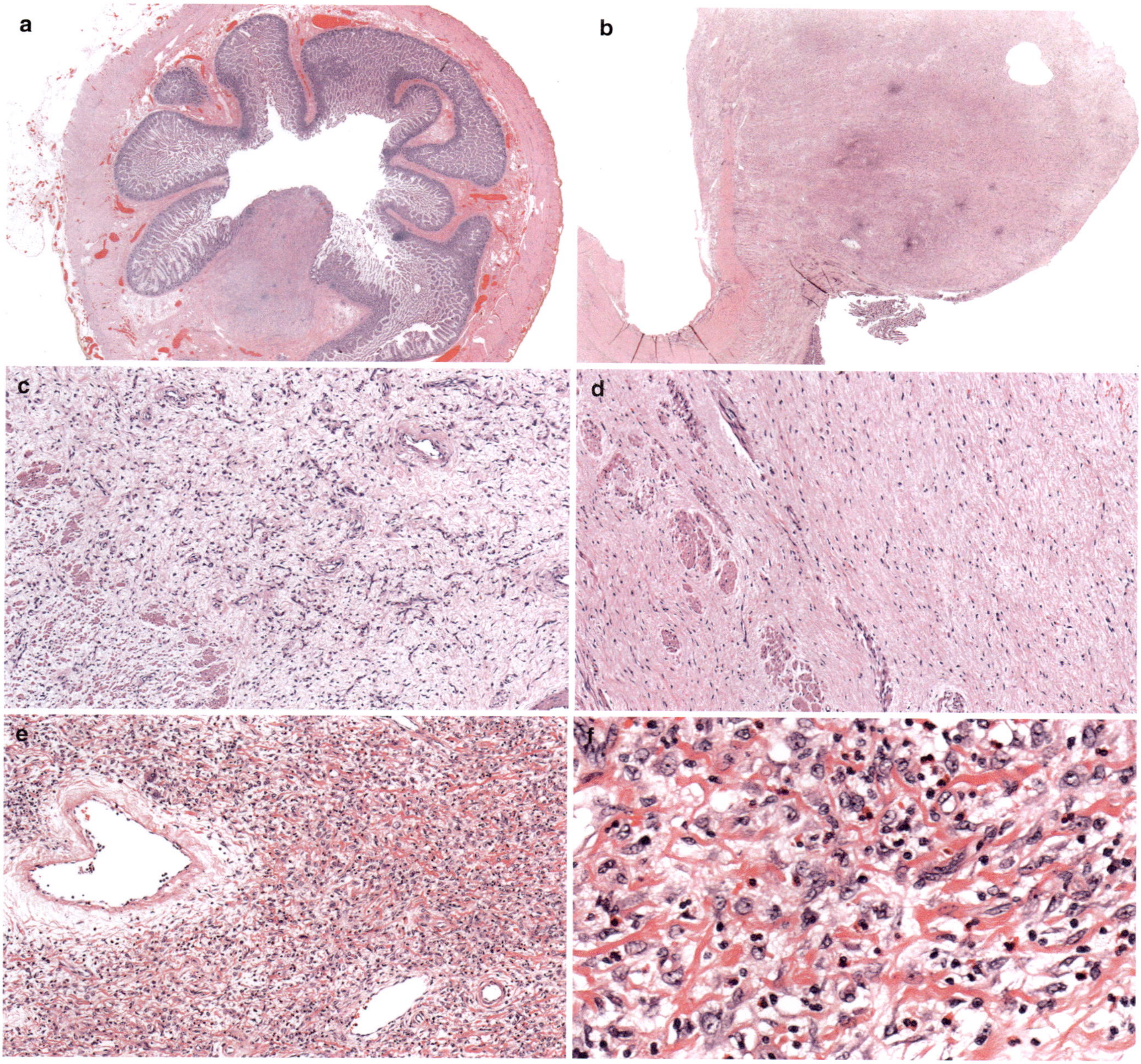

Inflammatory fibroid polyps (IFPs). These polyps may occur anywhere in the GI tract, but they are most common in the stomach, followed by the small intestine and the colon. They are grossly centered in the submucosa and range from small sessile or polypoid lesions (**a**) to very large masses, which can infiltrate through the muscularis propria and extend onto the serosa (**b**). Mucosal involvement with associated ulceration is a common feature. Small intestinal IFPs frequently present with intussusception. The typical appearance is a proliferation of cytologically bland, ovoid, spindled or stellate cells in a loose edematous-myxoid stroma (**c**), but in some cases the stroma is more collagenous (**d**, **e**). There is often a prominent inflammatory infiltrate rich in eosinophils (**e**, **f**). Prominent vascularity with interlacing vascular channels (**c**), perivascular edema (**e**), and concentric cuffing (onion-skinning) of spindle cells around vessels (**g**, **h**) are characteristic features, though onion-skinning is often absent or inconspicuous in small-bowel IFPs. Some tumors are quite cellular (**i**), whereas others are hypocellular, with more fibrous stroma and less inflammatory cells in the background (**d**). Other features that may occasionally be seen include a fascicular growth pattern (**j**), lymphoid aggregates (**k**), and multinucleated giant cells (**k**). The mitotic rate is low and atypical mitoses are absent. In spite of their sometimes infiltrative appearance, IFPs are benign lesions considered to have no metastasizing potential. Approximately 50–60% of cases have *PDGFR-α* gene mutations. CD34 immunohistochemistry is positive in the spindle-cell component in approximately 85% of cases [32]

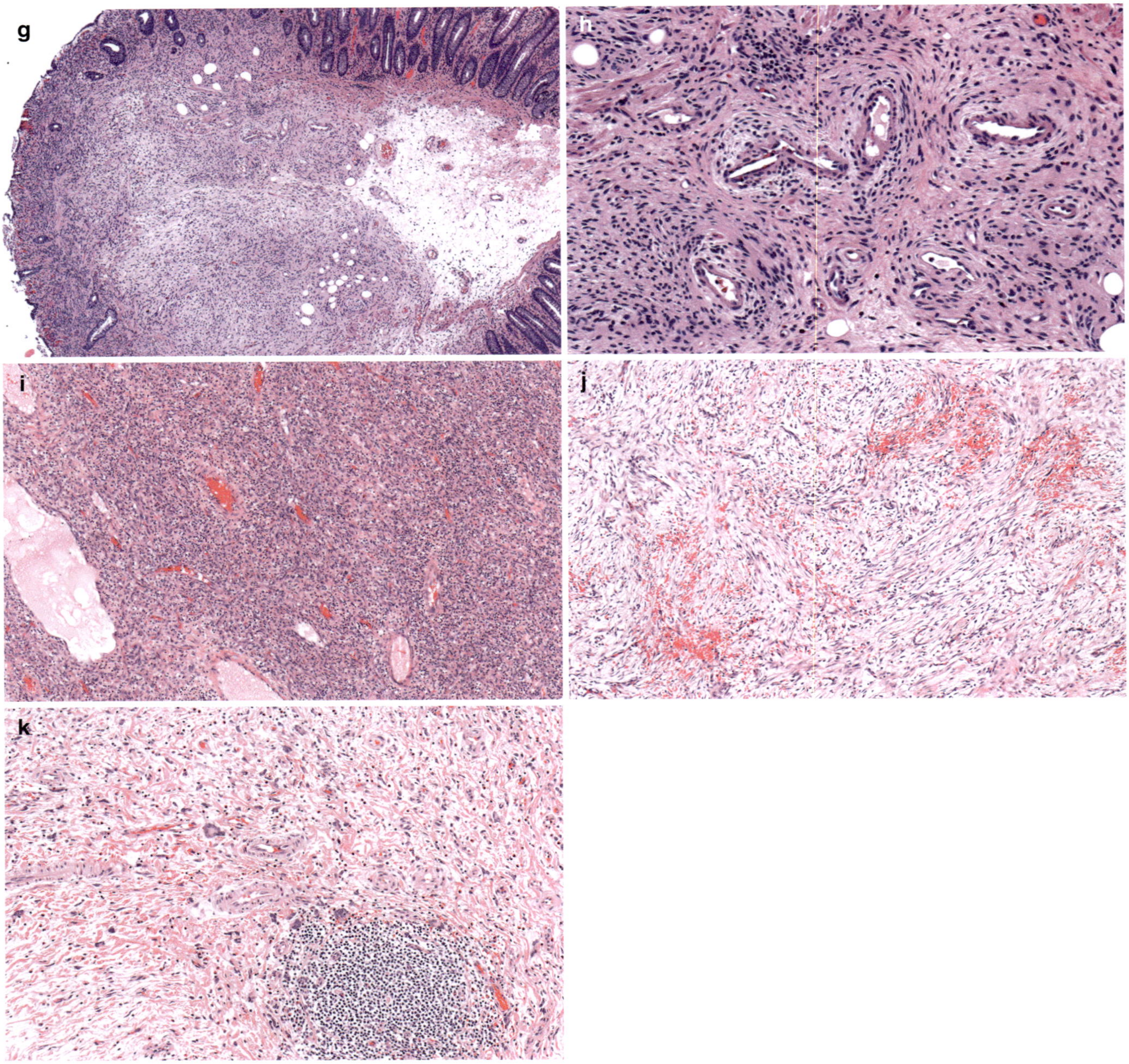

(continued)

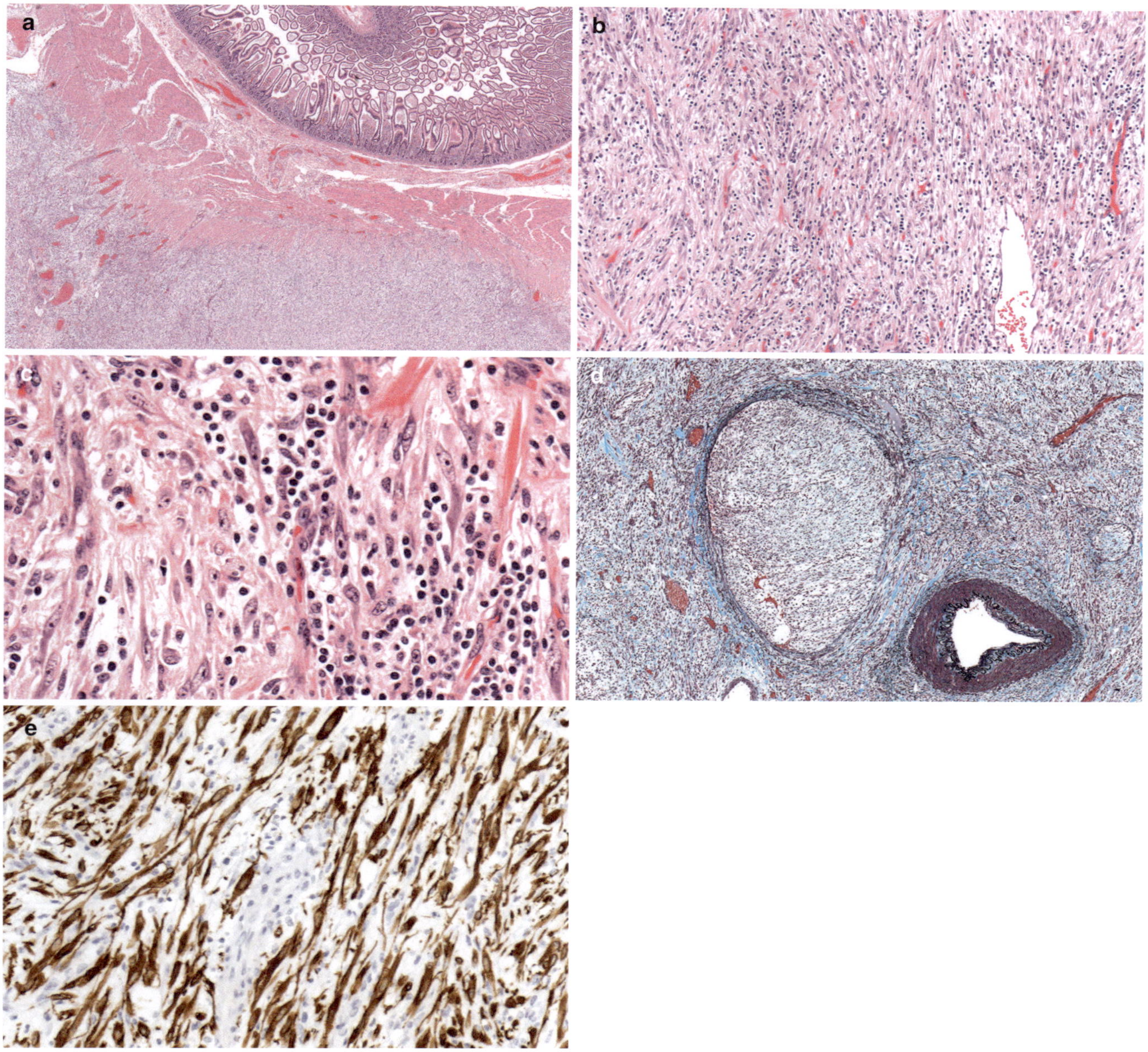

Inflammatory myofibroblastic tumor (IMT). This is an uncommon mesenchymal neoplasm, which most often involves the lung. The mesentery is a common extrapulmonary site, but primary involvement of the intestine is extremely rare. IMTs are usually well-circumscribed and range in size from lesions measuring less than a centimeter to large tumors exceeding 35 cm. A variety of morphologic patterns can be seen, even within the same tumor, including myxoid stroma, compact areas with dense spindle cells, and hypocellular/sclerotic areas. The histologic differential diagnosis depends upon the pattern(s) seen. (**a**), This IMT arising in the small bowel shows infiltration into the muscularis propria. (**b**), The tumor is composed of cytologically atypical myofibroblasts admixed with an inflammatory infiltrate composed predominantly of plasma cells and lymphocytes. (**c**), Higher-power magnification shows moderately atypical spindle to ovoid cells with large vesicular nuclei and prominent nucleoli. Note the abundance of inflammation in the background. Mitoses are readily identified. (**d**), An elastic-trichrome stain highlights venous invasion. (**e**), Approximately half of cases are positive for ALK expression by immunohistochemistry, usually due to clonal rearrangements involving the *ALK* gene. ALK expression can be diagnostically useful when present, although sensitivity is low [33]. Expression of SMA and/or keratin can be seen and should not be misinterpreted as evidence of a smooth muscle neoplasm or a carcinoma. IMT has intermediate malignant potential. Most cases are benign, although approximately a quarter recur locally; distant metastasis can occur but is rare

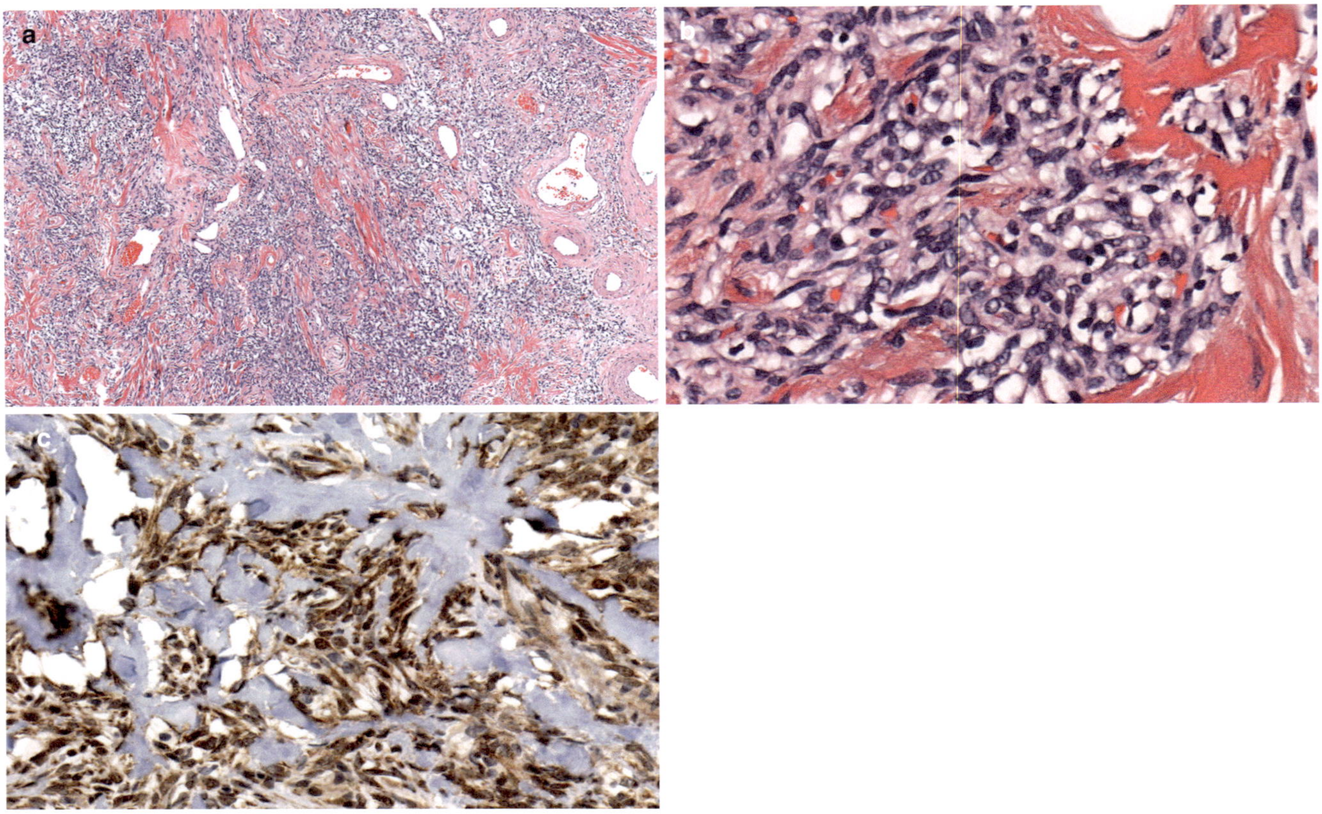

Solitary fibrous tumor (SFT). This tumor arises most often in the pleura, but extrapleural sites of involvement, including the peritoneum and retroperitoneum, are fairly common. When adherent to the visceral peritoneum, SFT can present clinically as an intestinal tumor. (**a**, **b**), This incompletely excised SFT was attached to the rectosigmoid colon. There are bland, ovoid to spindle-shaped tumor cells with a patternless arrangement and variable cellularity. Other typical features shown are markedly collagenous stroma, including keloid-like collagen, and thick-walled staghorn vessels. (**c**), A fusion transcript, NAB2-STAT6, which drives nuclear expression of STAT6, is considered the pathognomonic hallmark of SFTs; it can be demonstrated by STAT6 immunohistochemistry [34]. SFTs are also positive for CD34, but this marker is much less specific than STAT6. Although most SFTs are cured by surgical resection, approximately 15% of cases metastasize or recur locally. Histologic features are not particularly reliable in predicting recurrence risk

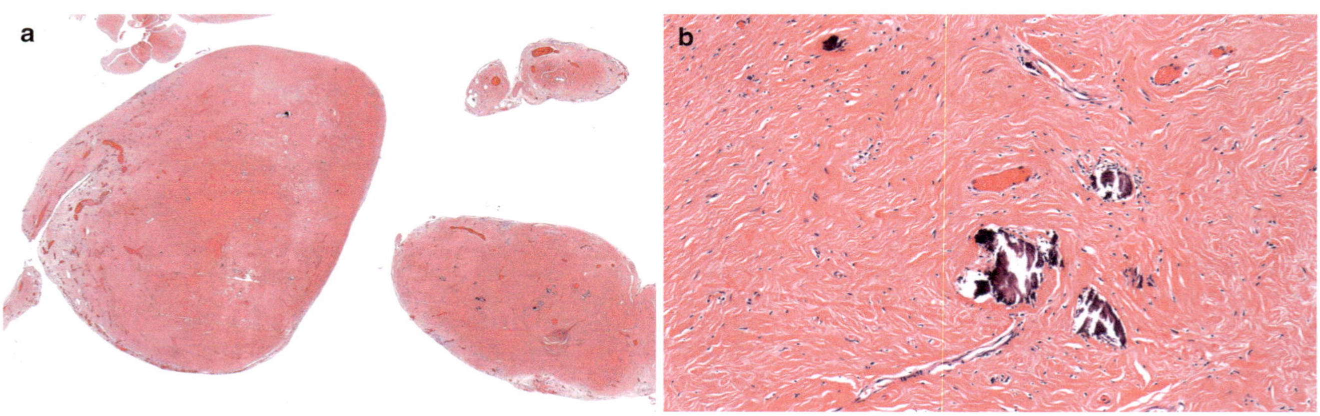

Calcifying fibrous tumor (CFT). This is a rare benign tumor which most often involves soft tissue, pleura or peritoneum. CFTs of the GI tract tend to be subserosal or submucosal in location. They are usually discovered incidentally, intraoperatively or at endoscopy. Grossly, CFT are well-demarcated, nonencapsulated, nodular or lobulated lesions with a size range of 0.5 to 11 cm (mean, 2.6 cm) [35]. Histologically, they are well-circumscribed, hypocellular lesions (**a**) composed of bland spindle cells embedded within a dense, hyalinized, collagenous stroma with interspersed psammomatous or dystrophic calcifications (**b**) and a variable perivascular lymphoplasmacytic infiltrate

3.5 Tumors of Vascular Origin

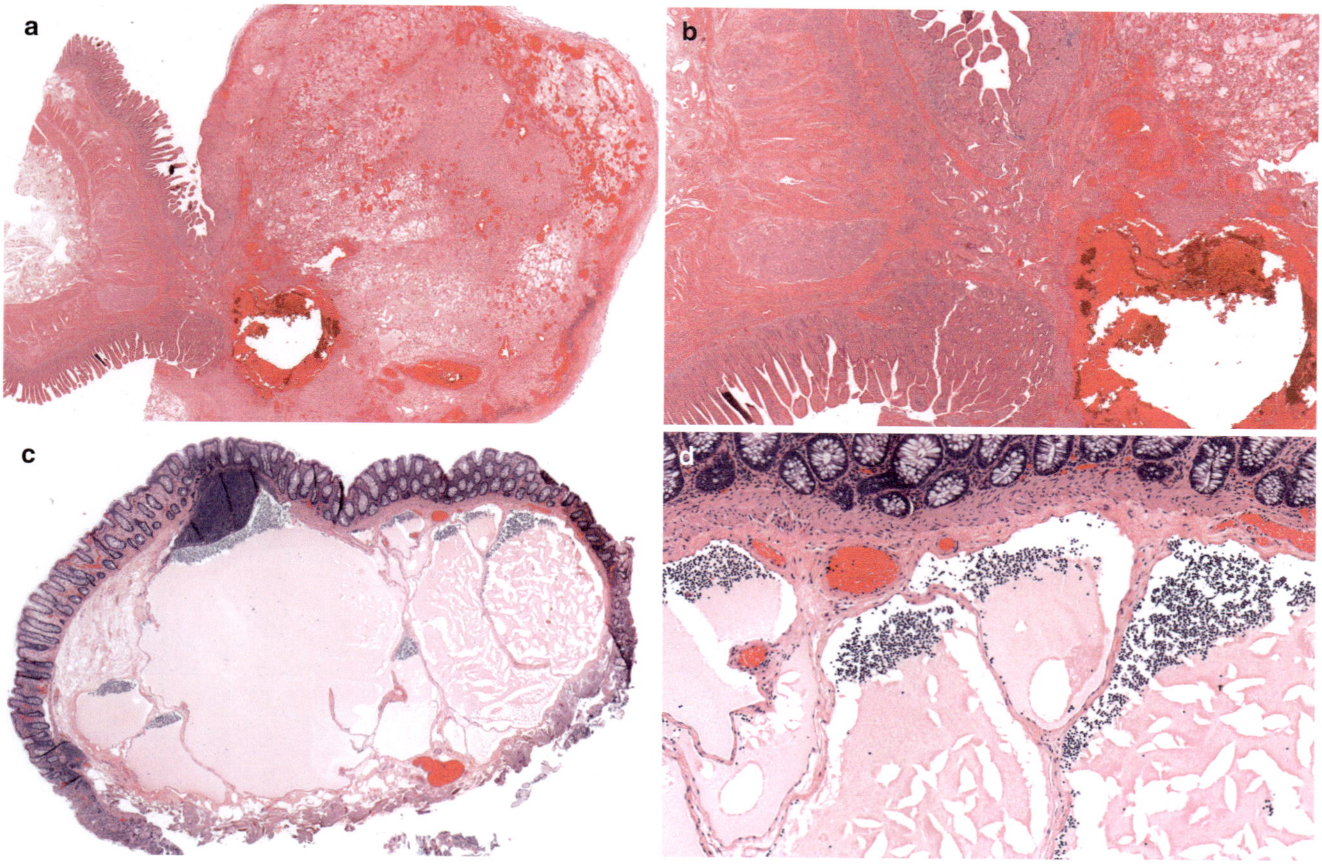

Hemangioma and lymphangioma. Hemangiomas and lymphangiomas can be seen throughout the GI tract and have similar morphology to their counterparts in soft tissue and other organs. (**a**, **b**), Small bowel hemangiomas may comprise both large and small, capillary-sized vessels. (**c**, **d**), This colonic lymphangioma includes numerous dilated lymphatic channels

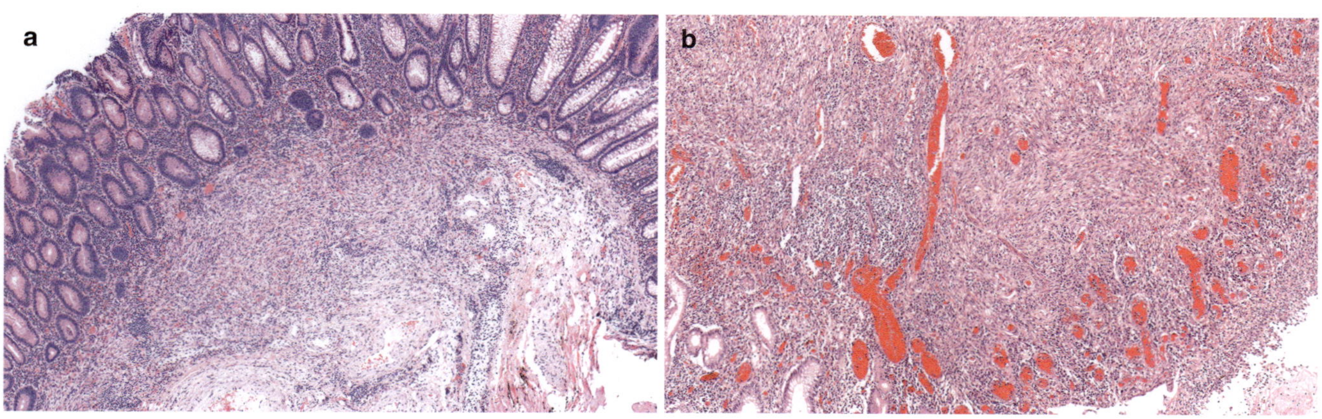

Kaposi sarcoma. (**a**, **b**), Examples of Kaposi sarcoma of the large bowel, one involving a tubular adenoma removed from an elderly man without known immunodeficiency, and the other from a patient with ulcerative colitis. Both tumors are composed of irregular fascicles of spindled cells lining slitlike vascular spaces containing erythrocytes (**a–c**). There is mild nuclear atypia and scattered mitotic activity. An associated plasma cell infiltrate (**c**, **d**) is characteristic and hyaline globules (**d**) are frequently observed. Lesional cells are immunoreactive for vascular endothelial markers and human herpes virus 8 (HHV-8)

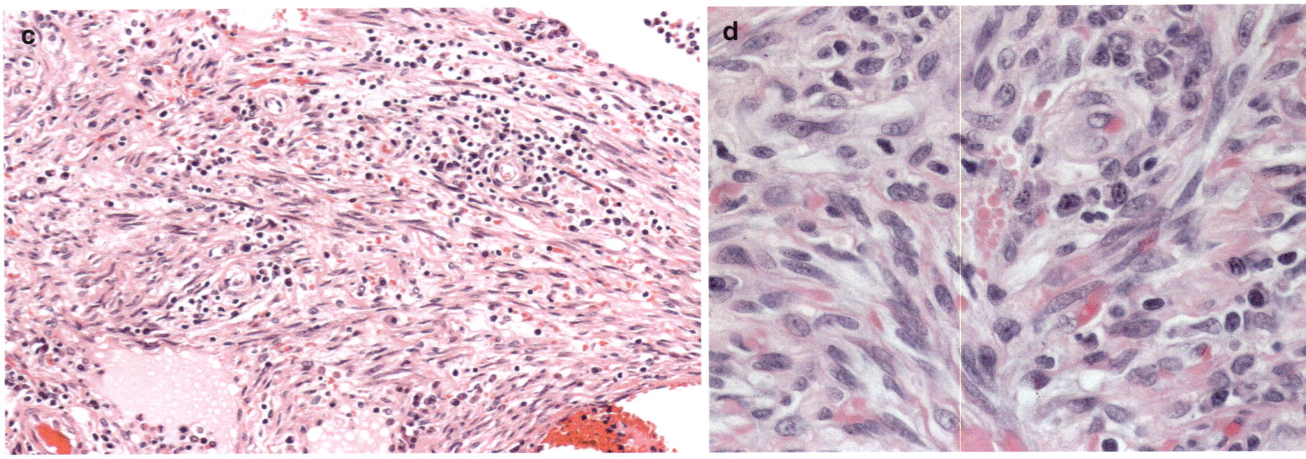

(continued)

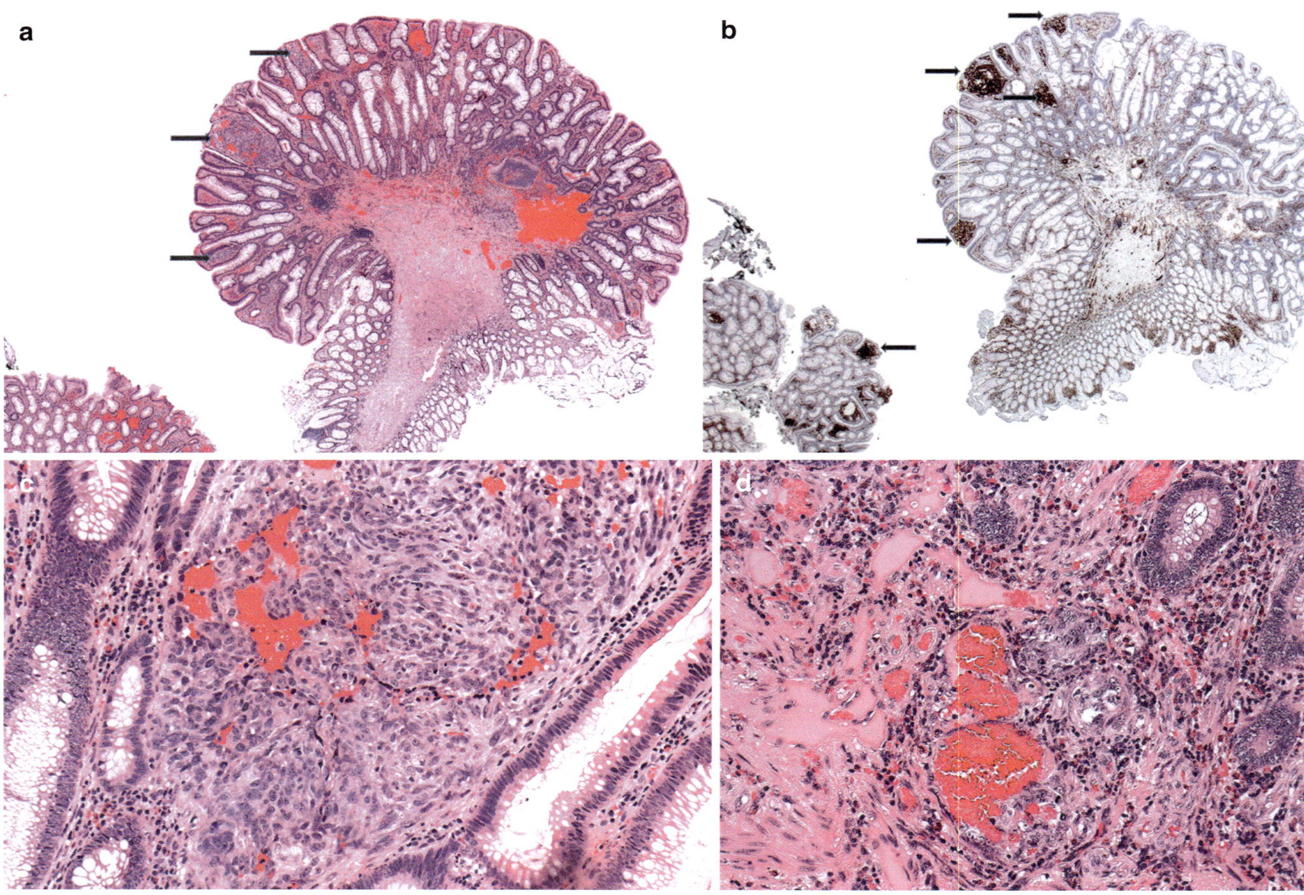

Angiosarcoma. Angiosarcoma uncommonly involves the GI tract and may represent primary or metastatic disease [36]. (**a**), Example of an angiosarcoma involving a tubular adenoma in the colon. The foci of angiosarcoma in this polyp are small and difficult to appreciate at scanning power (*arrows*) but are nicely highlighted by CD31 immunohistochemistry (*arrows*, **b**). (**c**, **d**), At higher magnification, a proliferation of atypical oval to spindle cells forming variably sized, irregular vascular channels can be appreciated. This patient had a history of breast carcinoma treated with mastectomy, radiotherapy, and chemotherapy. Amplification of the *c-MYC* oncogene, as evidenced by positive c-MYC immunohistochemistry in this case (**e**), is consistent with origin from a radiation-induced angiosarcoma [37]. Angiosarcomas may exhibit epithelioid morphology (**f**), immunoreactivity for cytokeratin, and, in some cases, only subtle vascular differentiation, so misdiagnosis as a carcinoma is potential pitfall

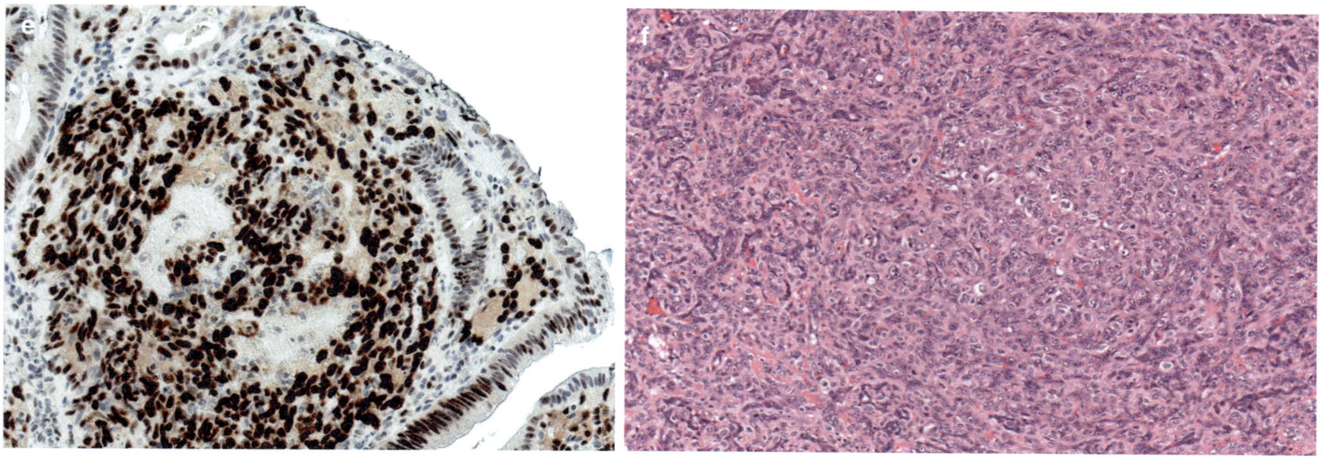

(continued)

3.6 Tumors of Adipocytic Origin

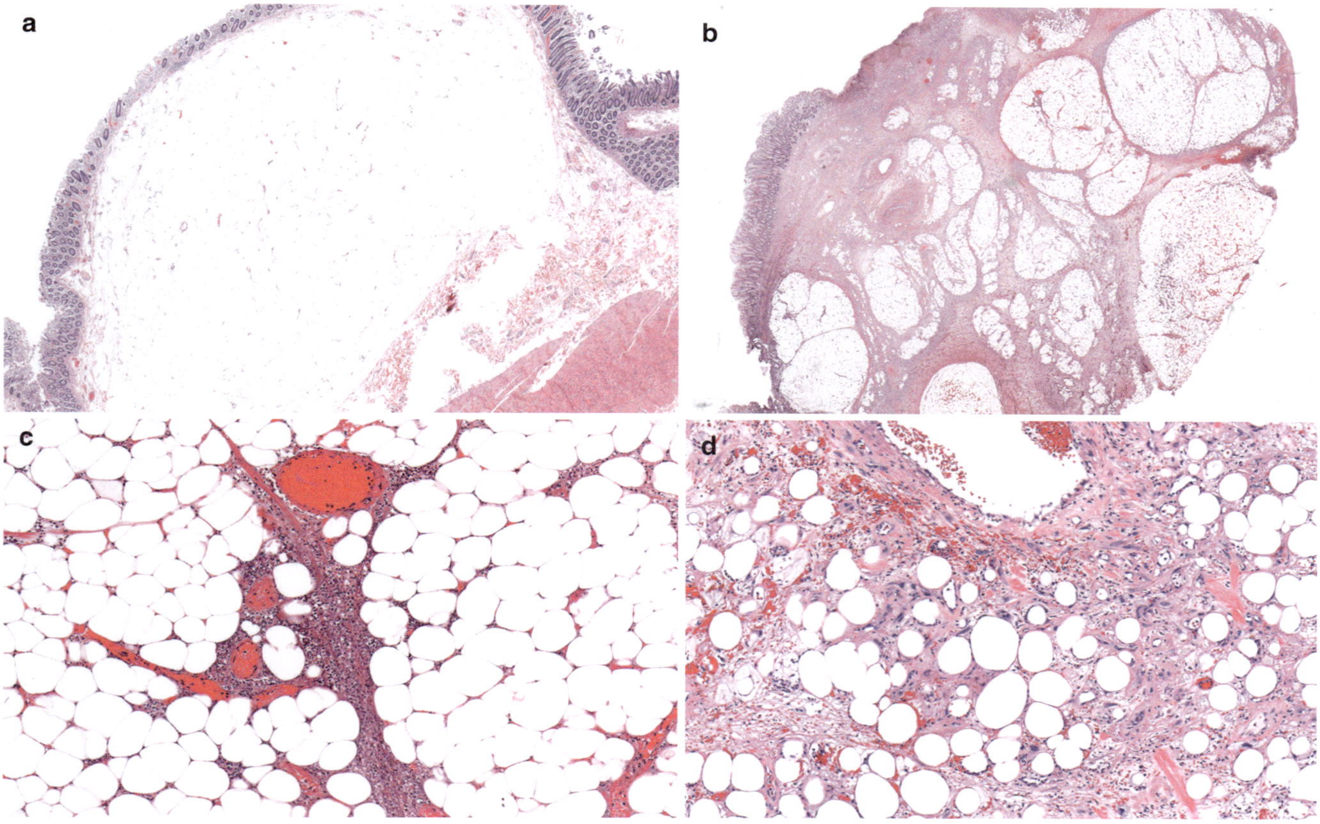

Submucosal lipoma. Submucosal lipomas usually present as incidental polyps at endoscopy, most frequently in the right colon. (**a**), Histologically, they are composed of mature adipocytes without cytologic atypia. (**b**), Larger lesions may cause intussusception, as was the case with this 8-cm lipoma. (**c**), Histologically, this example showed secondary changes related to intussusception, with lobules of mature adipose tissue separated by fibrous septa with areas of fat necrosis and acute inflammation. (**d**), Marked reactive atypia of stromal/myofibroblastic cells might raise a concern for liposarcoma or atypical lipoma, but the background necrobiotic and inflammatory changes and the absence of true lipoblasts should lead to the correct diagnosis

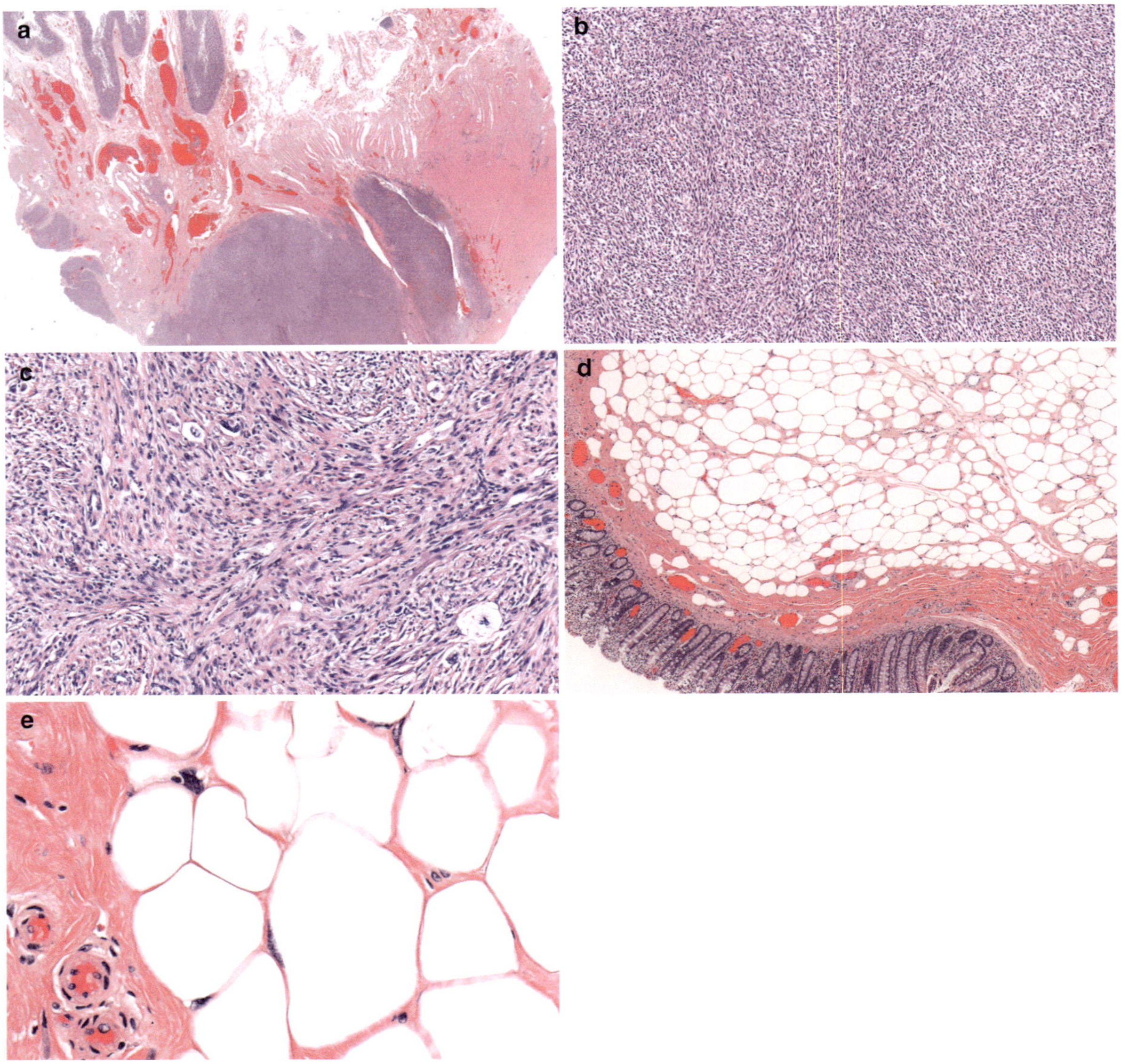

Liposarcoma. Primary liposarcoma of the GI tract is rare. Most cases involving the small or large bowel represent secondary involvement by a retroperitoneal liposarcoma. (**a**), An example of a retroperitoneal dedifferentiated liposarcoma, which infiltrates the wall of the large bowel. (**b**), The tumor is composed of pleomorphic spindle cells arranged in sheets and fascicles without overt adipocytic differentiation. (**c**), Another example of a liposarcoma involving the bowel wall with scattered large lipoblasts. In both examples, tumor cells were immunoreactive for MDM2 and CDK4 (with *MDM2* gene amplification confirmed by FISH), supporting the diagnosis of liposarcoma. (**d**), A focus of submucosal involvement by well-differentiated liposarcoma. (**e**), Lipoblast and atypical nuclei are detected on high-power magnification

3.7 Other Mesenchymal Tumors of the Small and Large Bowel

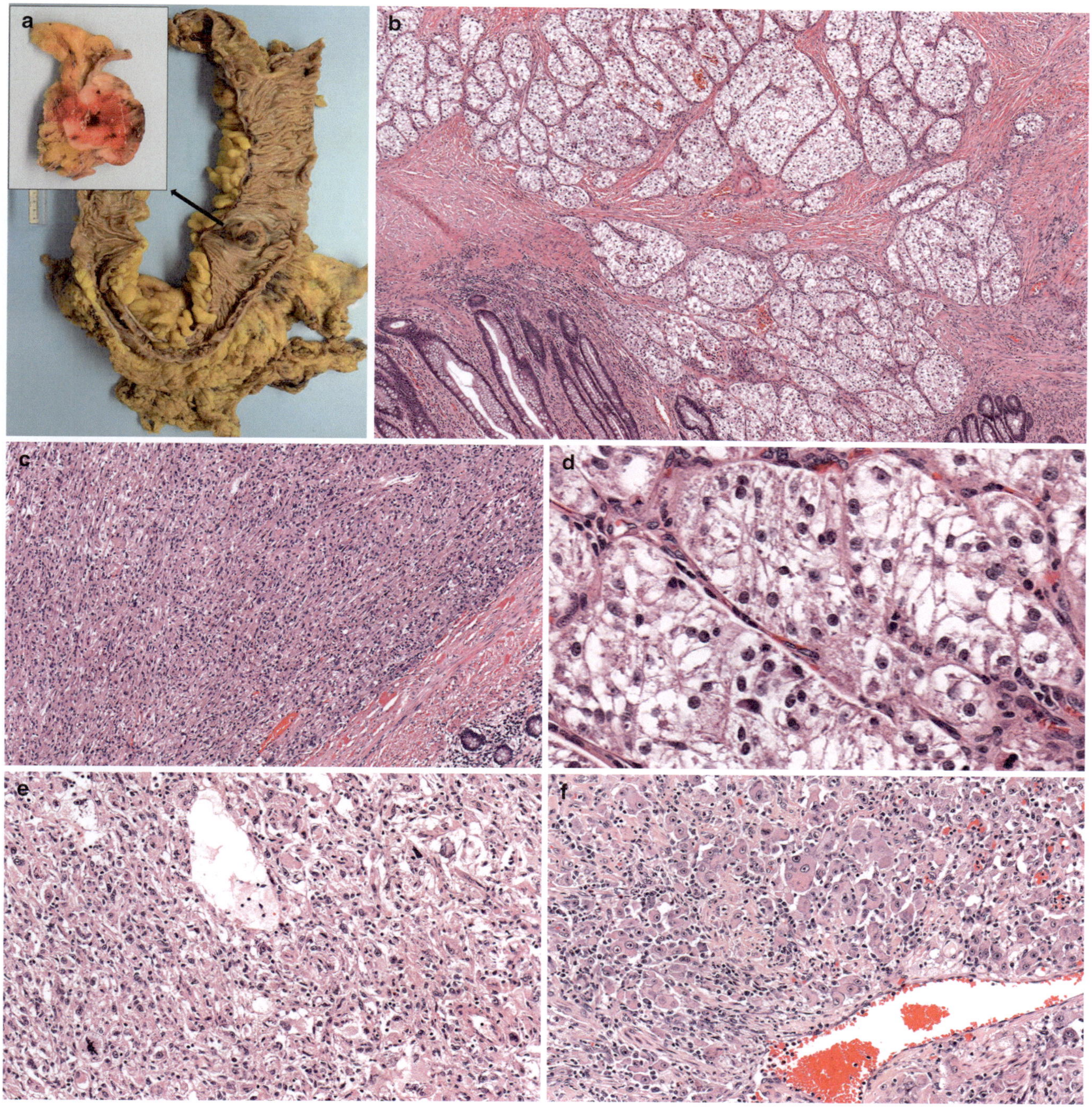

Perivascular epithelioid cell tumor (PEComa). PEComas belong to a family of tumors that includes angiomyolipoma, clear-cell ("sugar") tumor of the lung, and lymphangioleiomyomatosis, and are characterized by perivascular epithelioid cells with evidence of myomelanocytic differentiation. PEComas may occur at any anatomic site, including the GI tract [38, 39]. This example of a colonic PEComa presented as a polypoid mass involving the full thickness of the bowel wall (**a**). Tumor cells may be arranged in discrete nests (**b**) or in a diffuse, sheetlike pattern (**c**). The tumor cells are epithelioid to polygonal (although occasionally spindled), with abundant clear to granular eosinophilic cytoplasm, and round to oval nuclei with variable pleomorphism and mitotic activity (**d**–**f**). There is a close association with thin-walled vessels (**e**, **f**). Criteria for malignancy are less well established for GI PEComas than for the soft-tissue counterparts. The tumor cells are immunoreactive for melanocytic markers such as HMB45 and Melan A, as well as smooth muscle actin (typically focal/patchy)

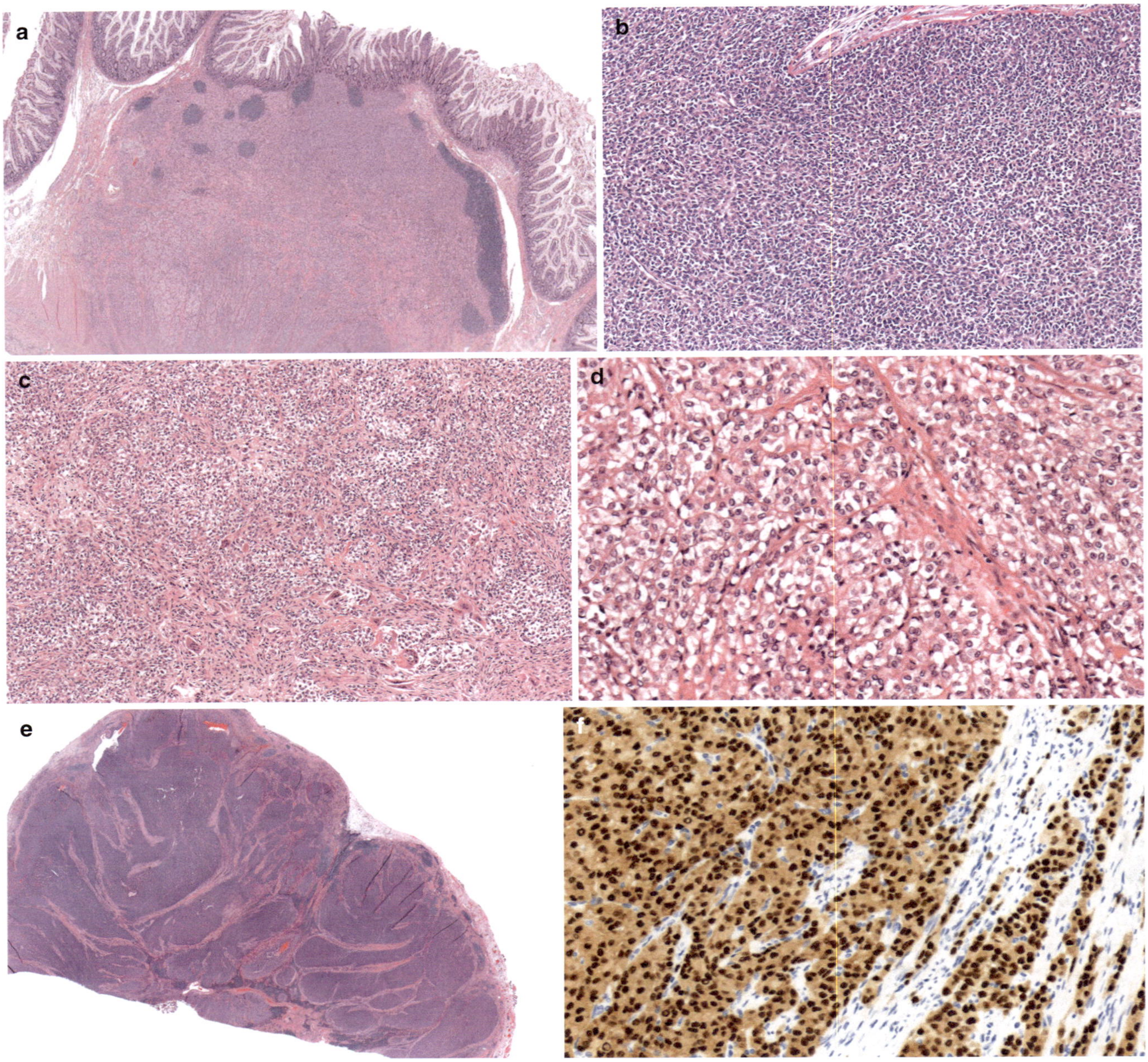

Clear-cell sarcoma-like tumor of the gastrointestinal tract (CCSLGT). This is an aggressive neoplasm with a poor prognosis [40]. This example in the small bowel (**a**) shows a cuff of lymphoid tissue resembling that seen in GI schwannomas. However, higher magnification shows a densely cellular, overtly malignant tumor arranged in diffuse sheets and focal, well-formed nested patterns (**b–d**). The tumor cells are relatively uniform, with central nuclei and pale eosinophilic to clear cytoplasm (**d**). Admixed osteoclast-like giant cells (**c**) are a frequent finding. Some cases may have a nodular architecture (**e**). CCSLGTs are immunoreactive for S100 and SOX 10 (**f**) but, unlike conventional clear-cell sarcomas, they are negative for markers of melanocytic differentiation (HMB45, Melan A, tyrosinase, MMTF-1). Immunostains for CD117 and DOG-1 are also negative. Because CCSLGTs show ultrastructural and immunohistochemical evidence of neural differentiation, some authors have termed these tumors *malignant gastrointestinal neuroectodermal tumor (GINECT)* [41]. These tumors are associated with *EWSR1-CREB1* and, less frequently, *EWSR1-ATF1* gene fusions

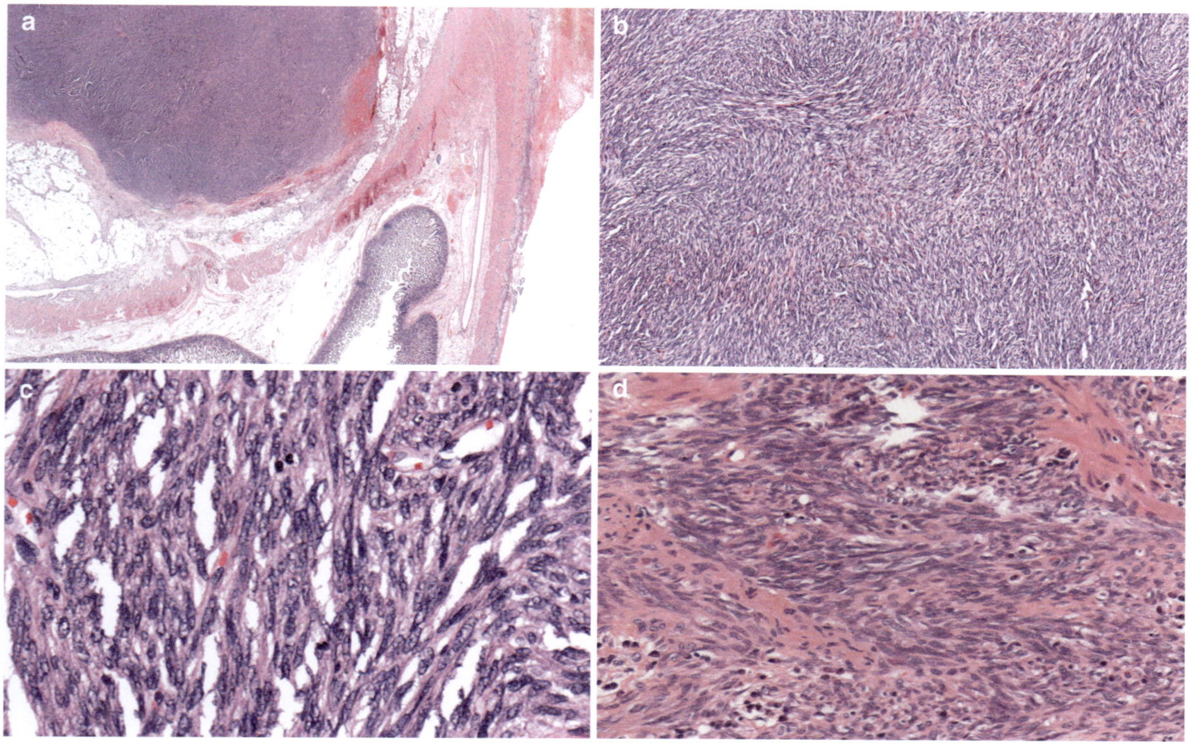

Synovial sarcoma (SS). Primary SS of the GI tract is rare and most frequently involves the stomach, but it also can involve the small bowel, large bowel, and esophagus. SS often involves the submucosa but can affect all layers of the bowel wall, as well as the mesentery. The morphology is similar to that of its soft tissue counterparts [42, 43]. (**a–c**), This example of a monophasic SS in the small bowel mesentery shows characteristic features including high cellularity, fascicular/herringbone pattern, and hyperchromatic (but relatively uniform) nuclei with frequent nuclear overlap. (**d**), A variable collagenous stroma may be present. SS typically shows focal immunoreactivity for pancytokeratin and EMA. The diagnosis can be confirmed by demonstration of *SYT-SSX* fusion transcripts. Occasional expression of CD117 and DOG1 may lead to confusion with a GIST, but expression of these markers tends to be focal in SS, and their co-expression is rare

3.8 Other Neoplasms and Reactive Conditions Mimicking Mesenchymal Tumors

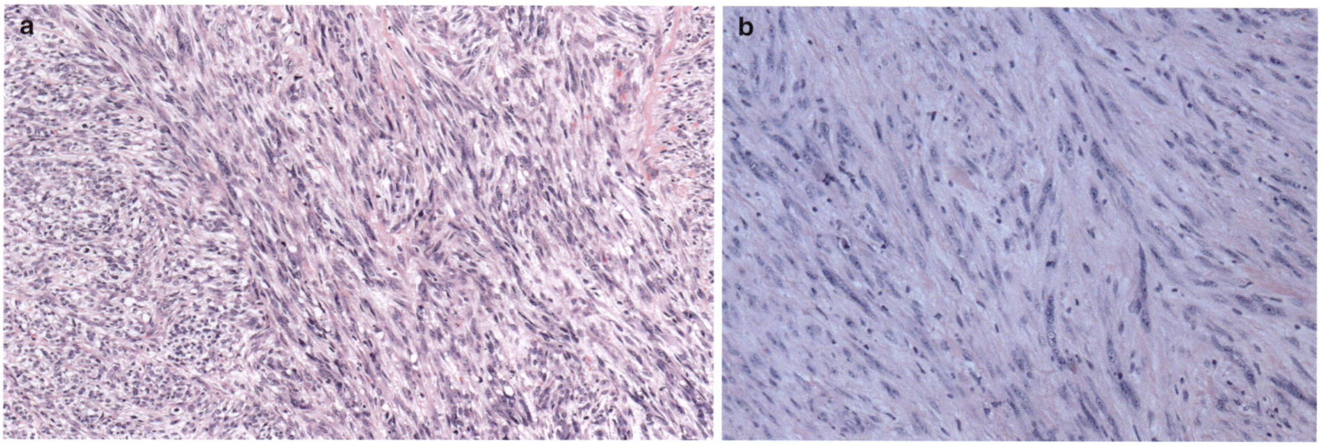

Malignant melanoma (MM). Amelanotic melanoma involving the GI tract can mimic a mesenchymal neoplasm. Most cases represent metastasis from cutaneous MM and most commonly involve the small bowel, but primary GI melanomas may occur, especially in the anorectal region and esophagus. (**a, b**), These two cases of anorectal amelanotic MM are composed of mitotically active, pleomorphic spindled cells. Nests of atypical melanocytes in the overlying epithelium can be a helpful diagnostic clue, and should always be sought. (**c**), These cases showed diffuse immunoreactivity for S100; they also showed focal reactivity for MART-1 and HMB-45. Up to 75% of MMs may be immunoreactive for CD117, representing a potential diagnostic pitfall. A small minority are immunoreactive for DOG1

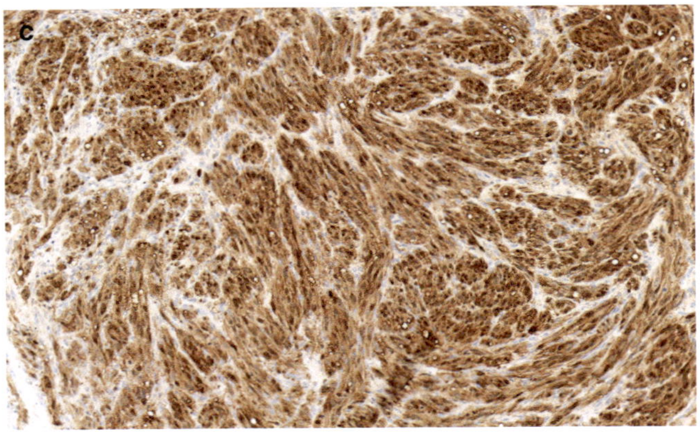

(continued)

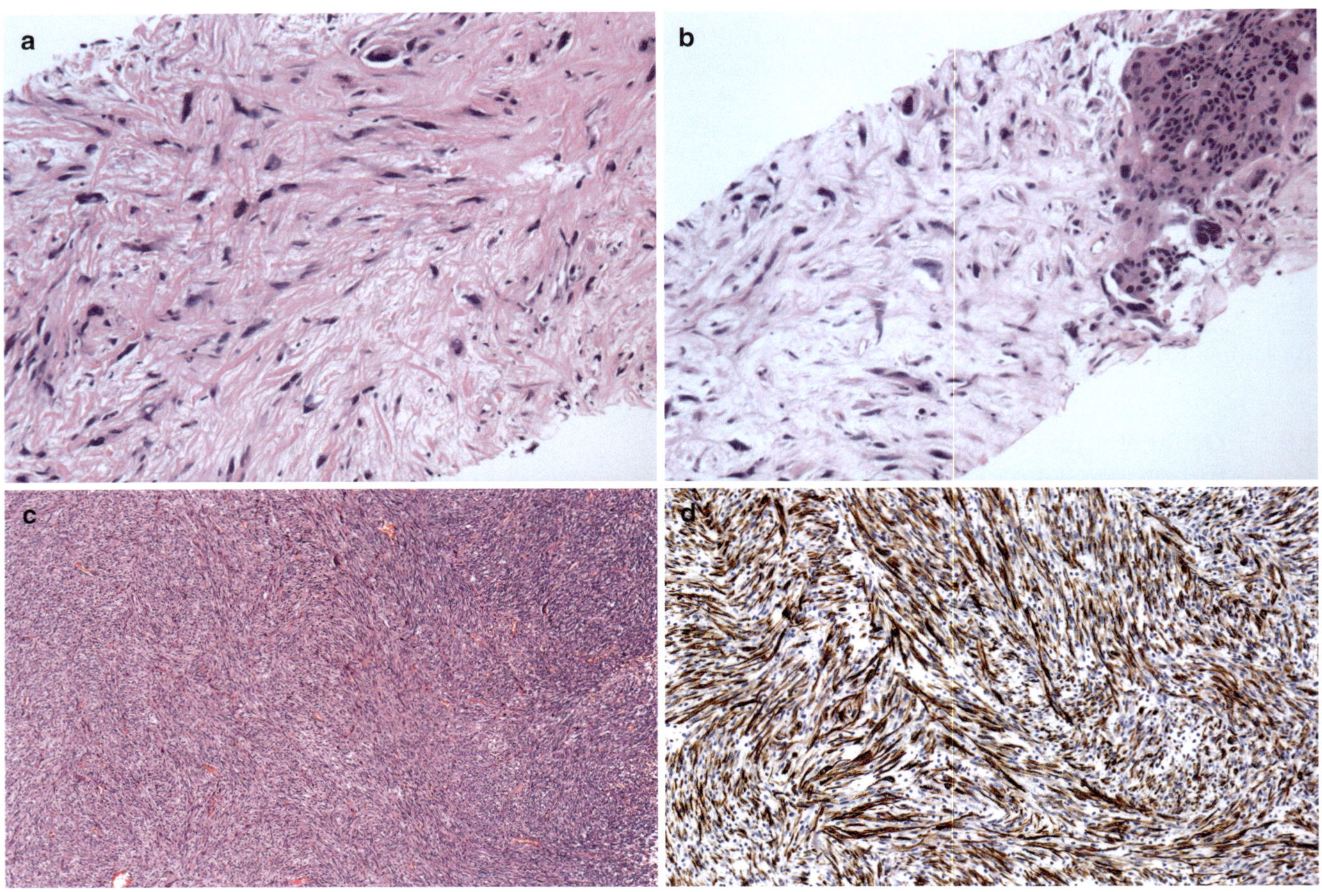

Sarcomatoid carcinoma. (**a**), Sarcomatoid carcinoma ("spindle cell carcinoma") of the large bowel may mimic a malignant mesenchymal neoplasm. The spindle cell component often loses markers of epithelial differentiation and may rarely differentiate along a specific mesenchymal lineage (osteoblastic, myogenic, etc.). (**b**), The presence of a focal overtly carcinomatous component in this case was helpful in arriving at the correct diagnosis. The finding of dysplastic epithelium in the overlying mucosa, when present, is another helpful clue. (**c**), This small bowel tumor is composed of atypical spindle cells arranged in fascicles. No carcinomatous component was identified. (**d**), The tumor was diffusely immunoreactive for pankeratin. It was negative with a broad panel of markers including melanocytic, myoid, neural, hematolymphoid, and vascular markers. Electron microscopy (EM) showed tight junctions. Based on the diffuse pankeratin immunoreactivity and the EM findings, this case was favored to represent a sarcomatoid carcinoma

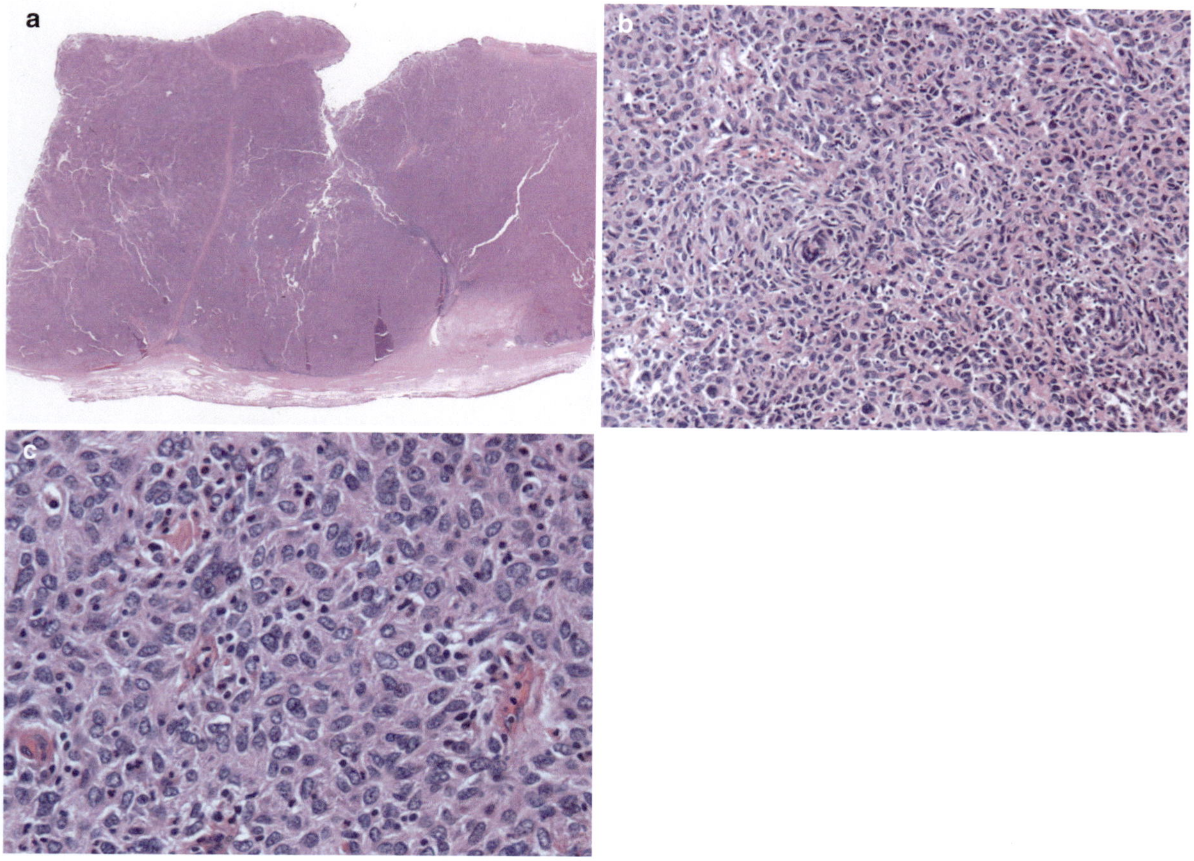

Follicular dendritic cell (FDC) sarcoma. FDC sarcoma is a rare tumor that typically arises within lymph nodes and only very rarely involves the GI tract. These tumors may pose a diagnostic challenge because they are usually not considered in the differential diagnosis of a spindle cell neoplasm in the GI tract [44, 45]. Histologically, tumor cells are arranged in fascicular, sheetlike, whorled, or storiform (**a**, **b**) patterns. The tumor cells are spindled, ovoid, or sometimes epithelioid with eosinophilic cytoplasm (**b**, **c**). Cell borders are often indistinct, owing to interwoven cell processes of adjacent cells, which impart a syncytial appearance. The nuclei have clear chromatin with distinct nucleoli. Admixed, small lymphocytes are a characteristic feature (**c**). Nuclear pleomorphism can be seen. The tumoral cells are immunoreactive for CD21, CD35, CD23, and clusterin, and are negative for cytokeratin, CD31, CD34, and CD1a

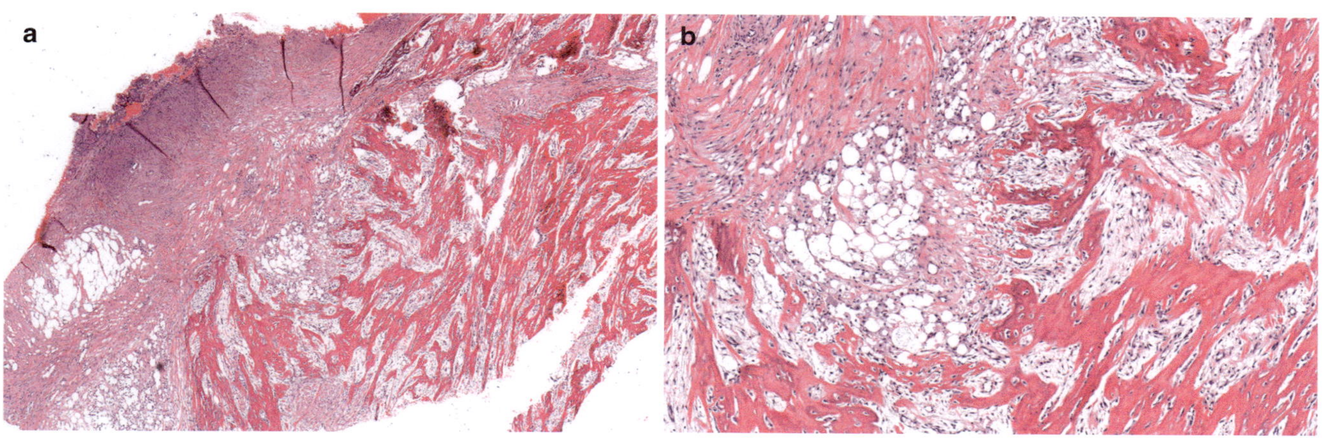

Heterotopic mesenteric ossification (HMO). HMO is a rare intraabdominal bone-producing pseudotumor, which may mimic a sarcoma (**a**). It is also known as *intraabdominal myositis ossificans*, *heterotopic ossification of the intestinal mesentery*, and *mesenteritis ossificans*. It typically occurs after surgery or abdominal trauma, and may present with small bowel obstruction [46]. Histologically, HMO shows distinct zonation with a central zone of prominent reactive myofibroblastic proliferation, fat necrosis, and peripheral ossification, frequently accompanied by lace-like osteoid (**b**). The presence of osteoid may lead to confusion with an extraskeletal osteosarcoma. Clues to the diagnosis of HMO include the clinical history (prior surgery, trauma), a zonation pattern identical to that of myositis ossificans, areas with a nodular fasciitis-like pattern, areas of fat necrosis (**b**), bland morphology, and absence of atypical mitosis and necrosis. If present, suture material and foreign body reaction (**c**) may be a helpful pointer to previous surgery

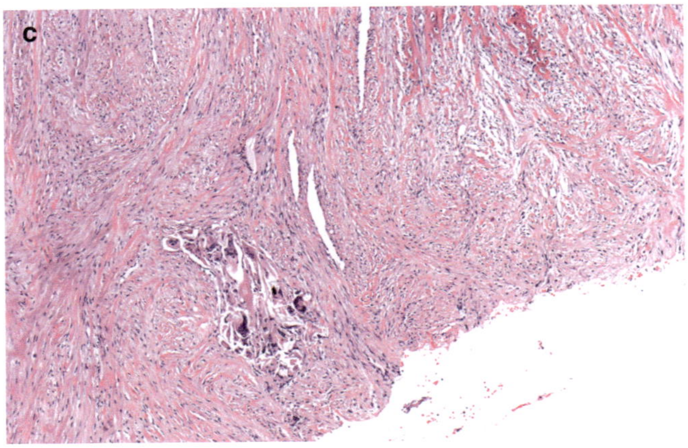

(continued)

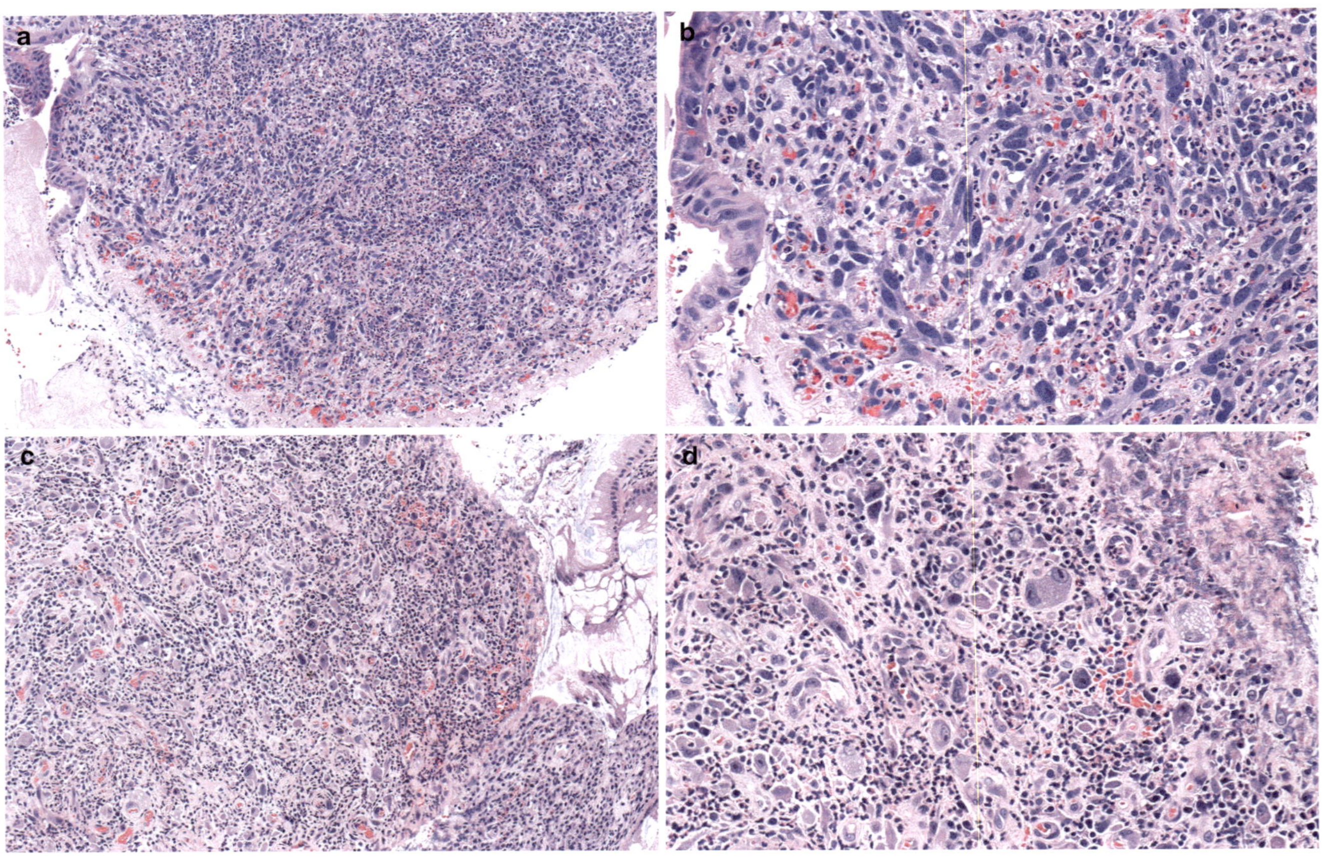

Reactive pseudosarcomatous changes. Highly atypical (sometimes bizarre) stromal and endothelial cells (so-called *ulcerocytes*) can be seen within the granulation tissue of GI ulcers and represent a reactive/regenerative phenomenon [47]. The atypical cells may be polygonal, spindled, or epithelioid in shape, with abundant amphophilic cytoplasm, vesicular nuclei, coarse chromatin, and large eosinophilic, inclusion-like nucleoli. Multinucleated and giant cell forms may also be seen. Mitotic figures are not uncommon, but atypical mitoses are not generally seen. (**a**), This duodenal biopsy specimen shows mucosal ulceration and pseudosarcomatous change. (**b**), Note the overlying restituting epithelium, overt inflammation, and mitosis. (**c–e**), Examples of colonic inflammatory polyps and a tubular adenoma (**f**), which show mucosal ulceration and associated atypical ulcerocytes. The differential diagnosis includes poorly differentiated carcinoma, sarcoma, and lymphoma. The ulcerocytes are immunoreactive with vimentin (diffusely) and are variably (usually focally) immunoreactive for SMA, CD10, and CD34. Despite their atypical features, these cells are entirely benign. Their association with heavily inflamed granulation tissue, concentration beneath regenerating epithelium or fibrin, and lack of atypical mitoses helps to distinguish these lesions from malignant neoplasms

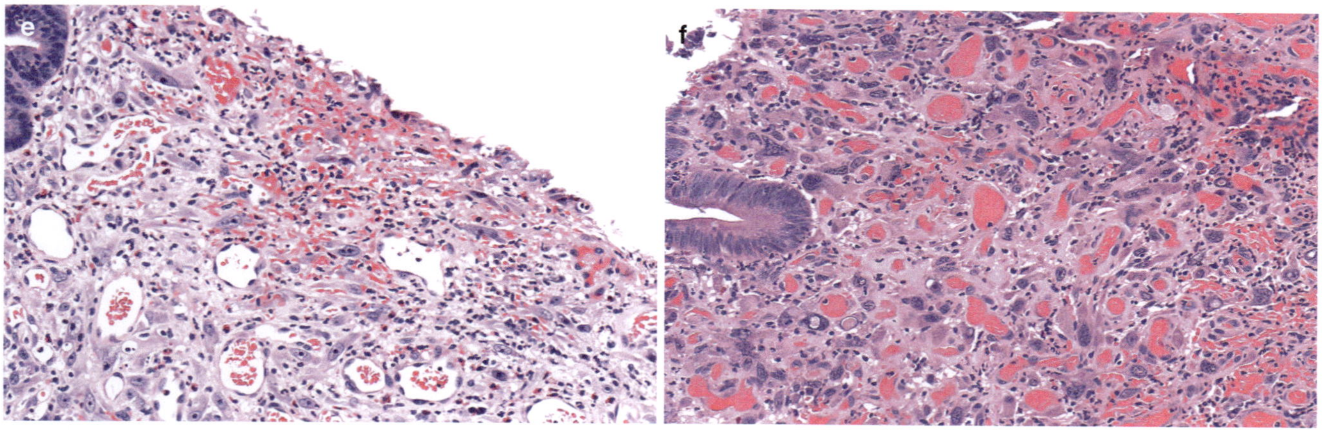

(continued)

References

1. Charville GW, Longacre TA. Surgical pathology of gastrointestinal stromal tumors: practical implications of morphologic and molecular heterogeneity for precision medicine. Adv Anat Pathol. 2017;24:336–53.
2. Miettinen M, Lasota J. Gastrointestinal stromal tumors: review on morphology, molecular pathology, prognosis, and differential diagnosis. Arch Pathol Lab Med. 2006;130:1466–78.
3. Ikemura M, Kunita A, Miwa Y, Jimbo K, Mori K, Seto Y, Fukayama M. Gut wall replacing type of gastrointestinal stromal tumor presenting as a perforation of the ileal diverticulum. Pathol Res Pract. 2015;211:892–5.
4. Agaimy A, Märkl B, Arnholdt H, Hartmann A, Schneider-Stock R, Chetty R. Sporadic segmental interstitial cell of cajal hyperplasia (microscopic GIST) with unusual diffuse longitudinal growth replacing the muscularis propria: differential diagnosis to hereditary GIST syndromes. Int J Clin Exp Pathol. 2010;3:549–56.
5. Dennis LK, Damjanov I. Evaluating and reporting gastrointestinal stromal tumors after imatinib mesylate treatment. Open Pathol J. 2009;3:53–7.
6. Hou YY, Tan YS, Xu JF, Wang XN, Lu SH, Ji Y, et al. Schwannoma of the gastrointestinal tract: a clinicopathological, immunohistochemical and ultrastructural study of 33 cases. Histopathology. 2006;48:536–45.
7. Kwon MS, Lee SS, Ahn GH. Schwannomas of the gastrointestinal tract: clinicopathological features of 12 cases including a case of esophageal tumor compared with those of gastrointestinal stromal tumors and leiomyomas of the gastrointestinal tract. Pathol Res Pract. 2002;198:605–13.
8. Liegl B, Bennett MW, Fletcher CD. Microcystic/reticular schwannoma: a distinct variant with predilection for visceral locations. Am J Surg Pathol. 2008;32:1080–7.
9. Chetty R. Reticular and microcystic schwannoma: a distinctive tumor of the gastrointestinal tract. Ann Diagn Pathol. 2011;15:198–201.
10. Trivedi A, Ligato S. Microcystic/reticular schwannoma of the proximal sigmoid colon, case report with review of literature. Arch Pathol Lab Med. 2013;137:284–8.
11. Lewin MR, Dilworth HP, Abu Alfa AK, Epstein JI, Montgomery E. Mucosal benign epithelioid nerve sheath tumors. Am J Surg Pathol. 2005;29:1310–5.
12. Miettinen M, Shekitka KM, Sobin LH. Schwannomas in the colon and rectum. a clinicopathologic and immunohistochemical study of 20 cases. Am J Surg Pathol. 2001;25:846–55.
13. Laskin WB, Fetsch JF, Lasota J, Miettinen M. Benign epithelioid peripheral nerve sheath tumors of the soft tissues: clinicopathologic spectrum of 33 cases. Am J Surg Pathol. 2005;29:39–51.
14. So JS, Epstein JI. GATA3 expression in paragangliomas: a pitfall potentially leading to misdiagnosis of urothelial carcinoma. Mod Pathol. 2013;26:1365–70.
15. Shekitka KM, Sobin LH. Ganglioneuromas of the gastrointestinal tract. Relation to Von Recklinghausen disease and other multiple tumor syndromes. Am J Surg Pathol. 1994;18:250–7.
16. Agaimy A, Stoehr R, Vieth M, Hartmann A. Benign serrated colorectal fibroblastic polyps/intramucosal perineuriomas are true mixed epithelial-stromal polyps (hybrid hyperplastic polyp / mucosal perineurioma) with frequent BRAF mutations. Am J Surg Pathol. 2010;34:1663–71.
17. Pai RK, Mojtahed A, Rouse RV, Soetikno RM, Kaltenbach T, Ma L, et al. Histologic and molecular analyses of colonic perineurial-like proliferations in serrated polyps: perineurial-like stromal proliferations are seen in sessile serrated adenomas. Am J Surg Pathol. 2011;35:1373–80.
18. Eslami-Varzaneh F, Washington K, Robert ME, Kashgarian M, Goldblum JR, Jain D. Benign fibroblastic polyps of the colon: a histologic, immunohistochemical, and ultrastructural study. Am J Surg Pathol. 2004;28:374–8.
19. Hornick JL, Fletcher CD. Intestinal perineuriomas: clinicopathologic definition of a new anatomic subset in a series of 10 cases. Am J Surg Pathol. 2005;29:859–65.
20. Gibson JA, Hornick JL. Mucosal Schwann cell "hamartoma". Clinicopathologic study of 26 neural colorectal polyps distinct from neurofibromas and mucosal neuromas. Am J Surg Pathol. 2009;33:781–7.
21. Celeiro-Muñoz C, Huebner TA, Robertson SA, Pittman ME, Singhi AD, Arnold CA, et al. Tactile corpuscle-like bodies in gastrointestinal-type mucosa: a case series. Am J Surg Pathol. 2015;39:1668–72.
22. Singhi AD, Montgomery E. Colorectal granular cell tumor: a clinicopathologic study of 26 cases. Am J Surg Pathol. 2010;34:1186–92.
23. Na JI, Kim HJ, Jung JJ, Kim Y, Kim SS, Lee JH, et al. Granular cell tumours of the colorectum: histopathological and immunohistochemical evaluation of 30 cases. Histopathology. 2014;65:764–74.

24. Fanburg-Smith JC, Meis-Kindblom JM, Fante R, Kindblom LG. Malignant granular cell tumor of soft tissue: diagnostic criteria and clinicopathologic correlation. Am J Surg Pathol. 1998;22:779–94.
25. Miettinen M, Sarlomo-Rikala M, Sobin LH. Mesenchymal tumors of muscularis mucosae of colon and rectum are benign leiomyomas that should be separated from gastrointestinal stromal tumors--a clinicopathologic and immunohistochemical study of eighty-eight cases. Mod Pathol. 2001;14:950–6.
26. Miettinen M. Smooth muscle tumors of soft tissue and non-uterine viscera: biology and prognosis. Mod Pathol. 2014;27(Suppl 1):S17–29.
27. Yamamoto H, Handa M, Tobo T, Setsu N, Fujita K, Oshiro Y, et al. Clinicopathological features of primary leiomyosarcoma of the gastrointestinal tract following recognition of gastrointestinal stromal tumours. Histopathology. 2013;63:194–207.
28. Miettinen M, Sobin LH, Lasota J. True smooth muscle tumors of the small intestine: a clinicopathologic, immunhistochemical, and molecular genetic study of 25 cases. Am J Surg Pathol. 2009;33:430–6.
29. Chen E, O'Connell F, Fletcher CD. Dedifferentiated leiomyosarcoma: clinicopathological analysis of 18 cases. Histopathology. 2011;59:1135–43.
30. Deyrup AT, Lee VK, Hill CE, Cheuk W, Toh HC, Kesavan S, et al. Epstein-Barr virus-associated smooth muscle tumors are distinctive mesenchymal tumors reflecting multiple infection events: a clinicopathologic and molecular analysis of 29 tumors from 19 patients. Am J Surg Pathol. 2006;30:75–82.
31. Zreik RT, Fritchie KJ. Morphologic spectrum of desmoid-type fibromatosis. Am J Clin Pathol. 2016;145:332–40.
32. Liu TC, Lin MT, Montgomery EA, Singhi AD. Inflammatory fibroid polyps of the gastrointestinal tract: spectrum of clinical, morphologic, and immunohistochemistry features. Am J Surg Pathol. 2013;37:586–92.
33. Coffin CM, Hornick JL, Fletcher CD. Inflammatory myofibroblastic tumor: comparison of clinicopathologic, histologic, and immunohistochemical features including ALK expression in atypical and aggressive cases. Am J Surg Pathol. 2007;31:509–20.
34. Yoshida A, Tsuta K, Ohno M, Yoshida M, Narita Y, Kawai A, et al. STAT6 immunohistochemistry is helpful in the diagnosis of solitary fibrous tumors. Am J Surg Pathol. 2014;38:552–9.
35. Larson BK, Dhall D. Calcifying fibrous tumor of the gastrointestinal tract. Arch Pathol Lab Med. 2015;139:943–7.
36. Allison KH, Yoder BJ, Bronner MP, Goldblum JR, Rubin BP. Angiosarcoma involving the gastrointestinal tract: a series of primary and metastatic cases. Am J Surg Pathol. 2004;28:298–307.
37. Laé M, Lebel A, Hamel-Viard F, Asselain B, Trassard M, Sastre X, Kirova YM. Can c-myc amplification reliably discriminate postradiation from primary angiosarcoma of the breast? Cancer Radiother. 2015;19:168–74.
38. Doyle LA, Hornick JL, Fletcher CD. PEComa of the gastrointestinal tract: clinicopathologic study of 35 cases with evaluation of prognostic parameters. Am J Surg Pathol. 2013;37:1769–82.
39. Chen Z, Han S, Wu J, Xiong M, Huang Y, Chen J, et al. A systematic review: perivascular epithelioid cell tumor of gastrointestinal tract. Medicine (Baltimore). 2016;95:e3890.
40. Wang J, Thway K. Clear cell sarcoma-like tumor of the gastrointestinal tract: an evolving entity. Arch Pathol Lab Med. 2015;139:407–12.
41. Stockman DL, Miettinen M, Suster S, Spagnolo D, Dominguez-Malagon H, Hornick JL, et al. Malignant gastrointestinal neuroectodermal tumor: clinicopathologic, immunohistochemical, ultrastructural, and molecular analysis of 16 cases with a reappraisal of clear cell sarcoma-like tumors of the gastrointestinal tract. Am J Surg Pathol. 2012;36:857–68.
42. Makhlouf HR, Ahrens W, Agarwal B, Dow N, Marshalleck JJ, Lee EL, et al. Synovial sarcoma of the stomach: a clinicopathologic, immunohistochemical, and molecular genetic study of 10 cases. Am J Surg Pathol. 2008;32:275–81.
43. Hostetter RB, Yan M, Vaghefi H, Pennington K, Cornette G. The first documented case of high-grade synovial cell sarcoma of the rectum. J Natl Compr Cancer Netw. 2012;10:947–50.
44. Chen T, Gopal P. Follicular dendritic cell sarcoma. Arch Pathol Lab Med. 2017;141:596–9.
45. Chang KC, Jin YT, Chen FF, Su IJ. Follicular dendritic cell sarcoma of the colon mimicking stromal tumour. Histopathology. 2001;38:25–9.
46. Patel RM, Weiss SW, Folpe AL. Heterotopic mesenteric ossification: a distinctive pseudosarcoma commonly associated with intestinal obstruction. Am J Surg Pathol. 2006;30:119–22.
47. Shekitka KM, Helwig EB. Deceptive bizarre stromal cells in polyps and ulcers of the gastrointestinal tract. Cancer. 1991;67:2111–7.

Appendiceal Tumors

4

Stephanie L. Reid and Robert H. Riddell

4.1 Introduction

Tumors occurring in the appendix have historically been regarded as similar to those in the large bowel, and the same terminology has been applied to both. Clinicians are familiar with many of these terms, and to some extent the morphologic characteristics have some similarities. However, studies from the literature, review, texts, and personal experience have shown that the majority of appendiceal neoplasms differ from the large bowel counterparts in their pathology, molecular pathogenesis, and behavior.

Morphologically, the single largest difference is that the adenoma-carcinoma sequence most frequently seen in the large bowel virtually never occurs in the appendix. These tubular adenomas are vanishingly rare, their occurrence being limited almost entirely to incidental changes in patients with familial adenomatous polyposis (FAP). Appendiceal carcinomas arising in tubular adenomas in FAP are therefore undescribed. Some lesions that have a resemblance to adenomas tend to be diffuse and associated with non-adenomatous lesions: for example, lesions having serrations; or appendiceal mucinous neoplasms (AMNs), whether low-grade (LAMNs) or high-grade (HAMNs). They can also be found in association with, or even giving rise to, infiltrating carcinomas. In contrast, in most infiltrating adenocarcinomas in which associated benign lesions can be found, the benign lesion is either serrated, with or without dysplasias, or a mucinous neoplasm, usually LAMNs [1].

The division between reactive and neoplastic lesions within the appendix is often not clear. Reactive lesions are not uncommon, especially following acute appendicitis or in appendixes resected following acute appendicitis. The most common of these is superficially serrated, but does not have the lesions at the crypt bases that are seen in hyperplastic polyps and are best called *serrated hyperplasia*. They have a well-formed lamina propria and the muscularis mucosae is present, although this may be duplicated as a result of prior ulceration and repair. These are often localized, sometimes being in only one section. It is therefore reasonable to regard them as reactive. The problem is that they are sometimes more diffuse, can have areas of dysplasia, and merge with either invasive neoplasms or LAMNs, which themselves can be associated with dysplasia, including lesions that can look very much like large bowel sessile serrated polyps with dysplasia. There is, therefore, a link between serrated lesions and LAMNs, which can merge and share common characteristics [1]. In many LAMNs, however, there is no trace of serrated lesion. It therefore appears that, in the appendix, in their pathways to carcinoma, there is a serrated pathway and a mucinous (LAMN/HAMN) pathway, but that these can co-exist and are therefore frequently related. While a pure serrated pathway likely exists, most neoplasms likely either go through a serrated/LAMN pathway, or LAMN de novo. Either of the latter may progress to dysplastic serrated or invasive lesions.

LAMNs confined to the appendix, and especially not extending beyond the muscularis propria (provided they have been completely excised), are benign and have virtually no risk of pseudomyxoma peritonei [2]. The nomenclature is also problematic, however, the use of the term "neoplasia" as part of LAMN is intrinsically ambiguous so causes consternation as to whether it can be fatal. Unless the surgeon is used to dealing with these tumors and understands the terminology and implications, a clear statement needs to be made that local excision is complete, that there is no evidence of perforation, and that the risk of subsequent pseudomyxoma peritonei (PMP) is virtually zero. Even if this is stated, one can often be expected to be summoned to an intermultidisciplinary tumor board review to explain the findings. Older terms such as mucinous cystadenoma, or any term that includes adenoma, is always interpreted as benign, whereas "neoplasia" leaves the

H. H. Li-Chang et al., *Atlas of Intestinal Pathology*, Atlas of Anatomic Pathology,
https://doi.org/10.1007/978-3-030-12379-6_4

element of doubt, and so may need an obsolete synonym such as mucinous cystadenoma for clarity.

Conversely, the term "mucocele" is purely descriptive and indicates an enlarged dilated appendix which, when opened, is full of mucin, but it gives no indication as to whether any epithelium, if present, is neoplastic (mucinous neoplasm/ "cystadenoma") or a variant of normal (benign mucocele). In a meta-analysis, the reported pathology associated with mucoceles was cystadenoma/low-grade appendiceal mucinous neoplasm (54%), unspecified/benign (25%), retention cyst (14.1%), cystadenocarcinoma (4.2%), and mucosal hyperplasia (2.9%) [3]. Treatment was appendectomy (52.1%), right hemicolectomy (17.6%), partial cecectomy (17.2%), and ileocecetomy (13.1%) [3]. Because there is invariably uncertainty as to whether the base of the appendix is involved or not, it makes sense to at least include the base of the appendix and cuff of cecum in any resection of a mucocele, so that the entire appendix has been removed; this has the added advantage of not transecting any underlying neoplasm.

A major problem with mucinous tumors is the diverticular-like outpouchings that can make them indistinguishable from invasive carcinomas [1]. Where outpouchings stop and carcinomas start is subjective, and it is particularly disconcerting when the outpouching penetrates the serosa and periappendiceal mucin is present, whether or not as part of an apparent diverticulum. The risk of subsequent PMP is presumably related to the extent of extra-appendiceal mucin and whether it is cellular; data for this specific circumstance, however, are lacking. Nevertheless, while confined to the appendix, mucinous tumors appear to be without metastasizing potential, despite the fact that what often appears to be an invasive infiltrating front is called "pushing."

The **carcinomas** arising from the appendix are mainly mucinous carcinomas, which are relatively common, and when they perforate they can cause pseudomyxoma peritonei (PMP). These lesions tend to expand, causing the lamina propria and muscularis mucosae to be initially lost or to become fibrotic. The same then happens to the submucosa and finally the muscularis propria, so that the wall of the appendix becomes thinner, and the muscle layers indistinct. Until they perforate, however, the risk of PMP is virtually zero, as is the risk of metastases [2]. It is assumed, in cases where mucin is found on the external surface of the appendix, that there has either been a true perforation that is inapparent or resealed, or that it is an artefact from the time that grossing occurred. Clearly inking the external surface of the appendix at the time of grossing would allow this distinction. Other useful features are organization and neovascularization of this mucin, and a peritoneal reaction, as these cannot happen unless genuine. However, if the perforation occurred very close to the time of appendectomy, there would not be time for this to occur; the presence of periappendiceal mucin can therefore be problematic. When there is only periappendiceal mucin, the risk of subsequent PMP depends on whether the mucin is acellular or cellular. PMP, however, can occur a decade or more after appendectomy, but such long-term data do not exist. Relatively short-term data suggest that the risk of PMP is about 5% if the periappendiceal mucin is acellular, but if it is cellular the risk increases to at least 33% [4–6].

Carcinomas arising from this pathway vary from mucinous through all of those described as intestinal type, which include all forming glands except those arising from goblet cell tumors. Rarely, even signet ring carcinomas, which usually arise goblet cell tumors, can also arise from this pathway.

Goblet cell carcinoid (GCC) is a poor term for a tumor that is virtually unique to the GI tract. They begin in the lamina propria but, like appendiceal NETs (carcinoids) have no preinvasive lesion. However, GCCs have a variety of cell types including goblet cells and a unique architecture of gland-forming epithelium with virtually no nuclear atypia. Interestingly, they are often the least well-differentiated in the lamina propria compared to when they are deeper in the wall of the appendix. These tumors do metastasize to nodes, but patients rarely die of disseminated metastatic disease; death is invariably caused by disease, via the peritoneal cavity, that involves any organ within the peritoneal cavity. In women, the ovaries are so frequently the location that prophylactic oophorectomy needs to be considered. Overt carcinoma can arise from GCCs, usually of signet ring type and with a variable mucin component, but occasionally poorly differentiated carcinomas occur [7]. Some have sought criteria to separate out those with more or less aggressive behavior [8].

Other, more conventional, adenocarcinomas are occasionally seen in appendixes with GCC. It is unclear, however, if all arise from the goblet cell or carcinomatous components, as occasionally mucinous tumors can co-exist, creating the potential for two pathways to co-exist in the same appendix.

The illustrations in the chapter attempt to highlight (1) the variety of lesions encountered in the appendix and (2) the spectrum of histologic changes that may be seen within them.

4.2 Normal Appendix and Serrated Hyperplasia, Dysplasia, and Carcinoma

The appendix is a distinct organ with many histologic features that are similar to those of the adjacent large bowel, but the tumors are distinctive (Figs. 4.1, 4.2, 4.3, 4.4, 4.5, 4.6, 4.7, 4.8, and 4.9). Serrated changes are seen in the appendix much more frequently than adenomatous lesions (the opposite is the case in the large bowel). In fact, in appendixes that are removed due to inflammation (appendicitis), serrated hyperplastic changes are often seen that are secondary to inflammation or injury. It is a source of frustration that the division between serrated lesions in the appendix—particularly hyperplastic polyps, serrated hyperplasia, and sessile serrated polyps/adenomas (SSP/A)—are poorly defined and differentiating between them is often subjective. This section illustrates the spectrum of serrated lesions in the appendix from the inflammation or injury-induced hyperplastic lesions to invasive adenocarcinomas.

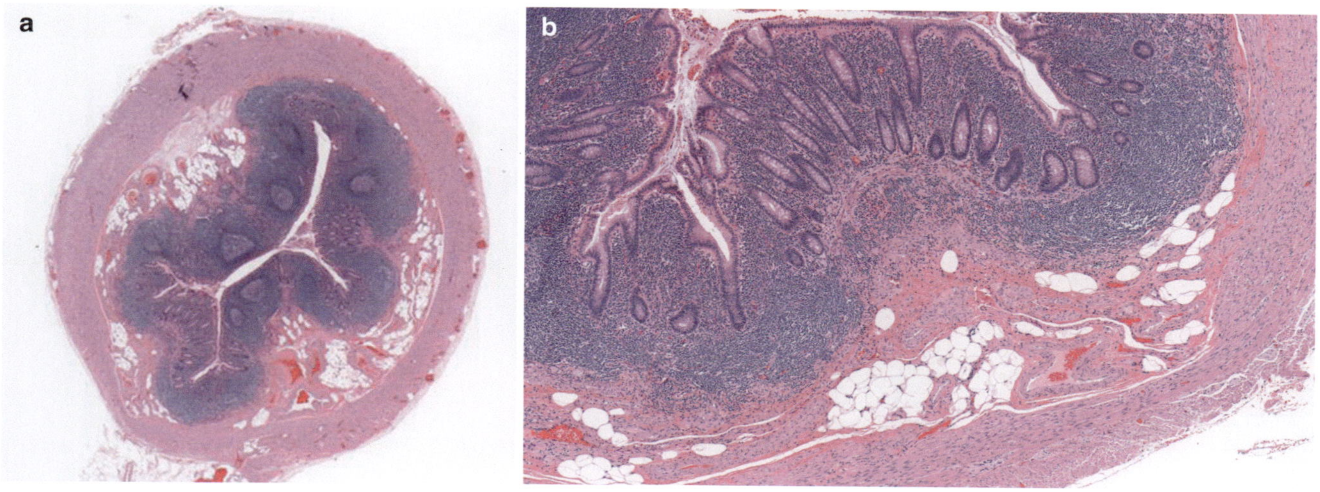

Fig. 4.1 Normal appendix. (**a**), Cross section of the appendix showing layers including colonic type epithelium, lamina propria, prominent lymphoid tissue, muscularis mucosae, submucosae, muscularis propria, and serosa. (**b**), Note the abundance of lymphoid tissue in this appendix, disrupting the muscularis mucosae focally (a common occurrence) and areas of fat and large blood vessels within the submucosa. The quantity of lymphoid tissue is variable and, in some appendixes, virtually absent. The muscularis propria has both circular and longitudinal muscle layers that are in continui with those in the large bowel. The mucosa has typical test-tube crypts but often more widely separated than in the right colon

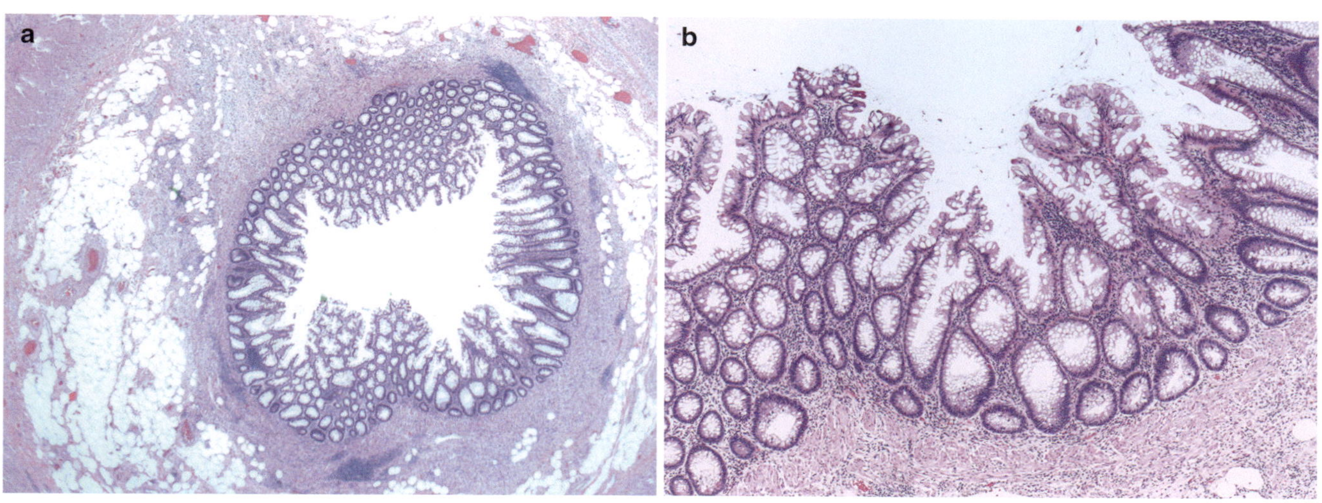

Fig. 4.2 Serrated hyperplasia. This is a common lesion thought by some to always be a reactive change following acute appendicitis. (**a**), The muscularis mucosae is present, but duplicated, although with a readily visible submucosa, while the epithelium has architectural distortion, both of which indicate previous mucosal destruction and repair. (**b**), There is a good lamina propria. The superficial epithelium is overtly serrated, and when these changes are very focal, it can resemble a hyperplastic polyp; indeed, some would call this a hyperplastic polyp, to which there can be little objection. Note that the crypt bases and sides lack dysplasia

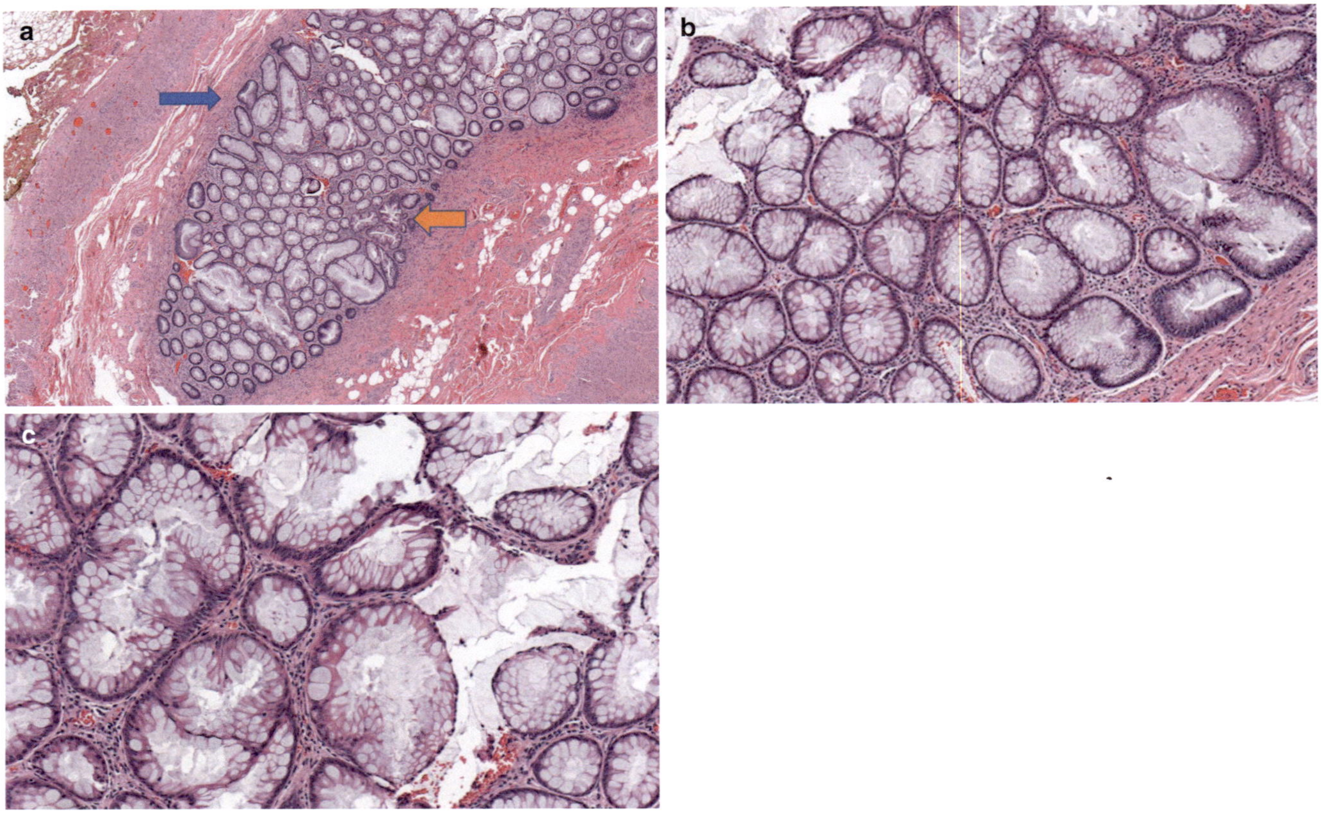

Fig. 4.3 A more extreme example of reactive (serrated) hyperplasia of the appendix. (**a**), Again, note the thickened duplicated muscularis mucosae and marked architectural distortion. In this case the latter has occasional boot-shaped crypts (*blue arrow*) and serrated crypts (*orange arrow*) as well as dilated crypts that are readily interpreted as being part of a sessile serrated polyp/adenoma (SSP/A), so are part of a spectrum of changes. This appendix has a thickened mucosa with abundant mucinous epithelium. (**b** and **c**), Detail of the mucosa that has luminal serrations and basally oriented small non-dysplastic nuclei, although in (**b**) they are slightly enlarged at the crypt bases. This type of reactive hyperplasia is commonly seen in appendectomies for acute appendicitis and the changes may be localized or occupy the entirety of the appendiceal lumen

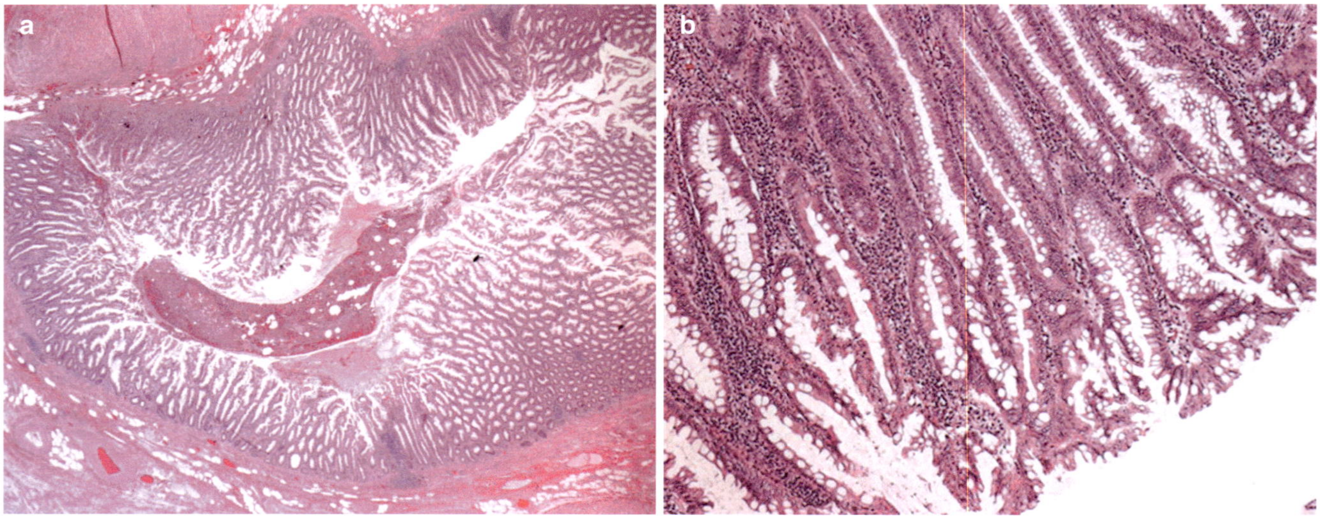

Fig. 4.4 Diffuse serrated hyperplasia. (**a**), The divide between hyperplastic polyps, serrated hyperplasia, and sessile serrated polyps/adenomas are often vague. However, note the thickened duplicated muscularis mucosae and presence of submucosal fat. Provided the lesion is removed in toto, there is no prognostic significance between them. (**b**), Diffuse serrated hyperplasia. Detail shows elongated crypts with a well-formed lamina propria and superficial serrations. The crypts at the top left are showing atypical changes

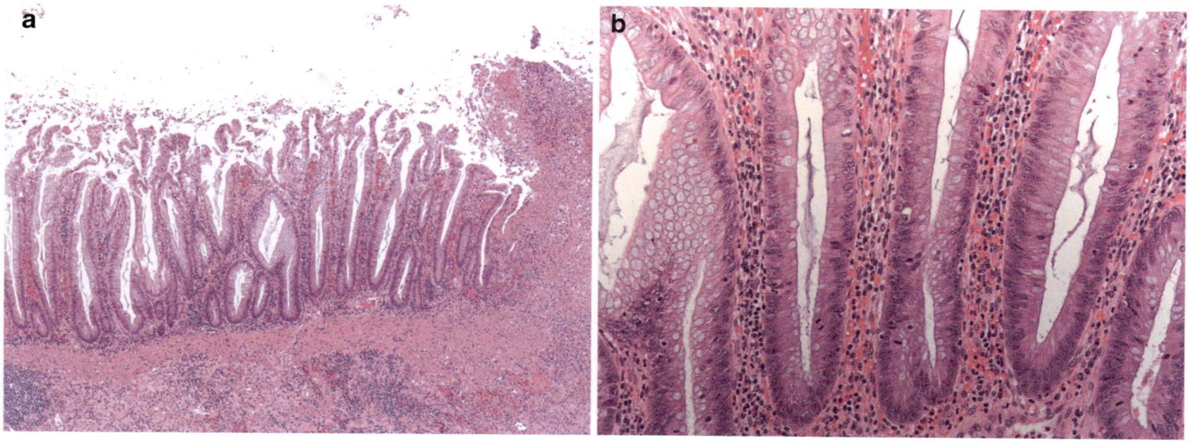

Fig. 4.5 Serrated hyperplasia with possible dysplastic changes. (**a**), Note the ulcer to the right; some could interpret these as being reactive. (**b**), Others might interpret these changes as being atypical, but provided the lesion has been completely excised and is entirely mucosal, the nomenclature matters little (as long as it cannot be interpreted as requiring any further treatment, as the lesion has been fully removed)

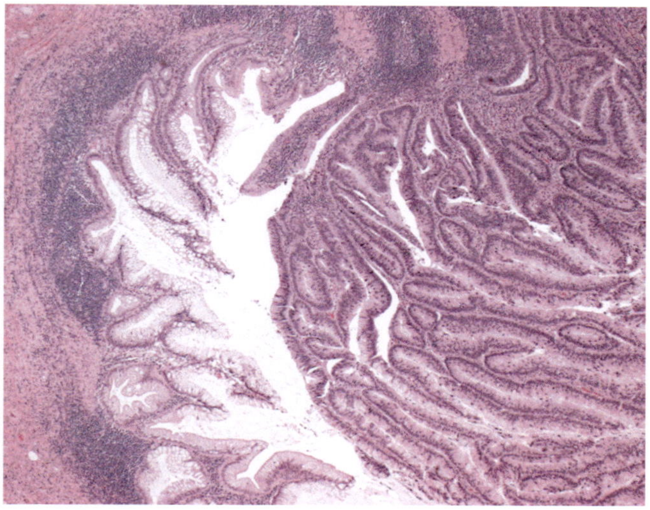

Fig. 4.6 Transition/junction from serrated hyperplasia (bottom left) in which no dysplasia is present to an overt adenoma, both of which have lamina propria, and which also had an infiltrating component. Carcinomatous architecture is present (top right), despite the nuclei still being confined to the crypt bases and without loss of polarity, so technically still low grade. The association of serrated hyperplasia with dysplasia and carcinoma suggests that at least some may be analogous to SSA/As in the large bowel and have the potential to transform into dysplastic and neoplastic variants

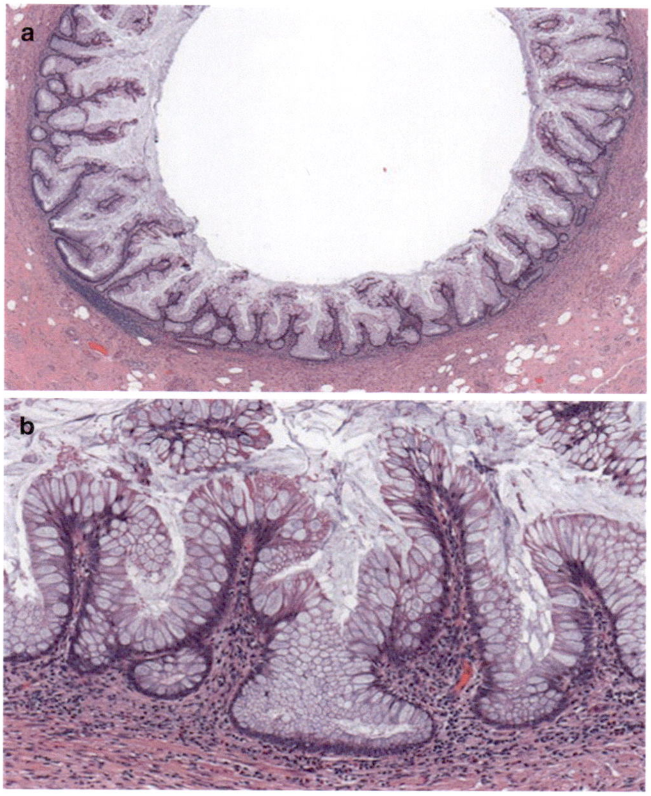

Fig. 4.7 Sessile serrated polyp/adenoma (SSP/A) without dysplasia. (**a**), The appendiceal lumen is lined by crypts resembling large bowel SSP/A, but if anything with more architectural distortion than usually seen in SSP/A; it appears to be an admixture of regenerating crypts and boots/anchors, walking legs seen in SSP/A. However, the crypt bases have a nuclear rim that is not increased in thickness, suggesting no dysplasia. Here the muscularis mucosae appears duplicated and fibrotic, and there is submucosal fibrosis, albeit with some remaining submucosal fat. (**b**), This detail has marked architectural changes including boot-shaped crypts and hypermucinous epithelium. The lamina propria and muscularis mucosae are maintained; this is a feature that differentiates SSP of the appendix from LAMNs

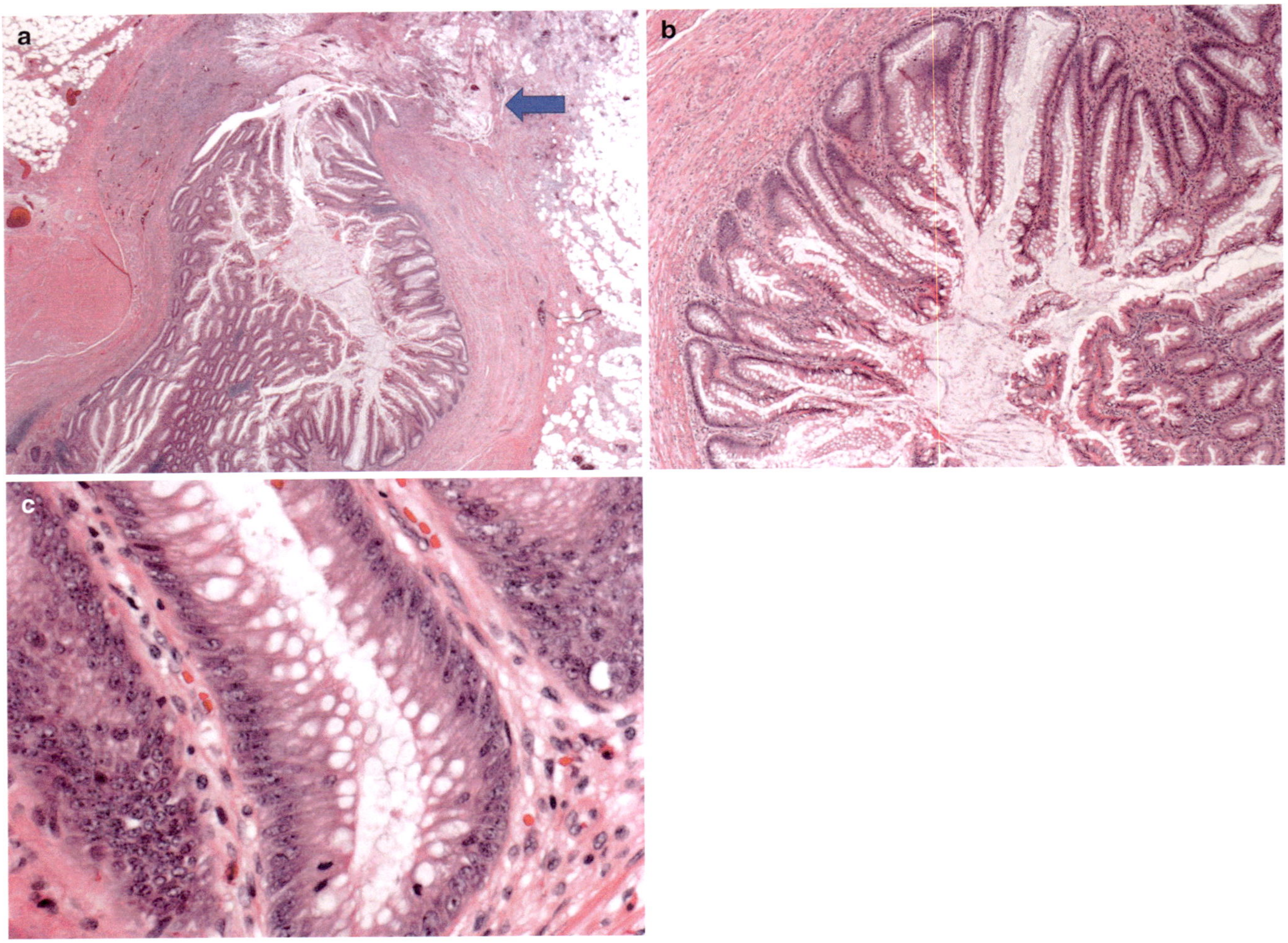

Fig. 4.8 (**a**), Sessile serrated adenoma/polyp (SSA/P) with low-grade dysplasia and perforation (arrow), possibly through a diverticulum. (**b**), The typical architecture of an SSA. (**c**), The typical serrated type dysplasia seen in dysplastic SSAs

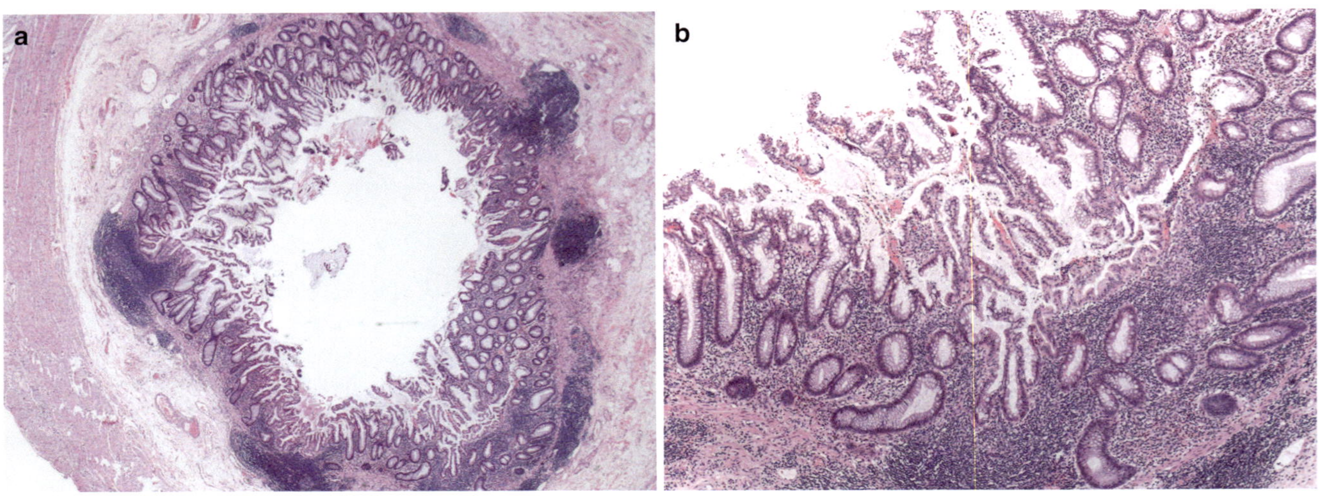

Fig. 4.9 Serrated hyperplasia, dysplasia, and carcinoma. All images are from the same appendix. (**a** and **b**), Serrated hyperplasia without dysplasia in one part of the appendix. (**c** and **d**), Dual population of serrated changes, one non-dysplastic and the other dysplastic. The two components are readily seen in (**c**). (**e–g**), Invasive adenocarcinoma. (**f**), Note the variety of dysplastic serrated components, including ectopic crypt formation especially toward the center of the field in (**f**) and shown in detail in (**g**)

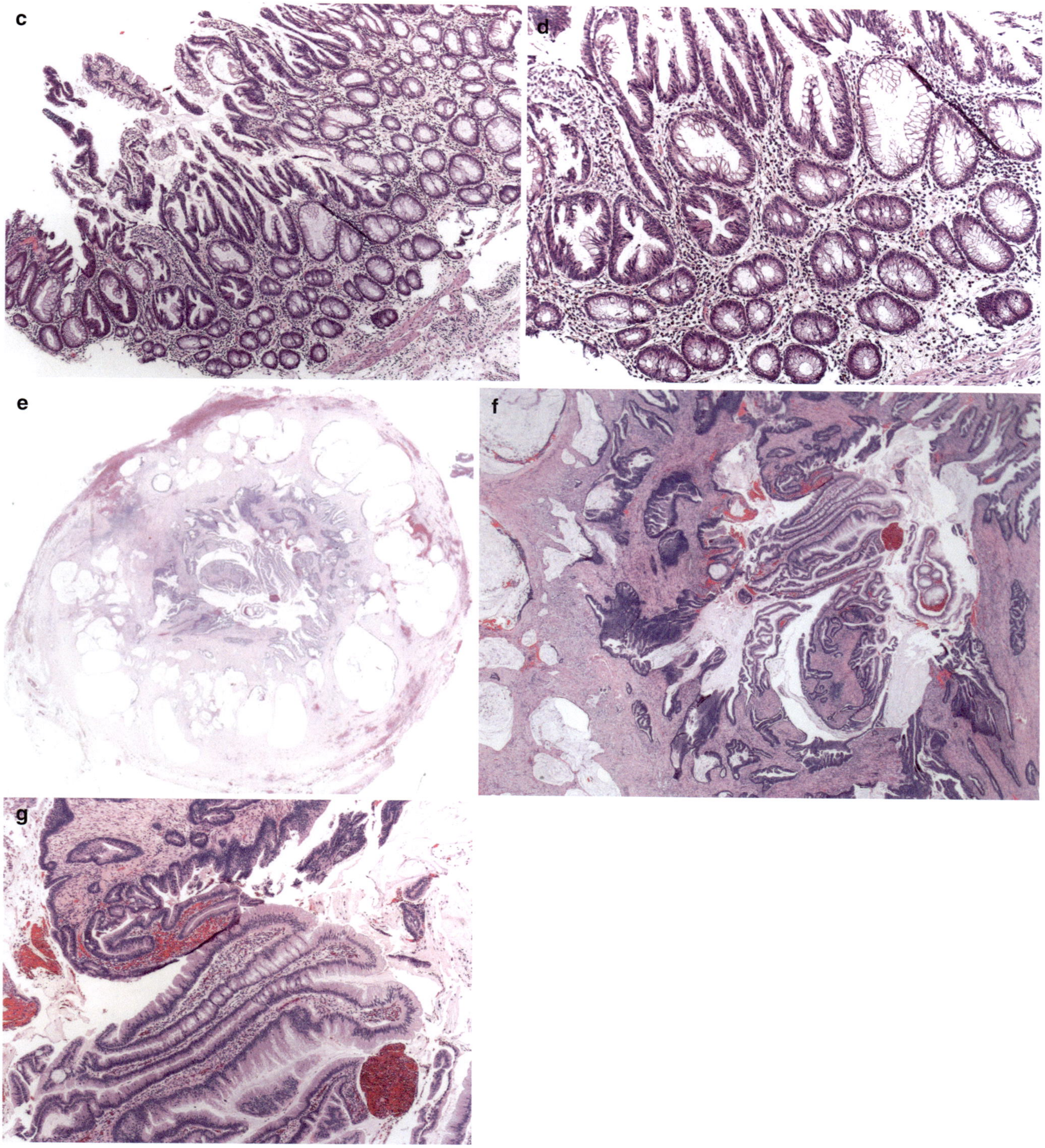

Fig. 4.9 (continued)

4.3 Mucinous Neoplasms

Like serrated changes discussed in Sect. 4.2, mucinous neoplasms are overwhelmingly more common in the appendix than are intestinal type adenomas/adenocarcinomas (Figs. 4.10, 4.11, 4.12, 4.13, 4.14, 4.15, 4.16, 4.17, 4.18, 4.19, 4.20, 4.21, 4.22, 4.23, 4.24, 4.25, 4.26, 4.27, 4.28, 4.29, 4.30, 4.31, 4.32, 4.33, 4.34, 4.35, 4.36, and 4.37). In addition to mucinous adenocarcinoma, there are distinct entities that are found solely in the appendix, including low-grade appendiceal mucinous neoplasm (LAMN) and high-grade appendiceal mucinous neoplasms (HAMN), which have overt architectural complexity or nuclear changes including marked atypicality and loss of polarity. The utility of the term HAMN is unclear, except that they may behave more aggressively. Mucinous neoplasms are important to recognize, as they have characteristic behaviors and prognostic implications. The most recent Cancer Staging Manual from the American Joint Committee on Cancer recognized this by their introduction of an in situ T stage (Tis) for LAMN and HAMN that includes invasion up to the muscular propria. This change acknowledges the low metastatic potential of these lesions until the serosal surface is breached. While LAMNs and HAMNs are distinct entities, it is worth noting that multiple neoplasms may arise within them, as also illustrated in this section.

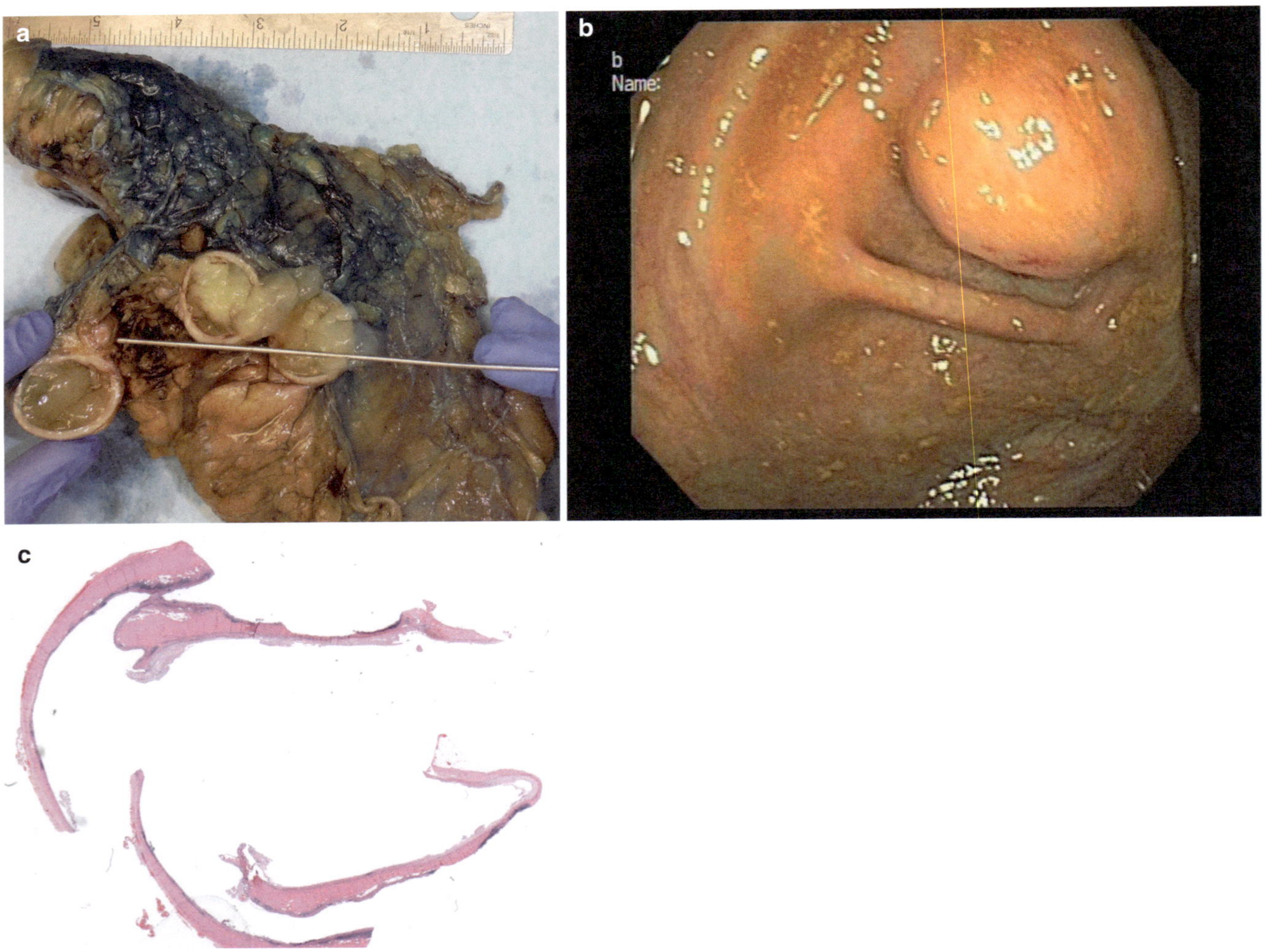

Fig. 4.10 (**a**), Gross illustration of a multiloculated benign mucocele. Sectioning of the entire appendix revealed no dysplastic epithelium. (**b**), Endoscopic image of a mucocele, which is bulging into the cecum. There is no way to distinguish a mucocele from a mucinous neoplasm on gross appearance. (**c**), Mucocele in which the appendiceal lumen is distended by mucin and the normal architecture of the appendix is lost. Mucoceles have no dysplastic epithelium

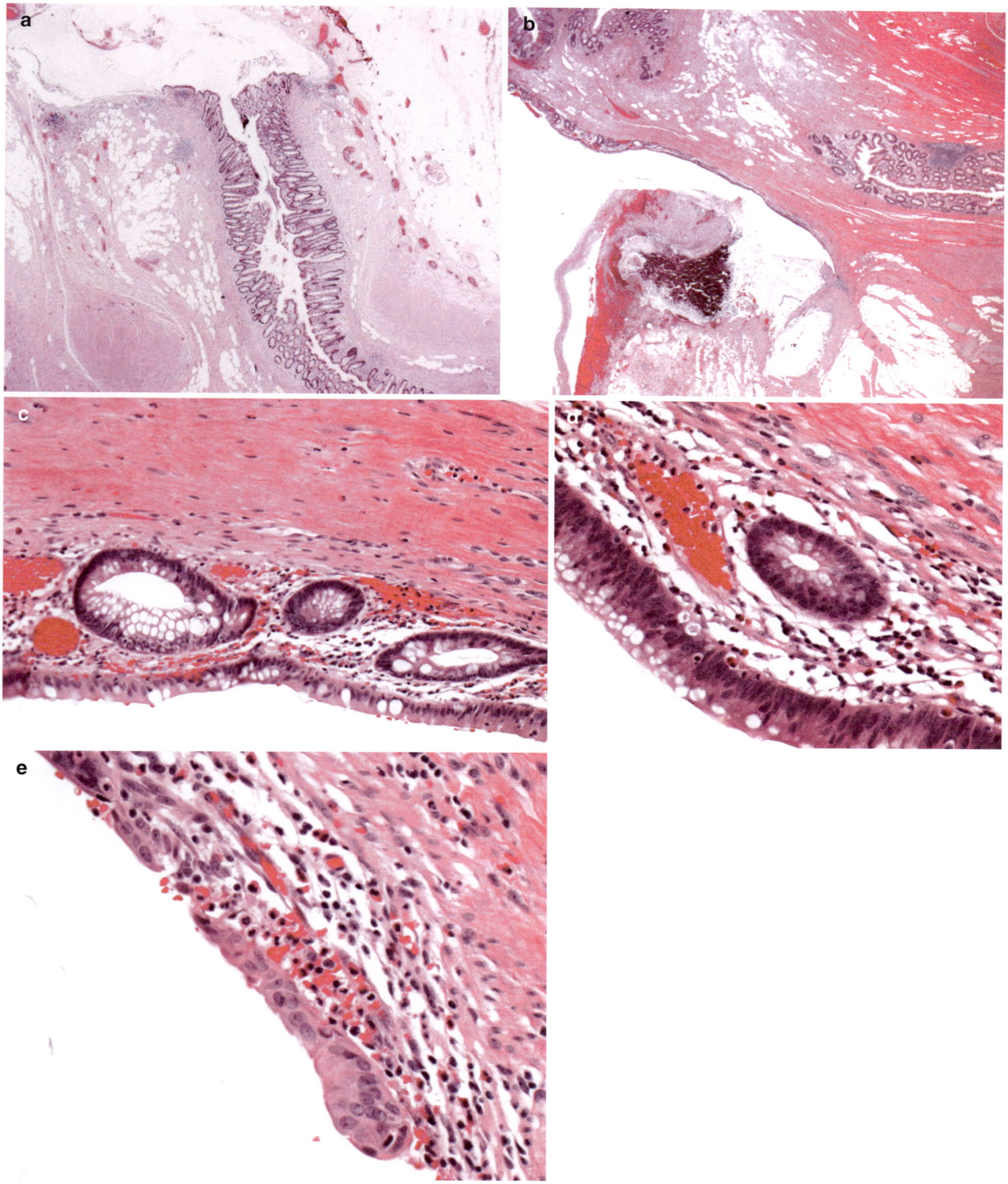

Fig. 4.11 Mucoceles. (**a**), Mucocele with an abrupt end to normal epithelium and a mucin pool in the upper part. (**b**), An overtly dilated appendix with mucin that has dystrophic calcification. (**c**), The epithelium is typical appendiceal mucosa but the luminal mucosa (**d**) is mucin-depleted and has large reactive nuclei. The inflammatory cells, and normal crypt nuclei help to make the diagnosis as dysplastic epithelium growing only across the surface is rare, and would also result in overt junctions with non-dysplastic mucosa. (**e**), The restituting epithelium at the growing edge is syncytial. It is the mucosa proximal to this (**d**) that can appear atypical and potentially be misinterpreted as neoplastic. It is helpful when the underlying crypts are not dysplastic

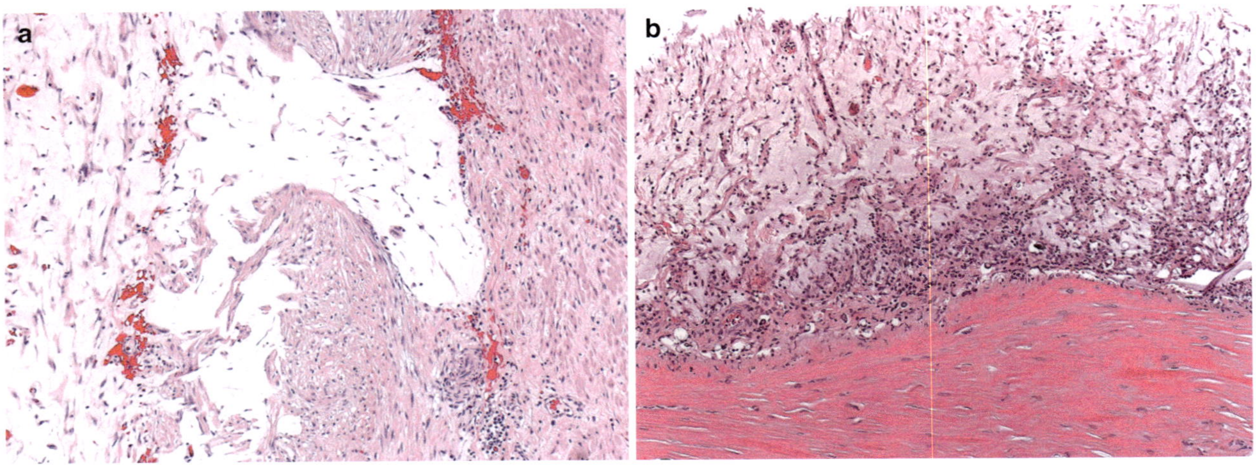

Fig. 4.12 (**a**), When no epithelium is found, the mucin has a variety of appearances, here engendering no reaction even though it has cells growing into it, and it is dissecting into the underlying muscle. The lack of lamina propria is part of having no mucosa, and therefore is of no help in differentiating between mucoceles and mucinous tumors. Mucin sometimes rests on fibrotic muscle, which is typically thick. As there is no mucosa, there is no lamina propria. (**b**), Detail showing a histiocytic reaction

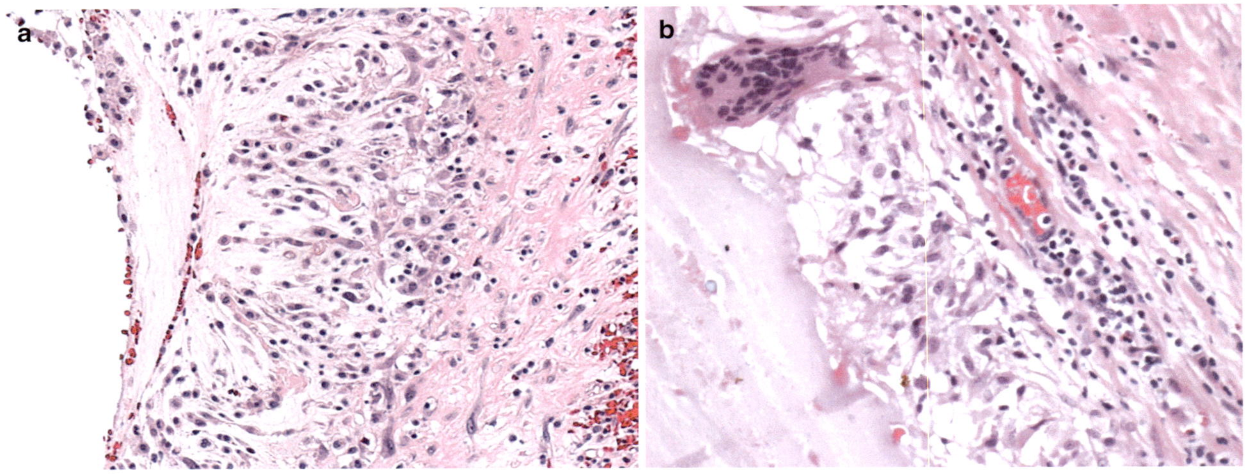

Fig. 4.13 (**a**), Detail of muciphages which can also form giant cells, as seen in (**b**), and undergo dystrophic calcification. Both features occur in benign mucoceles and neoplastic mucin

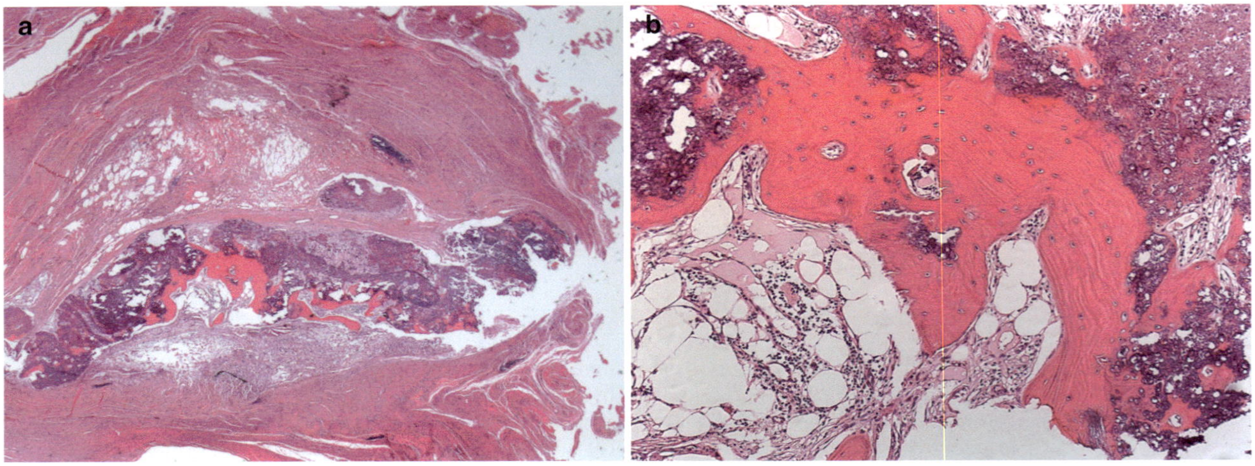

Fig. 4.14 (**a**), Mucin-filled appendix in which the mucin has undergone both dystrophic calcification and heterotopic bone formation. (**b**), Detail of dystrophic calcification (right and top left) and heterotopic bone formation

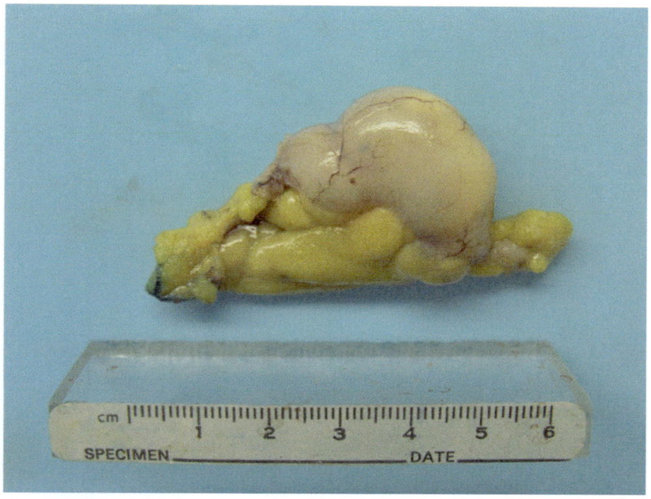

Fig. 4.15 Gross appearance of mucinous tumors. This appendix is dilated and was a secondary finding during a right hemicolectomy surgery for Crohn's disease. They are often found incidentally

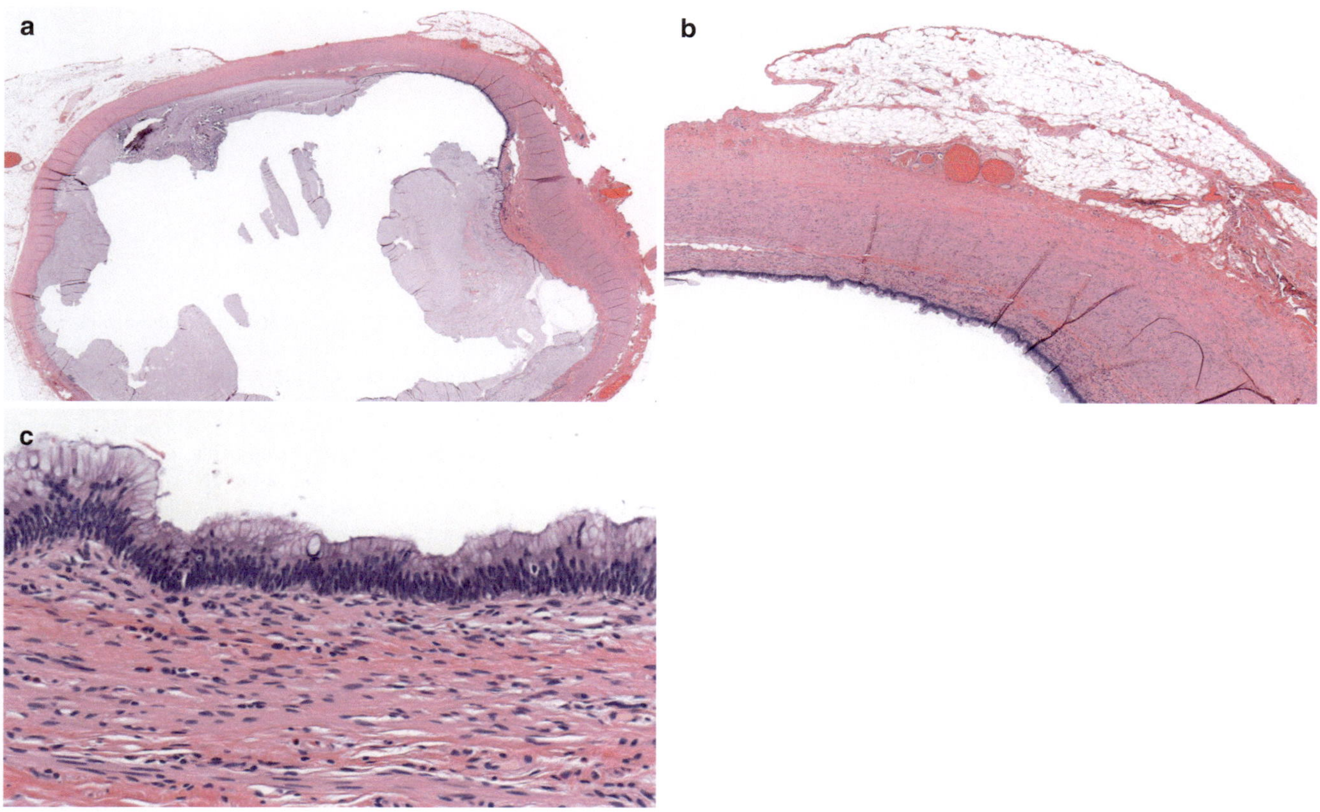

Fig. 4.16 (**a**, **b**), Low-grade appendiceal mucinous neoplasm (LAMN). There is loss of lymphoid tissue, lamina propria, and muscularis mucosae. The loss of these last two structures in particular are a key feature in LAMNs. (**c**), Detail of the neoplastic epithelium with mucin vesicles and occasional goblet cells. The nuclei are hyperchromatic and stratified, characteristic of low-grade dysplasia. This also highlights the loss of lamina propria, lymphoid follicles, and muscularis mucosae, as well as fibrosis of the underlying appendiceal wall

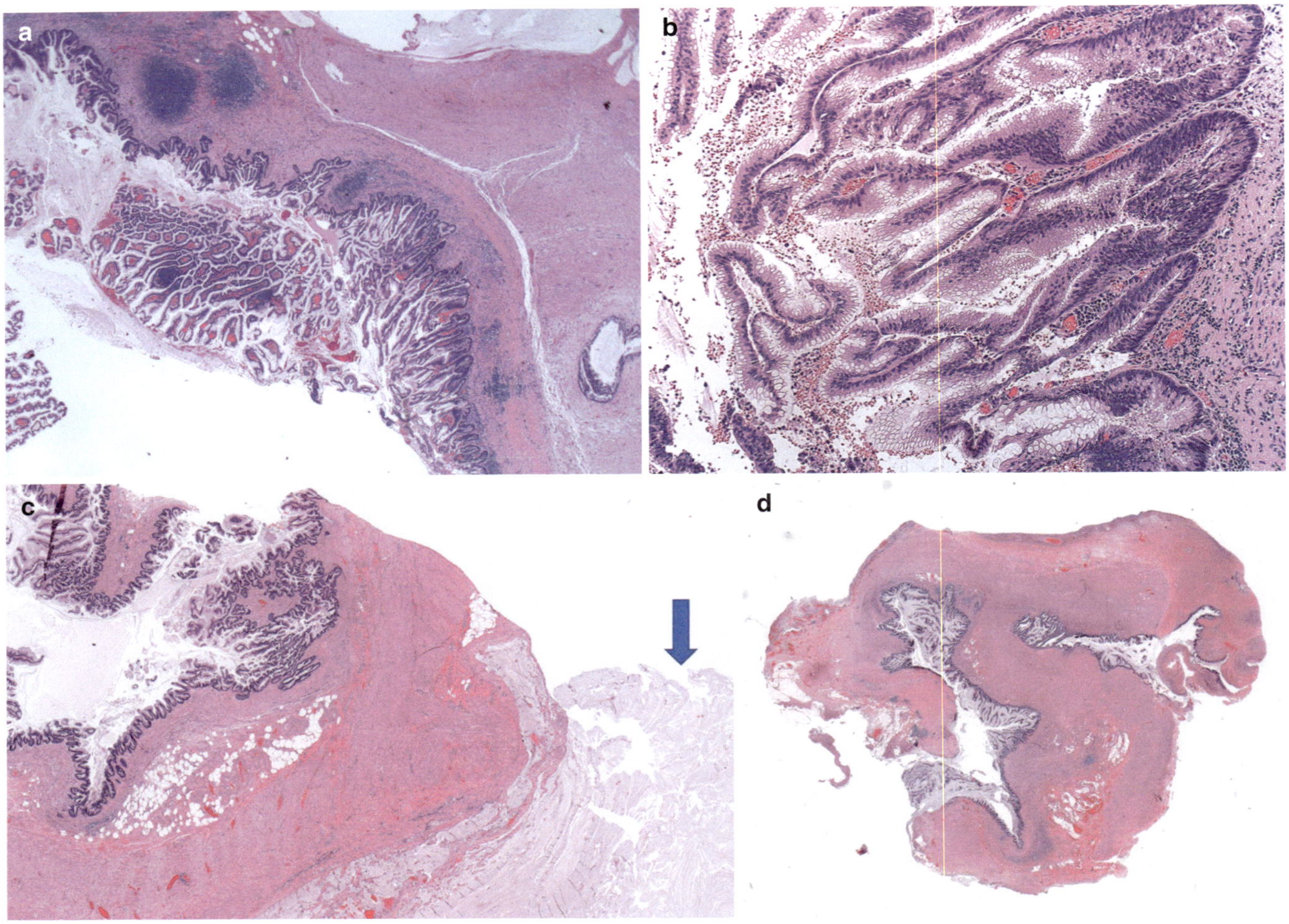

Fig. 4.17 (**a**), Typical mucinous neoplasm with an irregular pushing border surmounted on a typically thickened fibromuscular submucosa/muscularis propria. But note the gland in the muscle (right)—pushing or infiltrating? (**b**), Detail shows the crypts to have architectural high-grade dysplasia. (**c**), LAMN with extra-appendiceal mucin (arrow). This exemplifies the diverticular-like (pushing) growth pattern that characterizes LAMNs. The submucosa is focally lost, and mucin is seen on the serosal surface. The presence of localized extra-appendiceal mucin without neoplastic cells results in a risk of recurrence of approximately 5%. The presence of extra-appendiceal mucin with neoplastic epithelium increases the risk to approximately 33%. (**d**), LAMN that infiltrates through the appendiceal wall with perforation. That on the left has a typical "pushing" border while that on the right has more complex outpouchings. The borderline between outpouchings and low-grade adenocarcinoma can be very subjective. However, when confined to the appendix, outpouchings tend to behave in a benign manner. These two examples illustrate the difficulty in being certain whether one is dealing with a LAMN or a low-grade mucinous adenocarcinoma, and the diagnosis has a subjective component. Once the serosa is breached, however, the risk of pseudomyxoma remains, the risk depending on whether the mucin is cellular or acellular

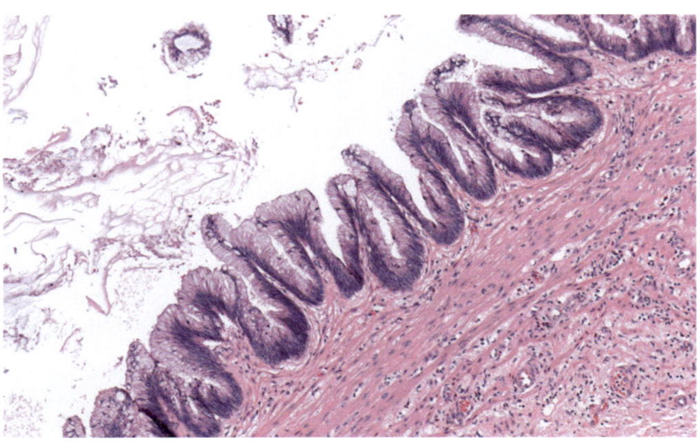

Fig. 4.18 LAMN. This detailed view of a LAMN with low-grade mucinous epithelium has lost its lamina propria and rests on a thickened duplicated but (at least in this example) well-preserved muscularis mucosae. However, submucosal fibrosis can be seen in the lower right corner

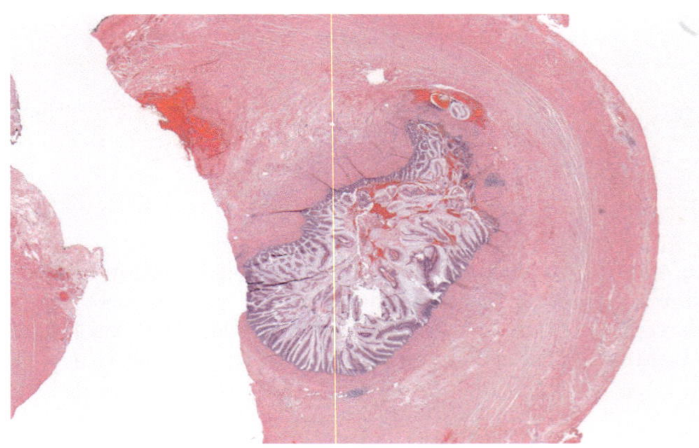

Fig. 4.19 LAMN. Appendix with thickened wall and neoplastic epithelium resting on a markedly thickened and duplicated muscularis mucosae, but with dense fibromuscular hyperplasia of the submucosal tissue

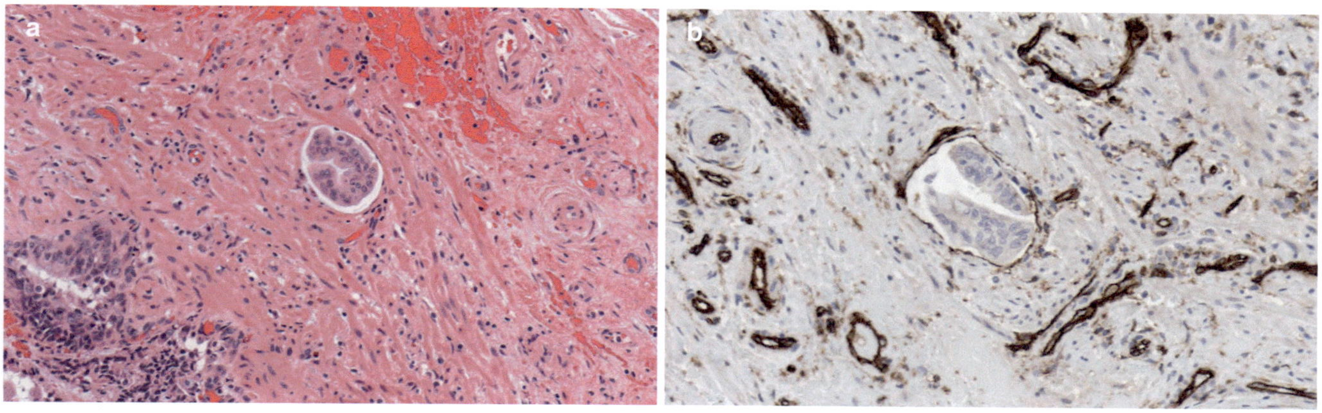

Fig. 4.20 (**a**), Lymphovascular invasion (LVI) in appendiceal wall. This is a rare finding in LAMNs and evidence for appropriate management of these patients is lacking. (**b**), Detail of CD31 immunohistochemical stain

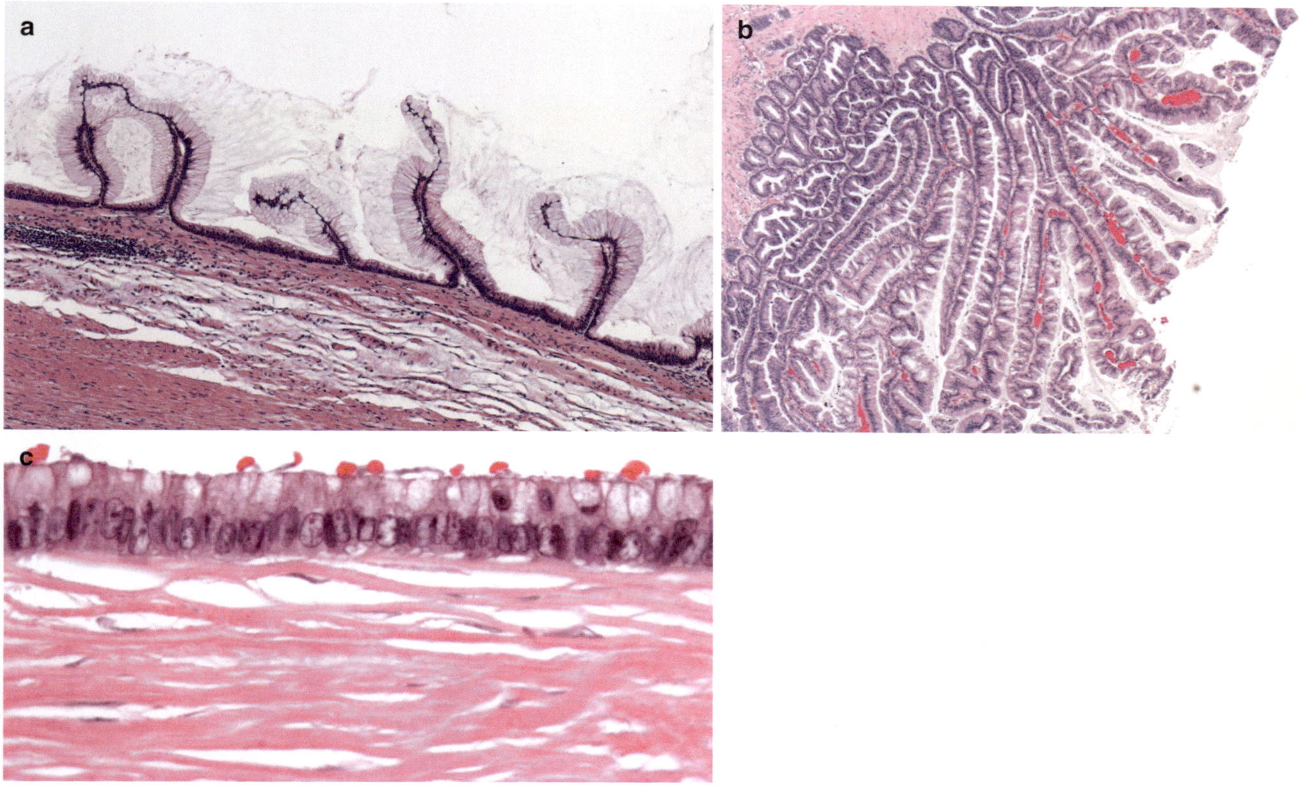

Fig. 4.21 Various epithelial types in LAMN. (**a**), Villous. (**b**), Undulating and serrated. (**c**), Flattened. Although the architecture of the epithelium varies, the characteristic features of LAMN remain, including loss of lamina propria, muscularis mucosae, and submucosal fibrosis with low-grade dysplastic epithelium resting on fibrous tissue

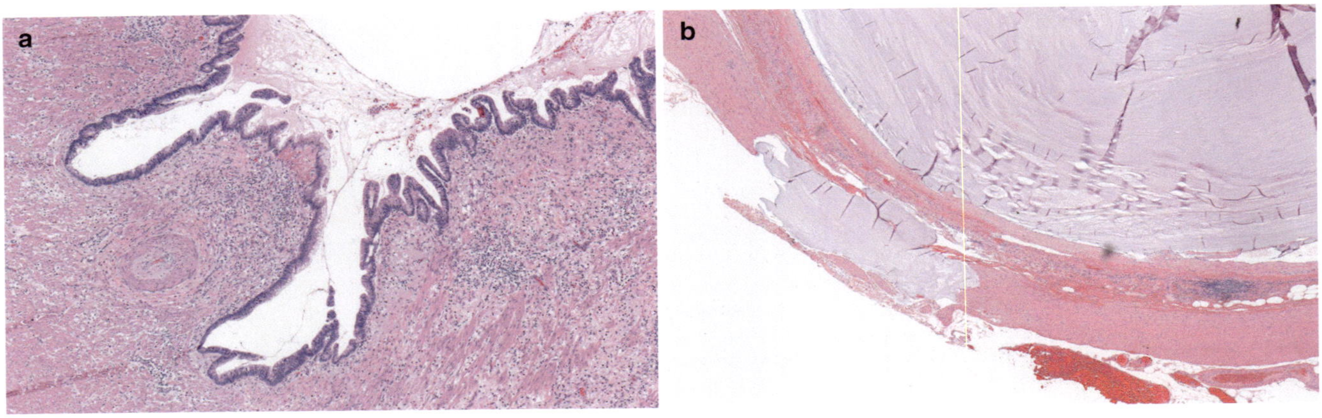

Fig. 4.22 Patterns of invasion in LAMN. Invasion in LAMNs is characterized by the AJCC 8th edition as non-destructive. It lacks the characteristic desmoplasia and destructive growth pattern seen in conventional adenocarcinomas. (**a**), LAMN may infiltrate surrounding tissues in two patterns. In this diverticular-like "pushing"/non-infiltrative growth pattern, the low-grade neoplastic epithelium has a broad pushing front without associated desmoplasia. They often resemble adenomatous epithelium growing along an appendiceal diverticulum. (**b**), Acellular mucin may also dissect through the appendiceal wall, and spread to the peritoneal cavity and organs. Here mucin is dissecting through the muscularis mucosae and penetrating the serosa. As the level of penetration of both mucin and neoplastic epithelium are used in assessing stage, this would be a Stage T4a

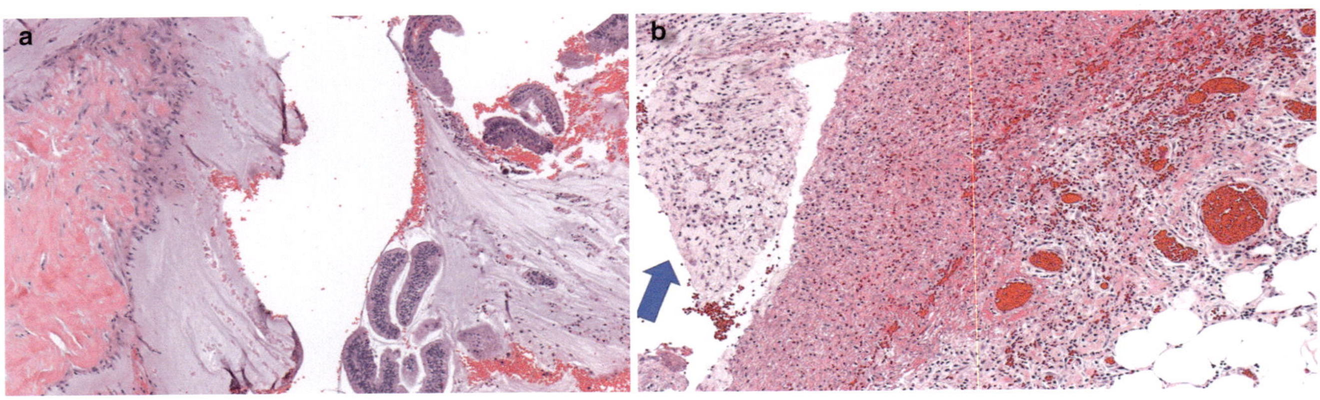

Fig. 4.23 Extra-appendiceal mucin. One of the most critical prognostic factors in LAMNs is the presence or absence of neoplastic epithelium cells in localized mucin outside of the appendix. (**a**), Cellular mucin is seen in this example with fragments of neoplastic mucinous epithelium. The risk of recurrence in this case would be in the region of 33%. (**b**), Acellular mucin (arrow) in this example has inflammatory cells as well as neovascularization. The risk of recurrence in LAMN cases with localized acellular extra-appendiceal mucin is approximately 5%

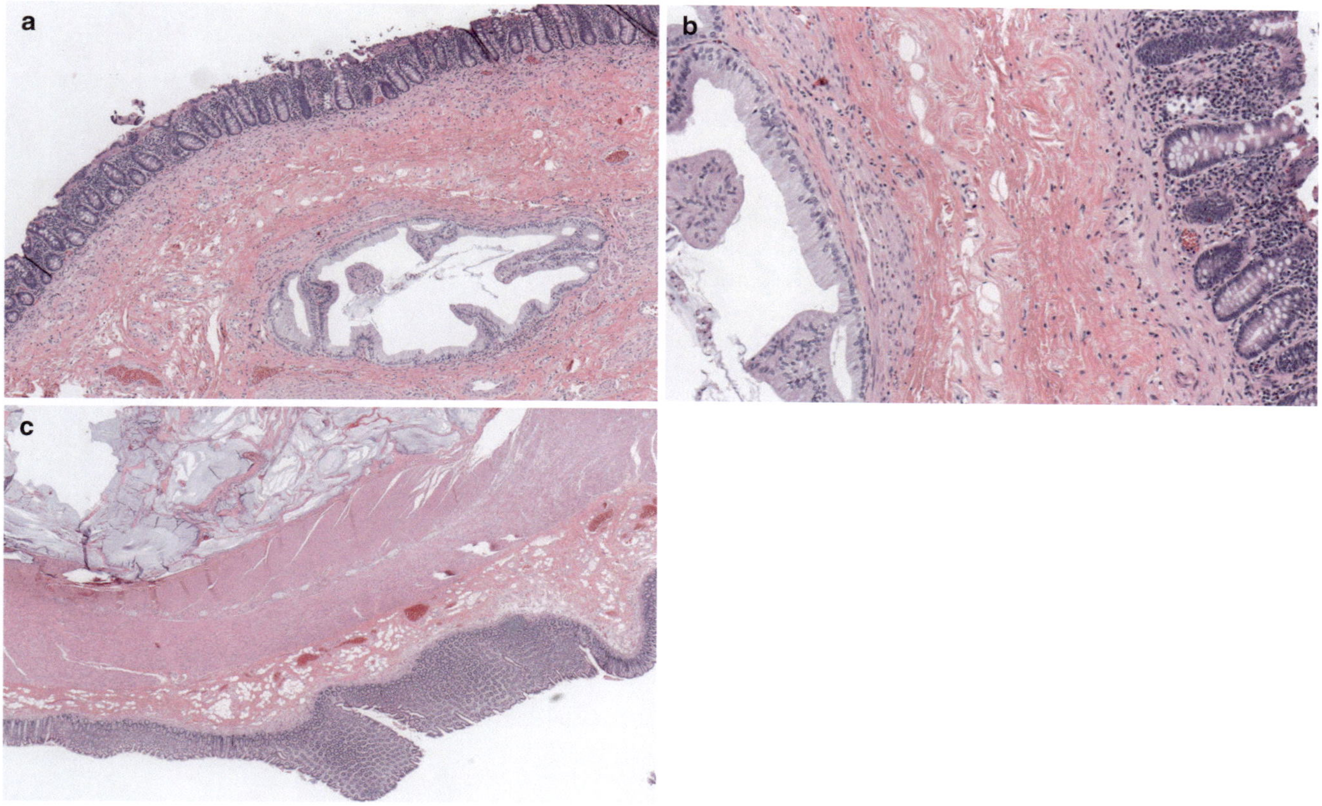

Fig. 4.24 Metastatic disease from LAMNs. LAMNs involve distant sites by invasion of organs/structures by neoplastic epithelium or by dissecting acellular mucin. (**a**, **b**), This section of large bowel has low-grade mucinous neoplasm invading through the bowel wall and encroaching on the overlying mucosa. (**c**), In contrast, this bowel contains acellular mucin only. In the AJCC 8th edition, M stage is determined by the presence or absence of neoplastic epithelium, as well as by the location of the metastases (intraperitoneal organs vs extraperitoneal). Cases in which only acellular mucin are found are classified as M1a, while those with neoplastic epithelium that is confined to the peritoneal cavity and organs are classified as M1b

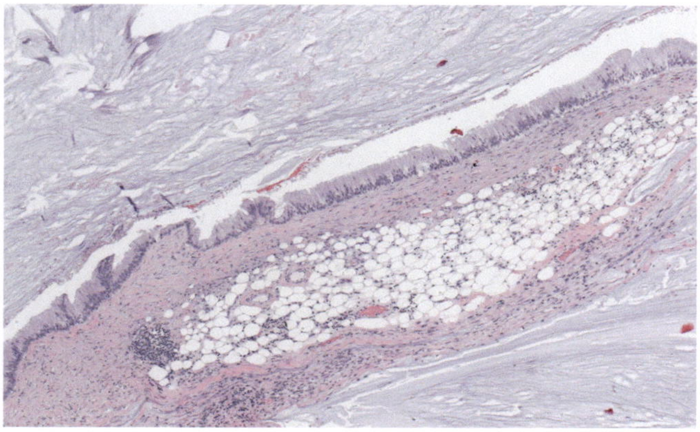

Fig. 4.25 LAMN involving omentum. Low-grade mucinous epithelium lines the surface of this omentum, which is also infiltrated by pools of mucin. Abundant mucin is also present outside the omentum. The findings in this example are frequently seen in pseudomyxoma peritonei

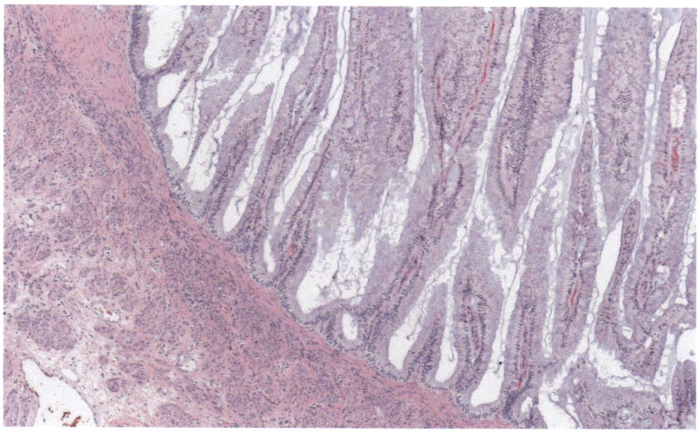

Fig. 4.26 LAMN metastatic to ovary. Low-grade mucinous epithelium with villous architecture infiltrating ovarian stroma. However, note the very bland nuclei. Involvement of the ovaries (often bilateral) frequently occurs in cases of disseminated intraperitoneal disease. Direct invasion into the ovary occurs in Stage T4b disease

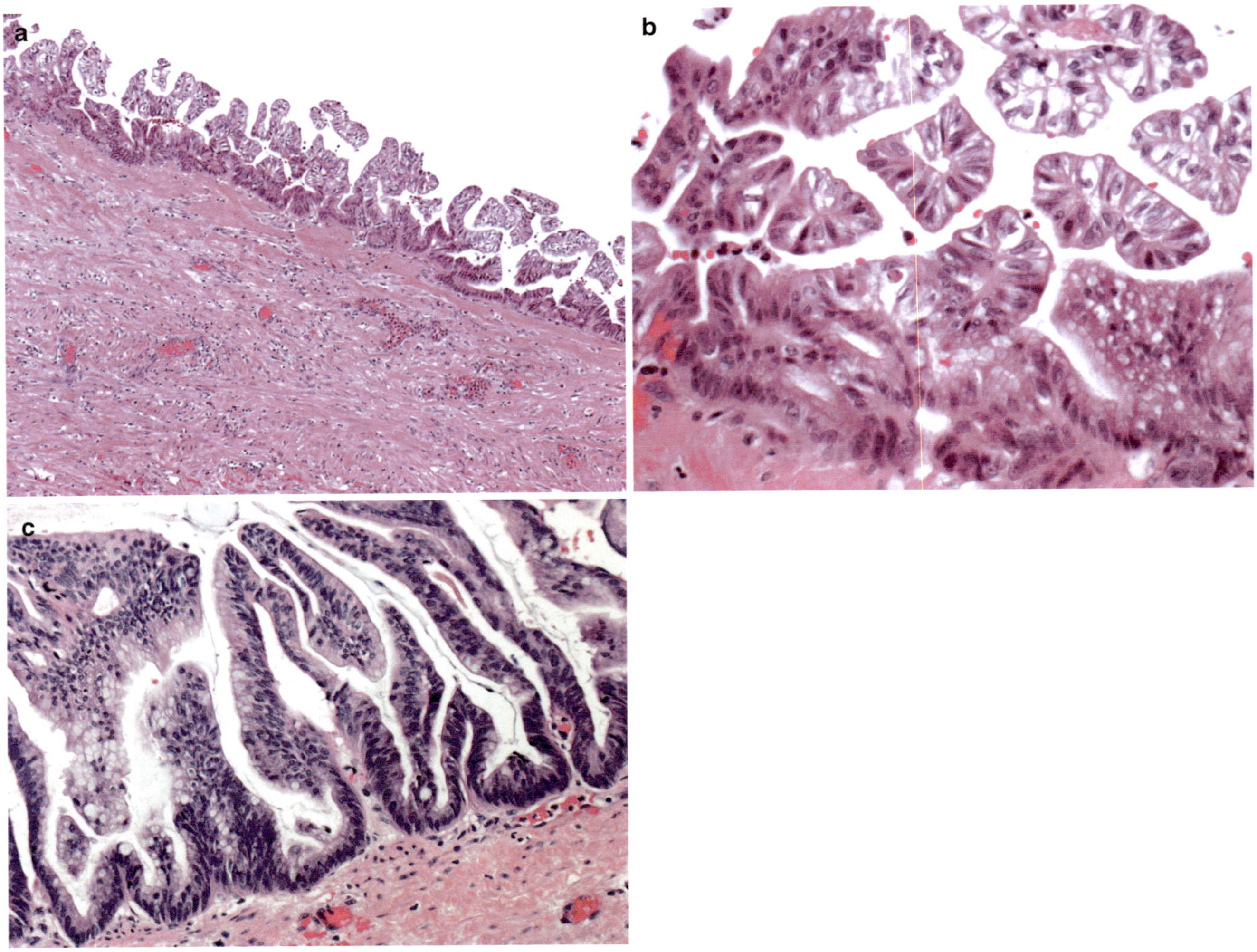

Fig. 4.27 High-grade appendiceal neoplasia (HAMN). (**a**, **b**), This lesion has a micropapillary appearance. (**b**), Detail shows nuclei that have lost polarity and reach the cell surface. (**c**), A further HAMN that co-existed with serrated dysplasia

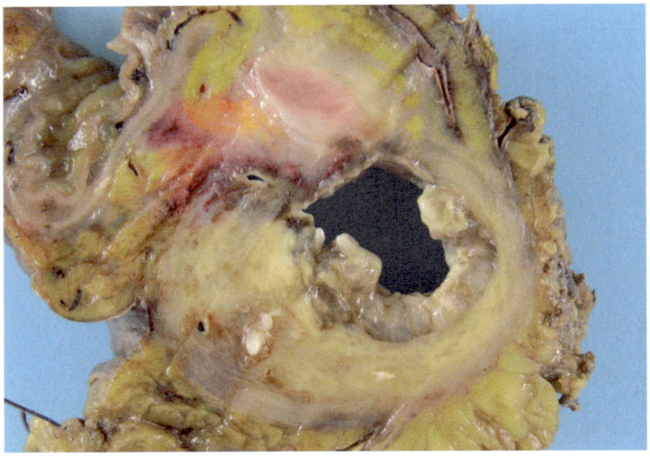

Fig. 4.28 Adenocarcinoma of appendix arising from a low-grade mucinous neoplasm. Tumor extends towards the cecum and ileum (top left)

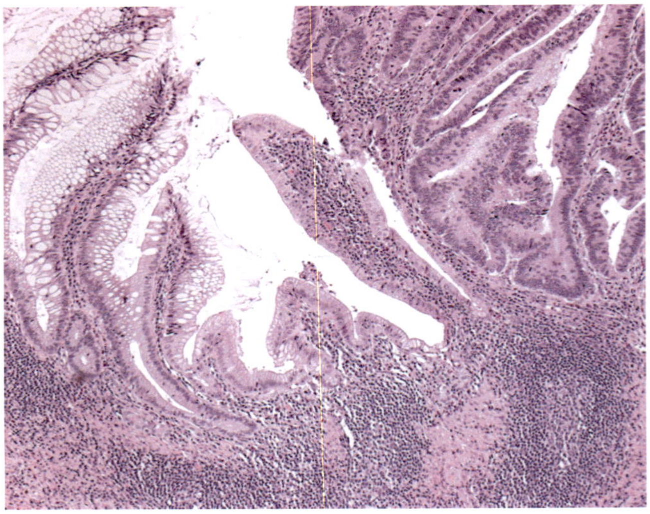

Fig. 4.29 Microscopic view of appendiceal lumen with junction between low-grade and high-grade mucinous epithelium

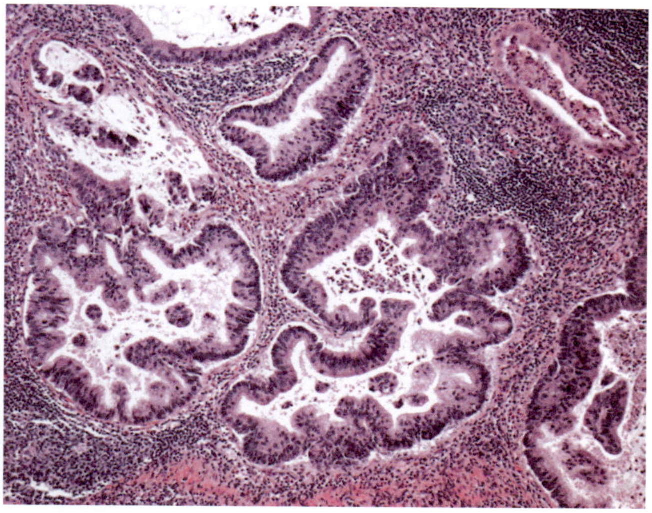

Fig. 4.30 Detail of the infiltrating component that arose from an area of high-grade dysplasia. The cytological features of this invasive component are similar to some serrated large bowel carcinomas and are sometimes referred to as "large bowel type"

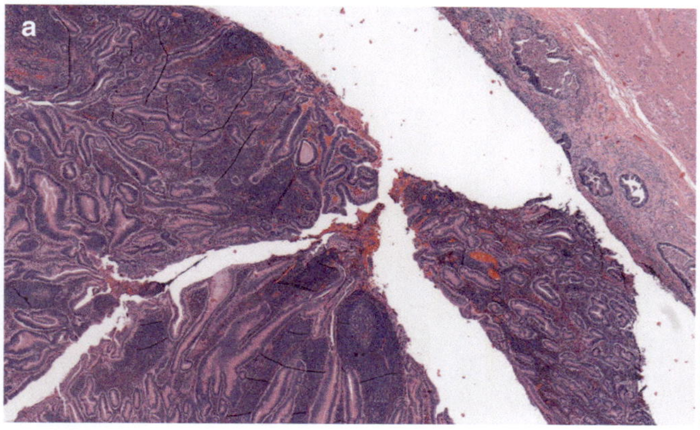

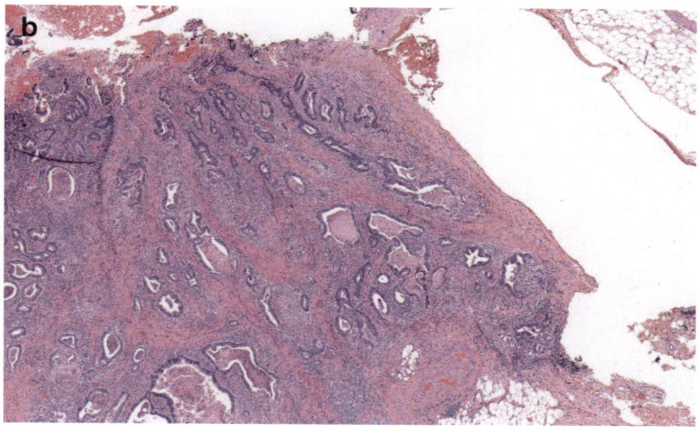

Fig. 4.31 (**a**), Adenocarcinoma arising from a LAMN via a tubulovillous adenoma. The appendiceal lumen is distended by the adenomatous component from which the invasive adenocarcinoma is arising. (**b**), Additional sections showed invasive adenocarcinoma, which is infiltrating adjacent cecal wall

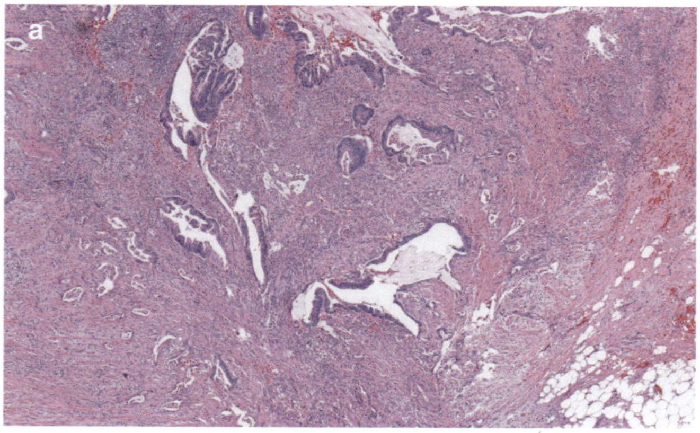

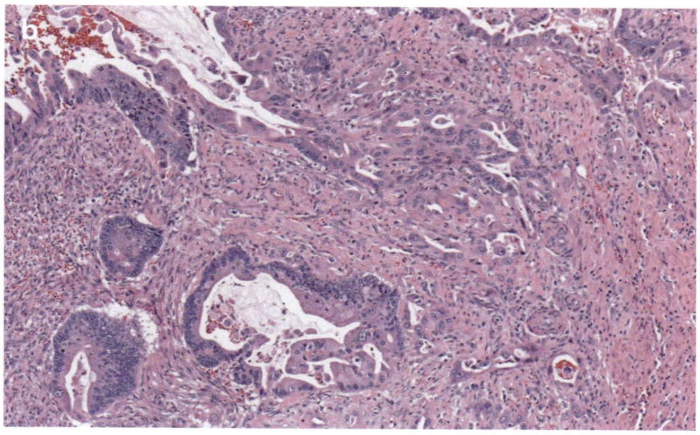

Fig. 4.32 (**a**), The architecture is obliterated by an infiltrative adenocarcinoma with no obvious residual precursor neoplasm. (**b**), A closer view highlights the irregular infiltrative glands in a desmoplastic stroma. There is a poorly differentiated component right of center with areas of infiltrative single cells ("budding")

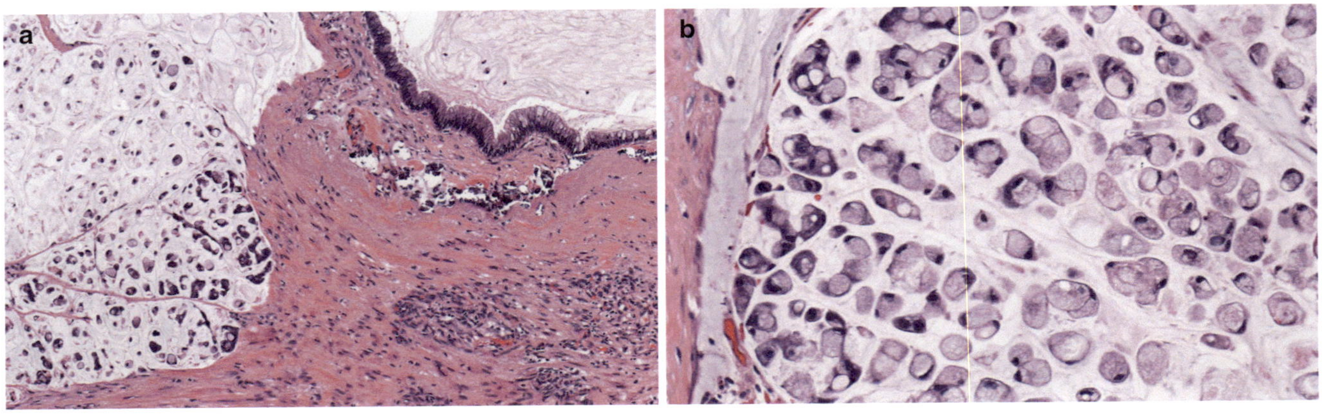

Fig. 4.33 Signet ring cell carcinoma arising from a LAMN. (**a**), The right side of the image consists of a LAMN with characteristic features including low-grade mucinous epithelium on a fibrosed appendiceal wall. Dystrophic calcifications are seen. A mucinous signet ring cell carcinoma is seen infiltrating the adjacent appendiceal wall. While signet ring cell carcinoma in the appendix most often arises ex goblet cell carcinoid (GCC), this is a reminder that they can also occur through the LAMN pathway. LAMNs and GCCs can occasionally arise in the same appendix; should this issue arise, therefore, sectioning of the entire appendix to exclude GCC, or demonstrating the transition between LAMN and carcinoma, is required to resolve the issue. (**b**), Detail of the infiltrative component consisting of single cells and groups of signet ring cells with prominent cytoplasmic mucin and displaced nuclei

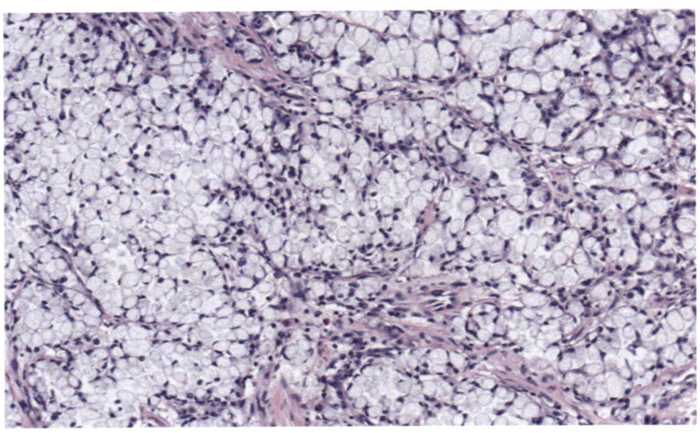

Fig. 4.34 Signet ring cell carcinoma. This example is from an appendiceal wall with sheets of cohesive signet ring cells. While signet ring cell carcinoma of the appendix often arises from a precursor lesion, it can also apparently arise de novo (possibly mimicking the stomach), as was the case in this example. When signet ring cell differentiation is seen, careful examination of the appendix for evidence of additional neoplasm (LAMN, goblet cell carcinoid) is required. While the pattern suggests a possible origin from a goblet cell tumor, no evidence of it could be found

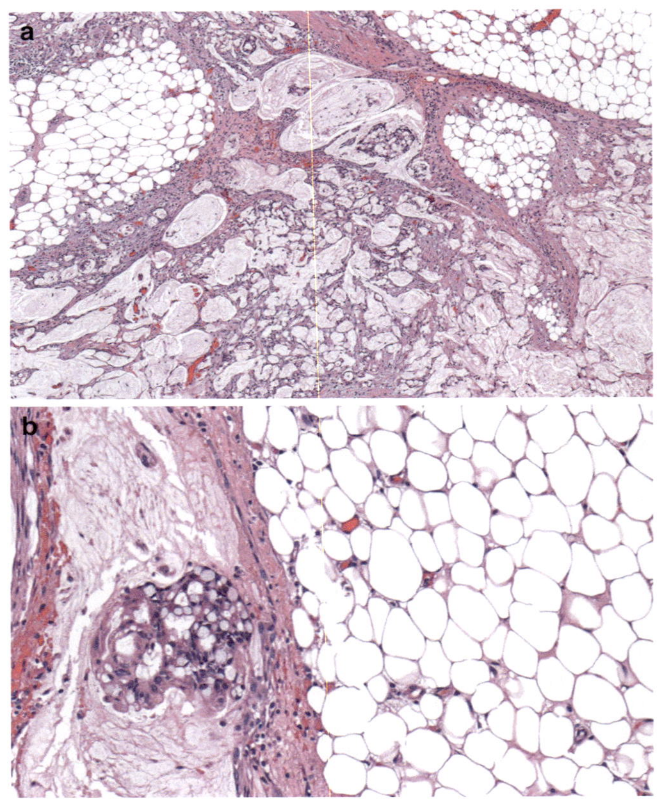

Fig. 4.35 (**a**), Omentum with high-grade mucinous adenocarcinoma. The omentum is infiltrated by pools of mucin and neoplastic cells. (**b**), Detail reveals mucinous adenocarcinoma with glandular architecture with foci of signet ring cell differentiation present in pools in mucin

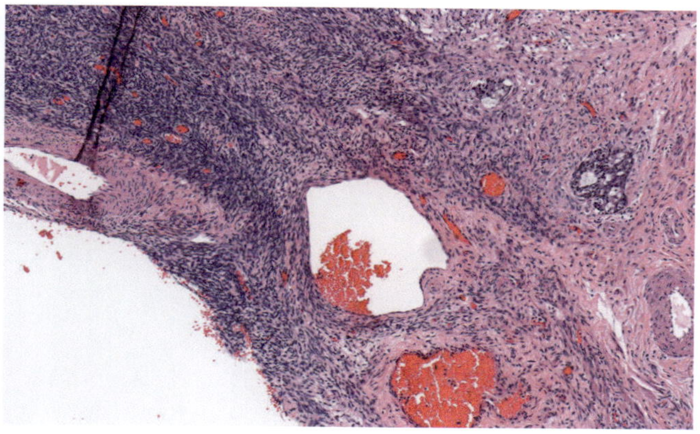

Fig. 4.36 Metastatic appendiceal adenocarcinoma in the ovary. This example contains small clusters of adenocarcinoma confined mainly to ovarian hilum

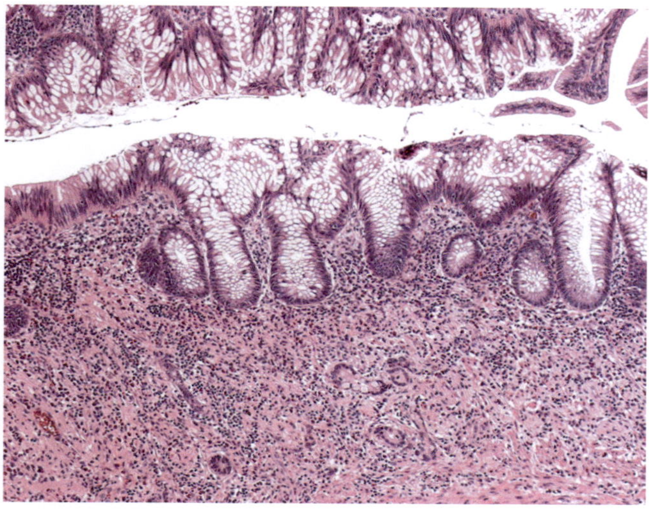

Fig. 4.37 LAMN with underlying goblet cell carcinoid. Combined tumors are rare

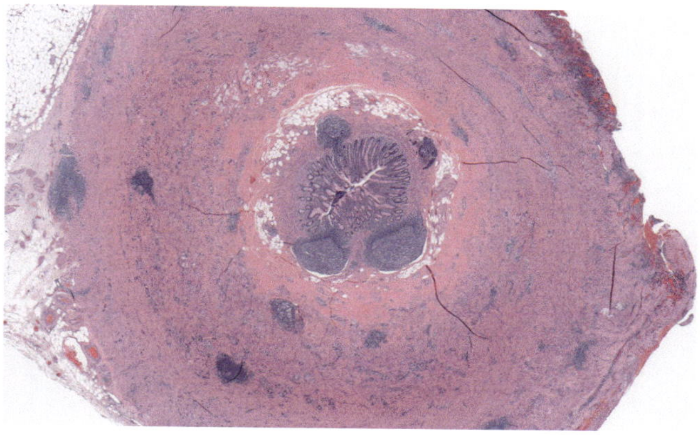

Fig. 4.38 Goblet cell carcinoid (GCC). Overview of an appendix with diffuse aggregates of cells visible within a thickened appendiceal wall. The mucosa, lymphoid tissue, and submucosa appear unremarkable at this view

4.4 Goblet Cell Carcinoids and Carcinomas ex Goblet Cell Carcinoid

Goblet cell carcinoid (GCC) is another neoplasm that occurs exclusively in the appendix (Figs. 4.38, 4.39, 4.40, 4.41, 4.42, 4.43, 4.44, 4.45, 4.46, 4.47, 4.48, 4.49, 4.50, 4.51, and 4.52). They are basically carcinomas from the onset, but do not usually exert any prognostic influence while limited to the appendix and are completely excised. These neoplasms are comprised of nests of cells resembling goblet or signet ring cells. They can also have endocrine cells (usually serotonin-producing with characteristic sub-nuclear orange-red granules) and Paneth cells with their characteristic larger supranuclear red granules. Hybrid cells are occasionally seen with goblet cells containing either or both of these granule types. Interestingly, there is no recognizable precursor lesion, and their infiltration can be notoriously subtle.

Small incidental GCCs are usually harmless. The real danger comes if the peritoneum or surgical resection margin is involved, when the risk of recurrence increases markedly. Until that happens, these tumors are largely benign. Once through the peritoneum, the prognosis should be much more guarded, even in the absence of carcinoma arising from them.

GCC as a group is more aggressive than its large bowel carcinoma counterparts, especially in any size-for-size comparison, and frequently have lymph node metastasis, perineural invasion, and diffuse infiltration into adjacent structures upon presentation. Occasionally they are diagnosed at an early stage, usually as an "incidentaloma" in appendectomy specimens for appendicitis. Although it is clear that GCCs can have nodal metastases, patients rarely die from systemic disease, but rather from the complications of intraperitoneal disease. Nodal metastases seem to occur more frequently when there is a carcinoma ex goblet cell, so the significance of nodal metastases, especially from pure GCCs, is unclear.

There are three variants of recognized GCC, including (1) the typical (conventional) type; and (2) signet ring cell adenocarcinoma ex goblet cell carcinoid: and (3) poorly differentiated carcinoma ex GCC. The signet ring is far more aggressive than regular GCC, and the poorly differentiated variant has an extremely poor prognosis [7]. However, when to make a diagnosis of carcinoma ex GCC, rather than just GCC is problematic and very subjective unless it is overt. Especially when small foci of carcinoma are present in a tumor that is composed largely of usual variant GCC, the significance of the carcinoma component is unclear [9, 10]. In this section, we will illustrate the spectrum of histological changes, as well as highlight the common findings within these lesions.

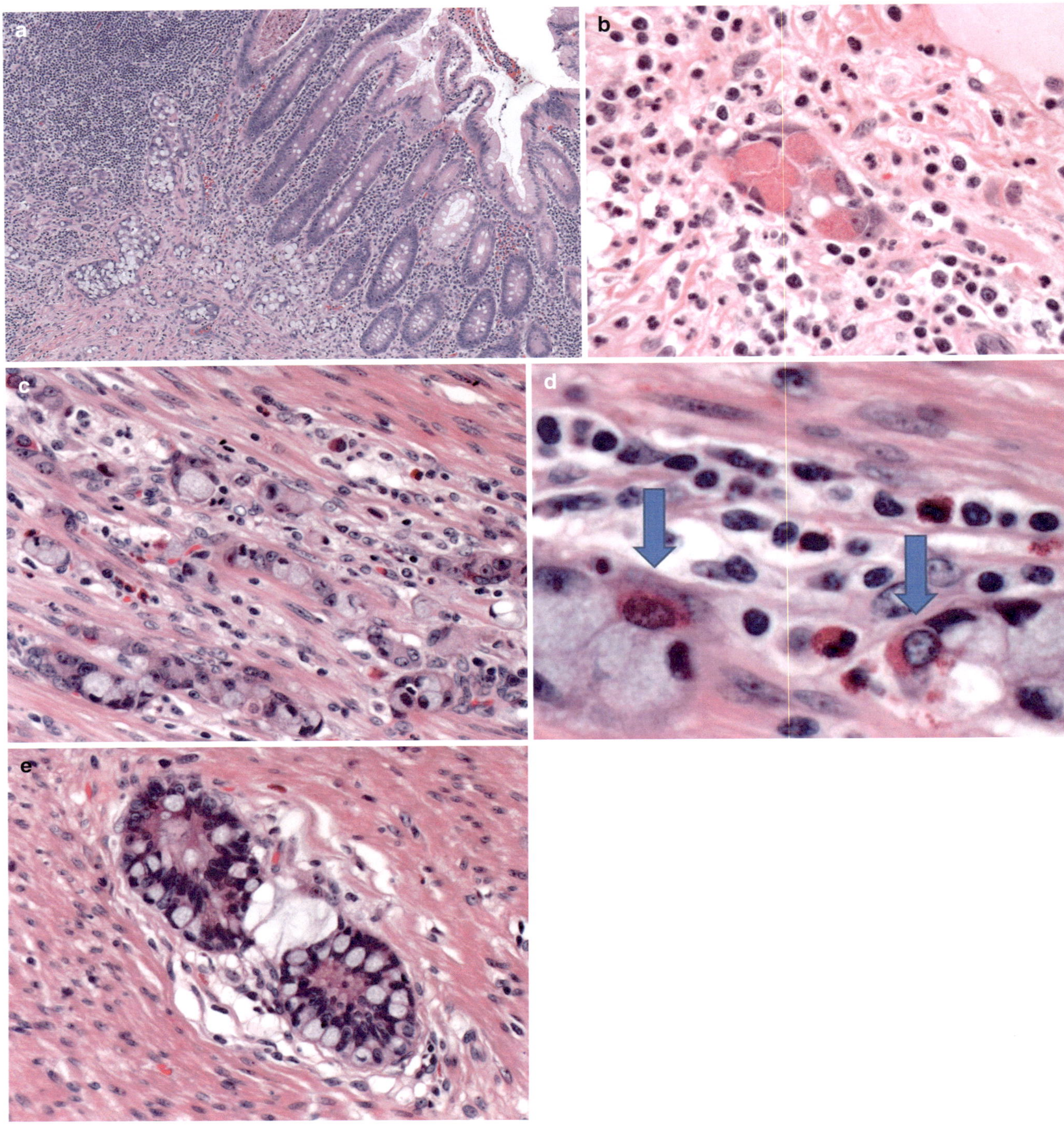

Fig. 4.39 (**a**), Goblet cell carcinoid (GCC). Appendiceal mucosa with aggregates of goblet cell carcinoid infiltrating the lamina propria. GCC frequently has areas of single cells when it involves the lamina propria. This is a common finding and should not be interpreted as a focus of poor differentiation or signet ring cell carcinoma. (**b**), Focus of Paneth cells. (**c**), Carcinoma ex GCC with focal enterochromaffin cell differentiation; detail in (**d**) in which the sub or perinuclear red granules can be seen. (**e**), Absorptive and goblet cells, many of which have lost their polarity (dystrophic goblet cells), and with a partial rim of dystrophic goblet cells reminiscent of gastric mucosa with in situ signet ring carcinoma seen in some patients with germline cdh-1 mutations

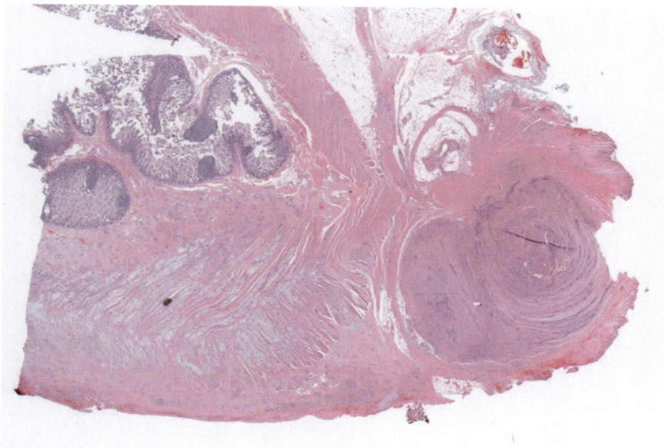

Fig. 4.40 Adenocarcinoma ex goblet cell carcinoid. An overview of appendix (right) and small bowel (left) which both contain infiltrating lesions within the wall. The appendix (at right) has loss of lumen and normal appendiceal musculature

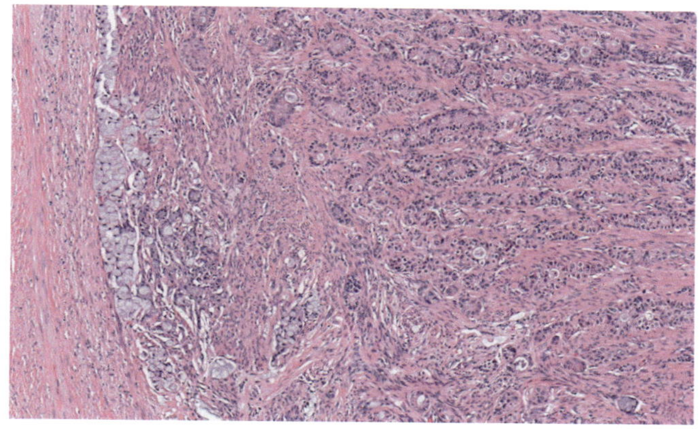

Fig. 4.41 Adenocarcinoma ex goblet cell carcinoid. Detailed view of the appendiceal wall with areas of typical goblet cell carcinoid at the right. At left, sheets of signet ring cells are starting to form. This is an example of adenocarcinoma ex goblet cell carcinoid–signet ring cell variant

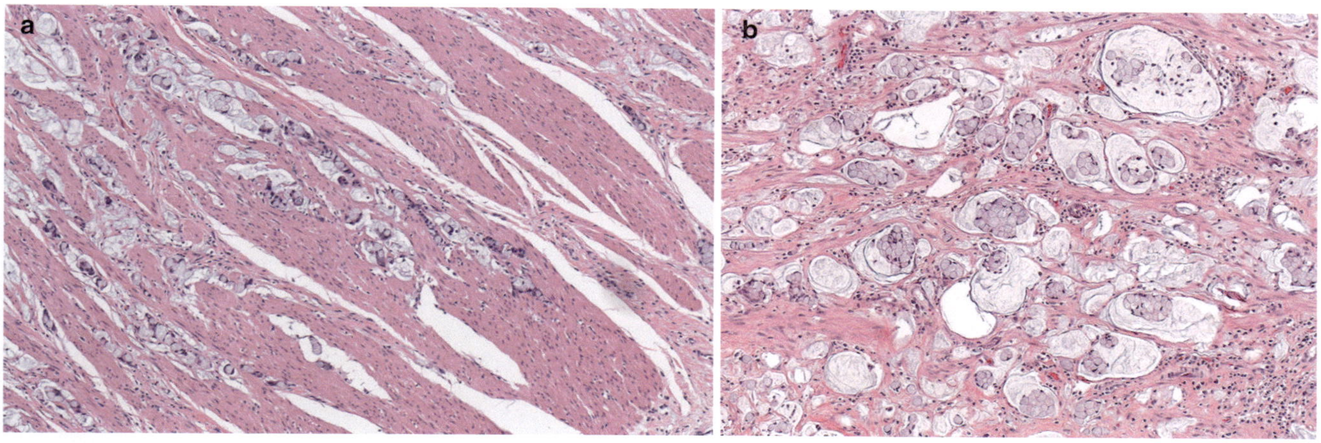

Fig. 4.42 Adenocarcinoma ex goblet cell carcinoid–signet ring variant. (**a**), Cords of signet ring cells with areas of cellular and acellular mucin within the small bowel muscularis propria. Often, the division between conventional goblet cell carcinoid and signet ring cell variants can be subjective, but features such as sheets of cells, abundant extracellular mucin, single cells, and nuclear size (increased in signet ring variant) may aid in making the distinction. (**b**), Signet ring carcinoma with pools of mucin, within which are clusters of signet ring cells

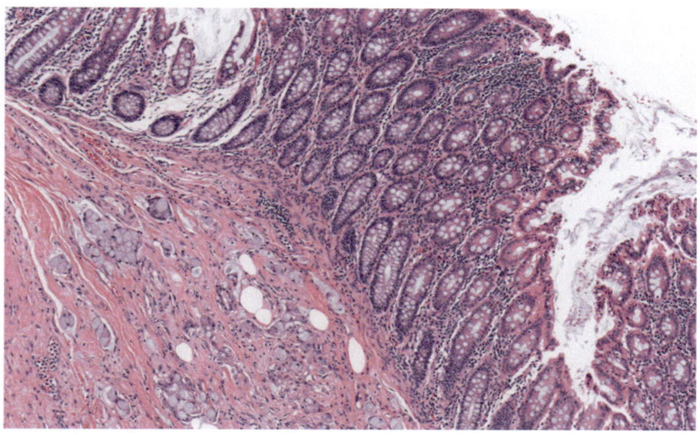

Fig. 4.43 Adenocarcinoma ex goblet cell carcinoid. A detailed view of large bowel (cecum) with foci of typical goblet cell carcinoid admixed with signet ring cell carcinoma, including larger sheets of cells and isolated single cells

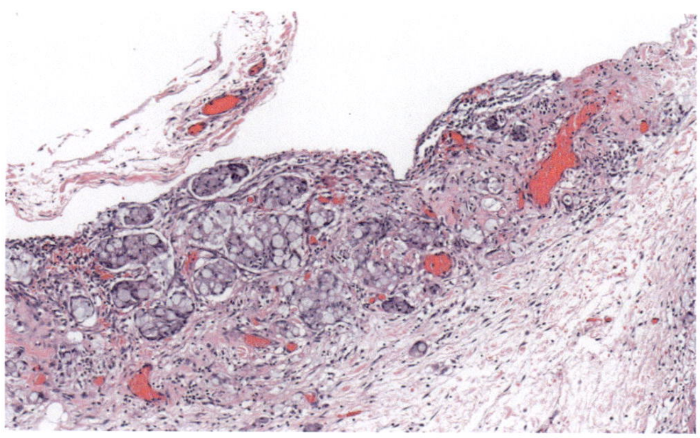

Fig. 4.44 Adenocarcinoma ex goblet cell carcinoid. Serosal involvement of the appendiceal wall. Death in goblet cell carcinoids (and variants) is invariably secondary to intraperitoneal spread, and not nodal or distant metastases. Involvement of the serosa therefore has significant prognostic implications

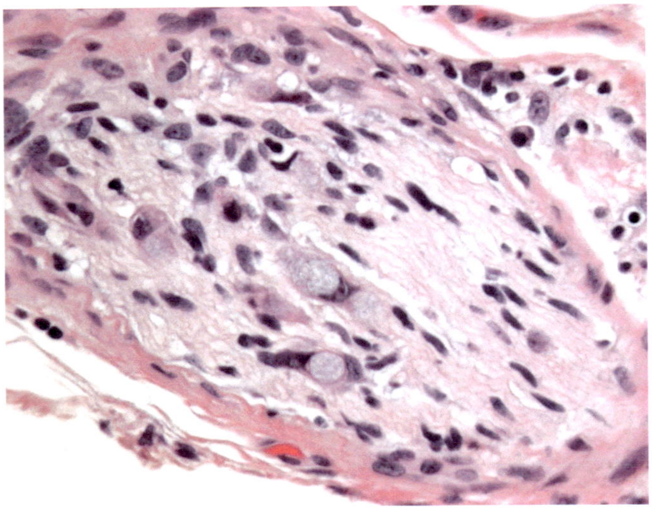

Fig. 4.45 Perineural invasion. Signet ring tumor cells within the nerve in mesoappendix. Involvement of nerves is a common finding in goblet cell carcinoid (and variants) and is often widespread involving nerves in the mesoappendix and soft tissue surrounding large or small bowel

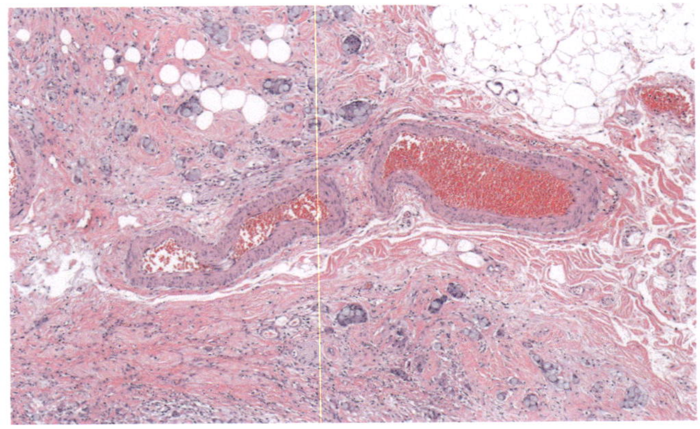

Fig. 4.46 Goblet cell carcinoid and signet ring adenocarcinoma infiltrating into the mesoappendix

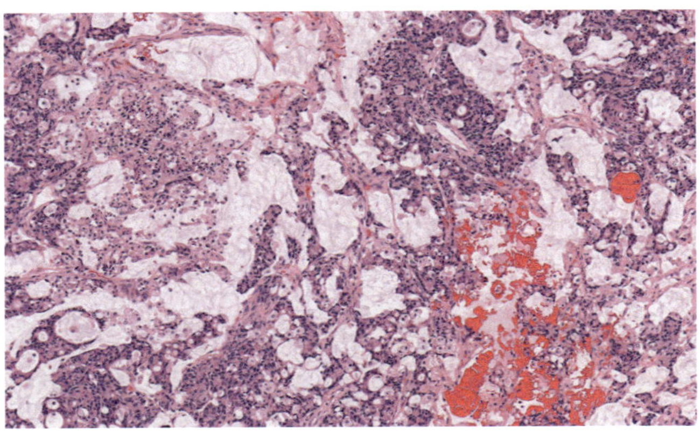

Fig. 4.47 Adenocarcinoma ex goblet cell carcinoid, poorly differentiated variant. This variant often presents with advanced disease and is aggressive, with a survival rate of 15% at 30 months

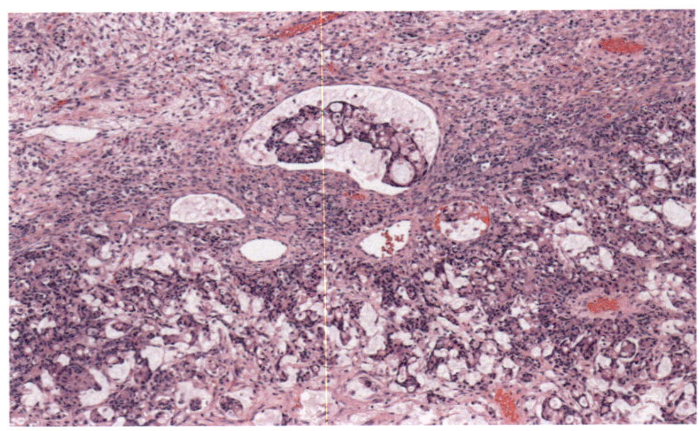

Fig. 4.48 The same tumor as in Fig. 4.47, with lymphovascular invasion. Lymphovascular invasion and lymph nodes metastases are a common finding in the poorly differentiated variant

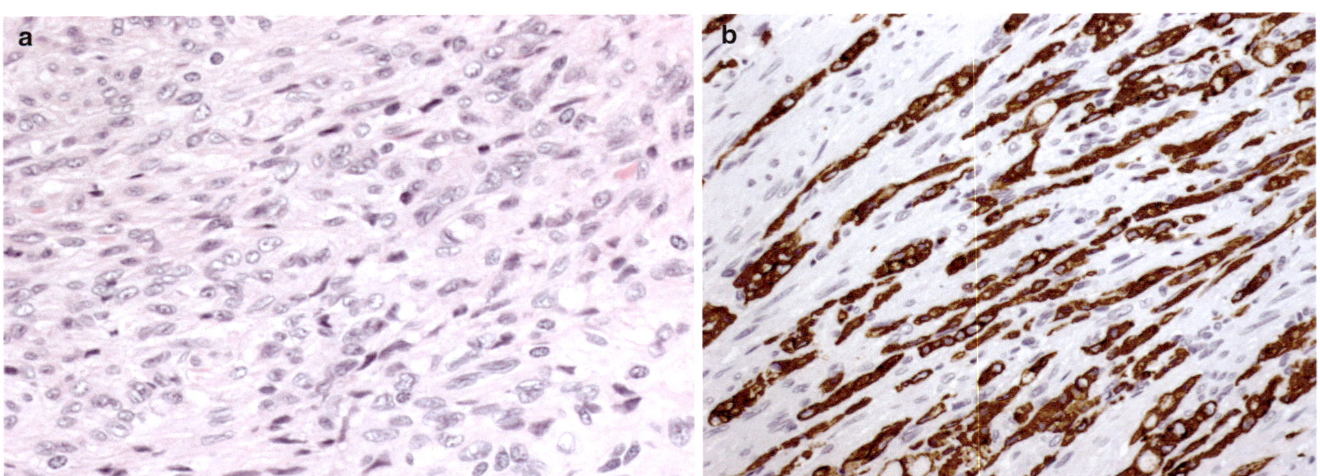

Fig. 4.49 Poorly differentiated carcinoma ex goblet cell carcinoid. (a), Tumor cells are difficult to discern from the desmoplastic stroma. (b), The cytokeratin stain showing an almost Indian file appearance of the infiltrating carcinoma

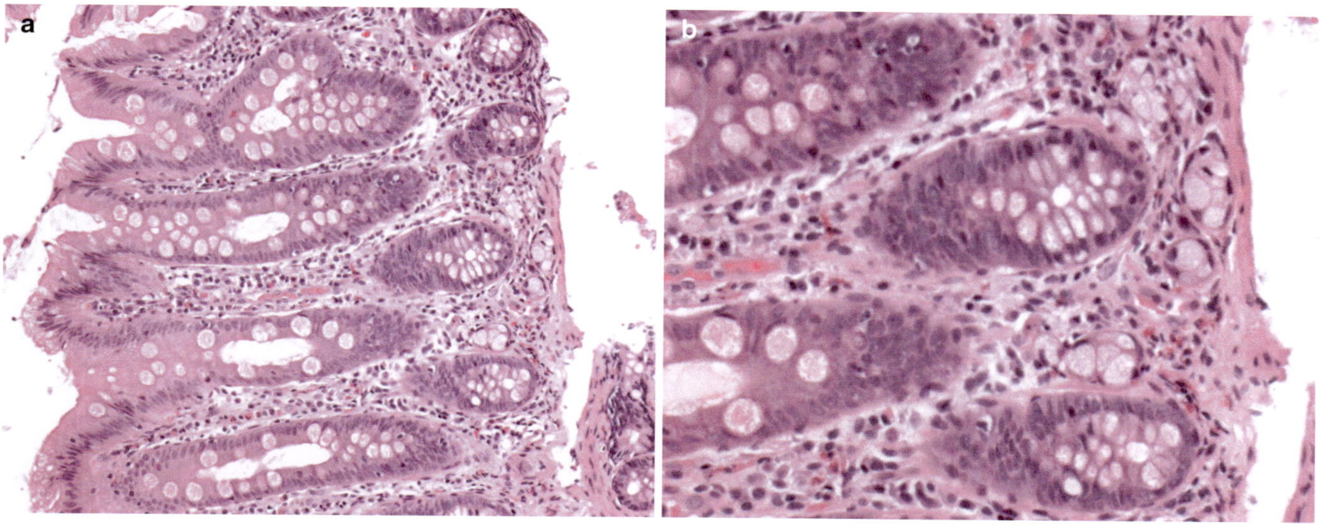

Fig. 4.50 (**a**, **b**). Local recurrence of GCC in a cecal biopsy

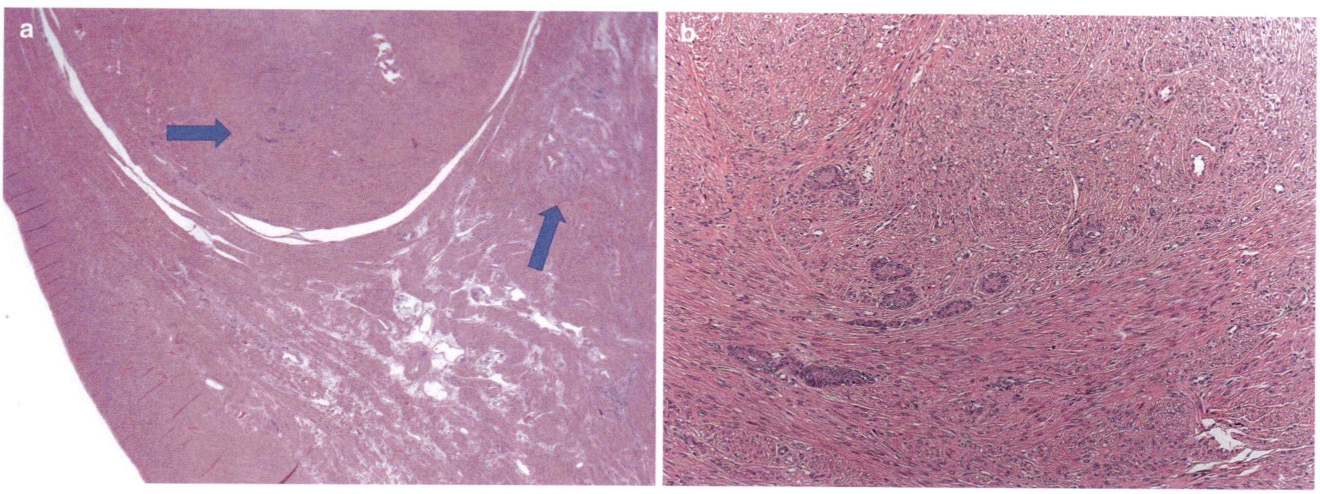

Fig. 4.51 (**a**), Endometrium with foci of GCC within the endometrium (bottom right) and within a leiomyoma (left arrow). (**b**), Detail of GCC within the leiomyoma

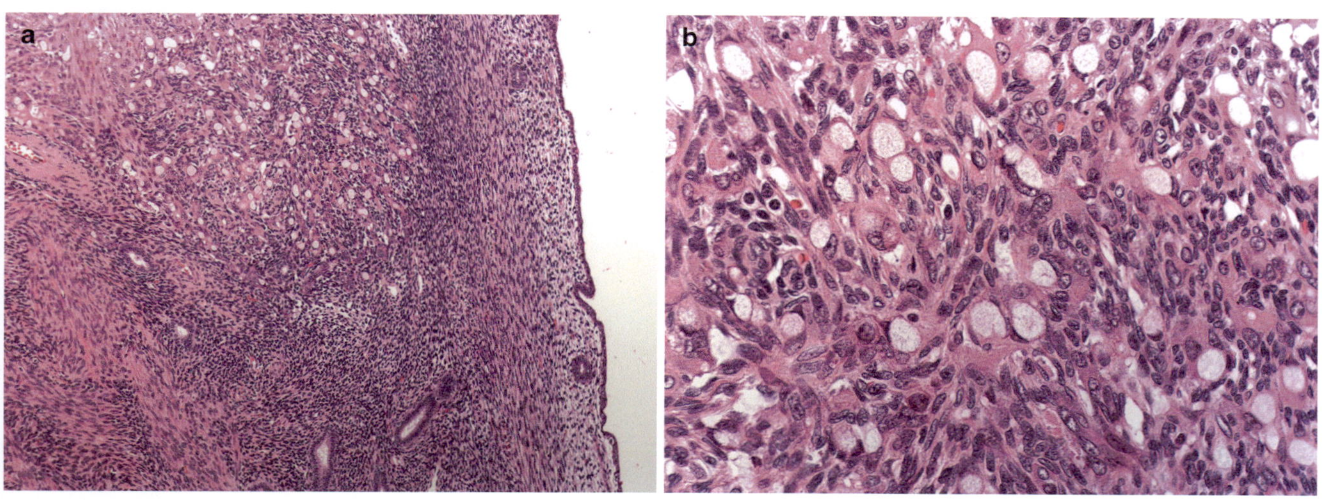

Fig. 4.52 (**a**), The same uterus as in Figs. 4.50 and 4.51, but with signet ring carcinoma infiltrating beneath an atrophic endometrium. (**b**), Detail of signet ring cells within the superficial myometrium

4.5 Other Primary Appendiceal Polyps

Other primary appendiceal polyps are rare and limited largely to appendiceal involvement in patients with polyposis syndromes, whether familial (adenomatous) polyposis syndrome, hamartomatous polyposis (juvenile/PTEN syndromes), or vanishingly rarely Peutz-Jeghers syndrome (Figs. 4.53, 4.54, 4.55, 4.56, and 4.57).

4.6 Other Diseases Involving the Appendix

Other diseases involving the appendix are relatively uncommon but include lesions usually associated with the peritoneum or female genital tract (Figs. 4.58, 4.59, 4.60, and 4.61). They can also include endosalpingiosis and Walthard's rests, reactive and malignant mesothelial proliferations,

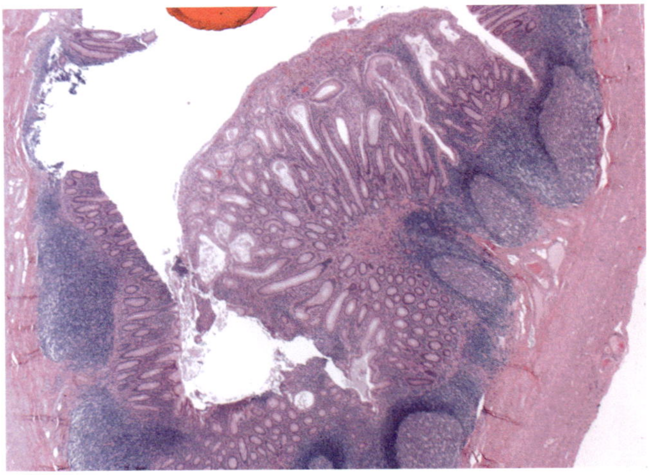

Fig. 4.53 Juvenile polyp of appendix. This polyp was present in an appendectomy specimen of a patient with juvenile polyposis syndrome. The changes are early with lymphoid follicles retained beneath, and minimal architectural distortion of the remaining appendix. The polyp consists of elongated crypts that superficially are becoming disorganized, with focal cystic dilatation and superficial erosion

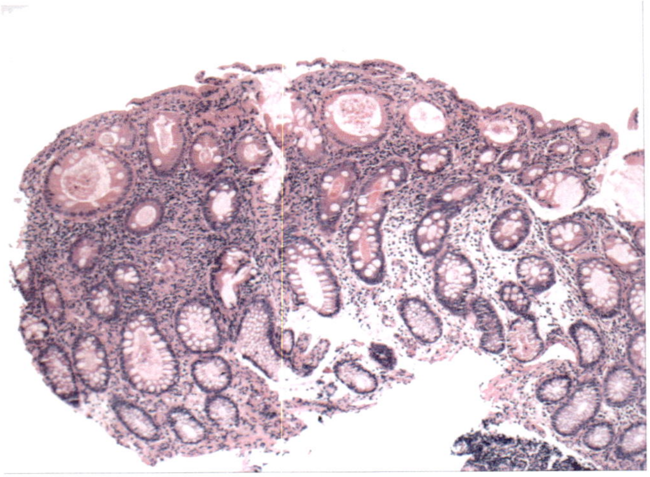

Fig. 4.55 Early appendiceal juvenile polyp. Superficial changes of a juvenile polyp are identified in this appendiceal mucosa with expansion of the lamina propria and cystic dilation of superficial glands. Note the relative preservation of the architecture

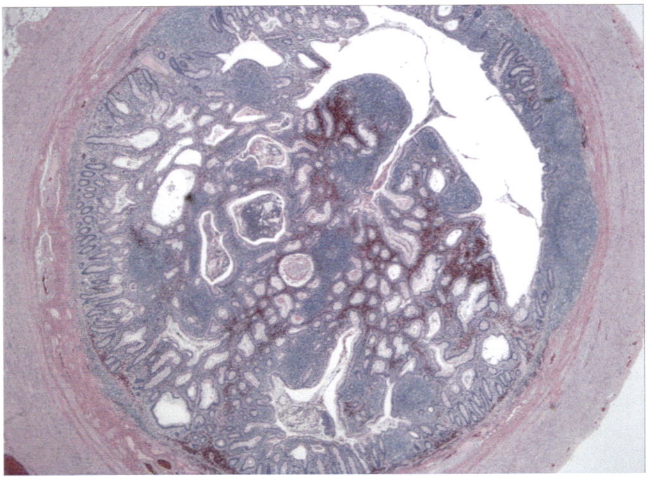

Fig. 4.54 Juvenile polyp. Cross-section of an appendix from a patient with juvenile polyposis syndrome. There is much greater architectural disarray in this polyp compared to the previous polyp

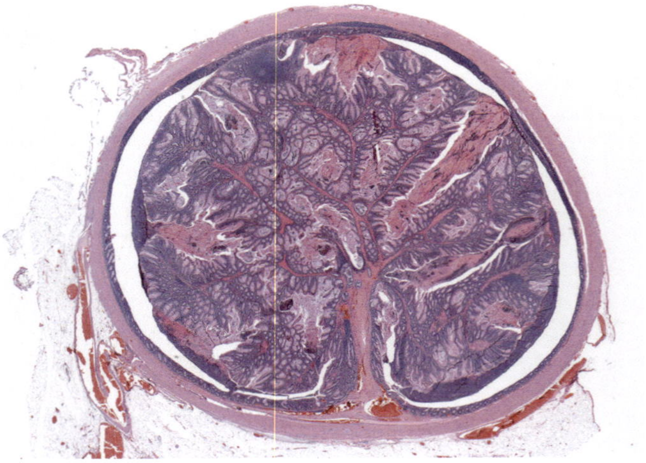

Fig. 4.56 Appendix with a spectacular Peutz-Jeghers polyp showing the characteristic arborizing strands of smooth muscle. (Courtesy Dr. Jolanta Jedrzkiewicz, Salt Lake City, Utah)

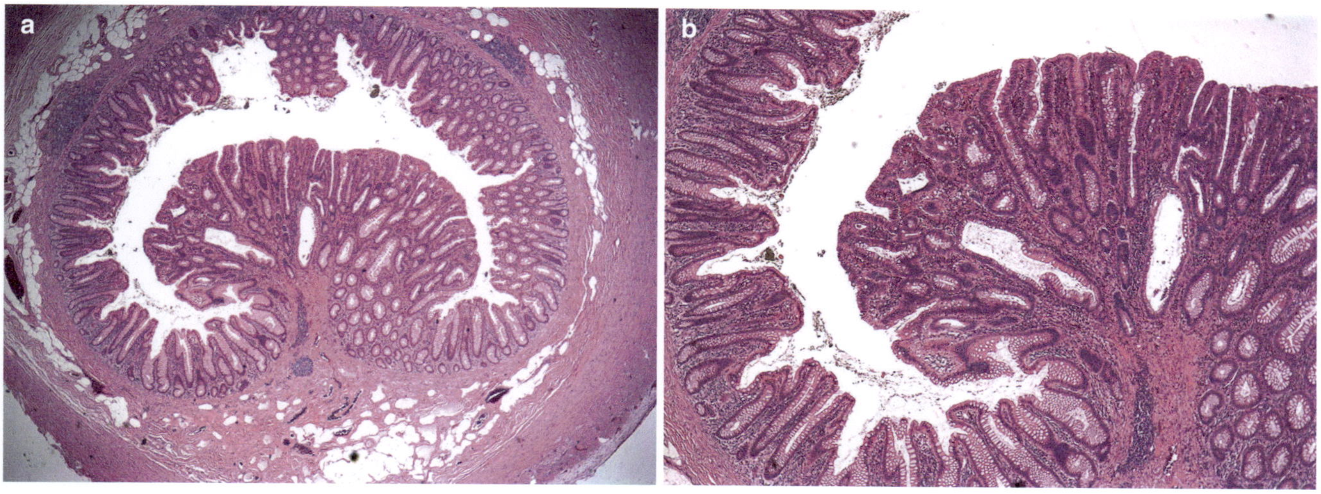

Fig. 4.57 (**a**, **b**), Tubular adenoma. This appendix from a patient with familial adenomatous polyposis (FAP) contains a polypoid tubular adenoma with characteristic polypoid shape and low-grade adenomatous dysplasia. Tubular adenomas are rare in the appendix but are sometimes seen as an incidental finding in the appendix of patients undergoing in colectomy for FAP

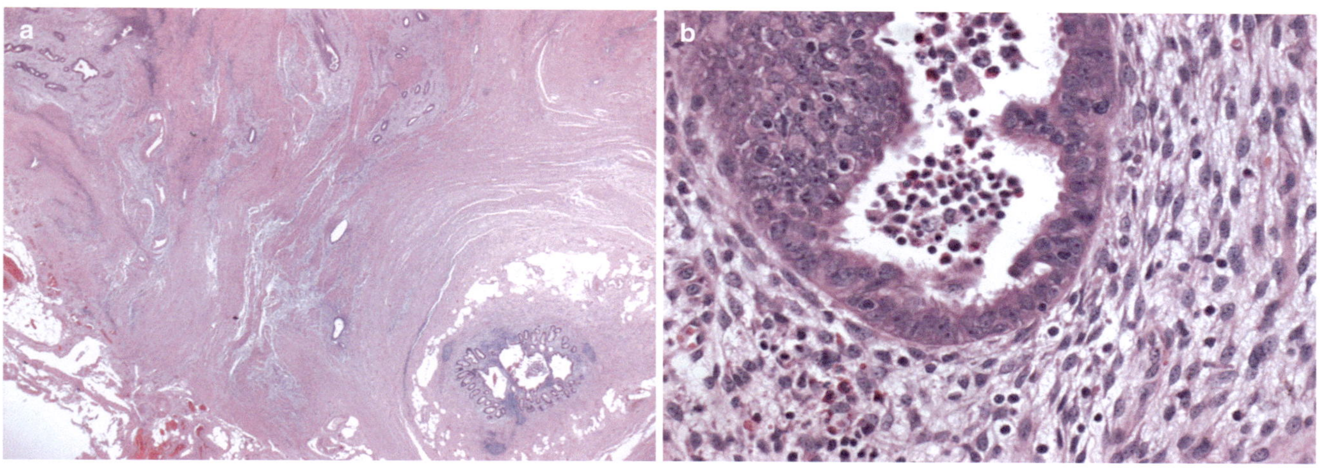

Fig. 4.58 Endometriosis involving the appendix. (**a**), The lumen is lower right and numerous glands surrounded by paler staining stroma can be seen coming in from the top left. (**b**), Detail showing classical gland and stroma

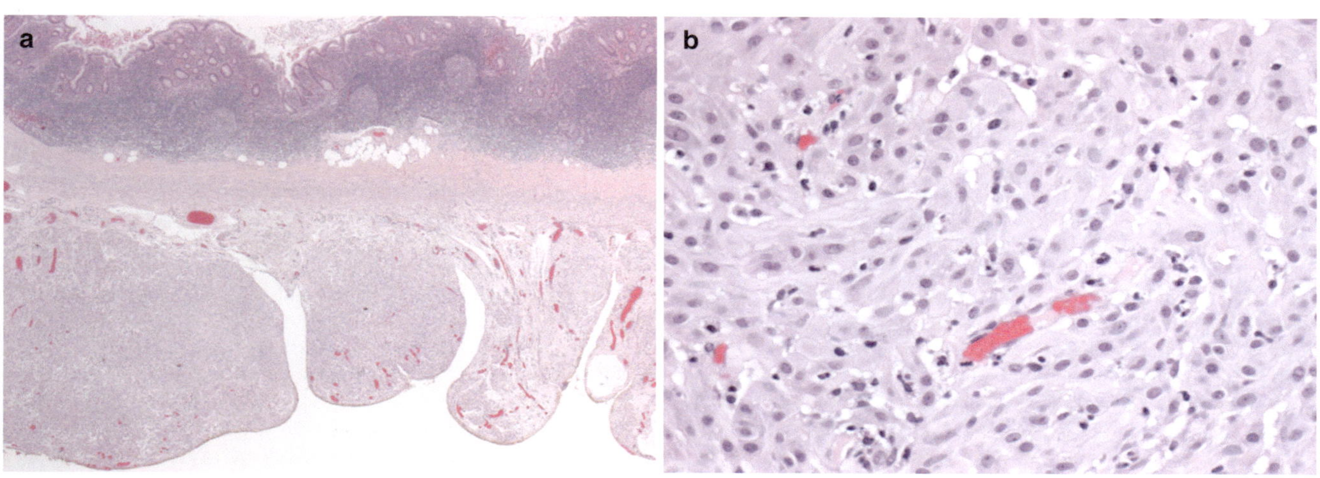

Fig. 4.59 Massive deciduosis of appendiceal serosa. (**a**), The appendix lumen is visible at the top. The subserosa is massively expanded by pale staining cells. (**b**), Detail shows typical decidual cells

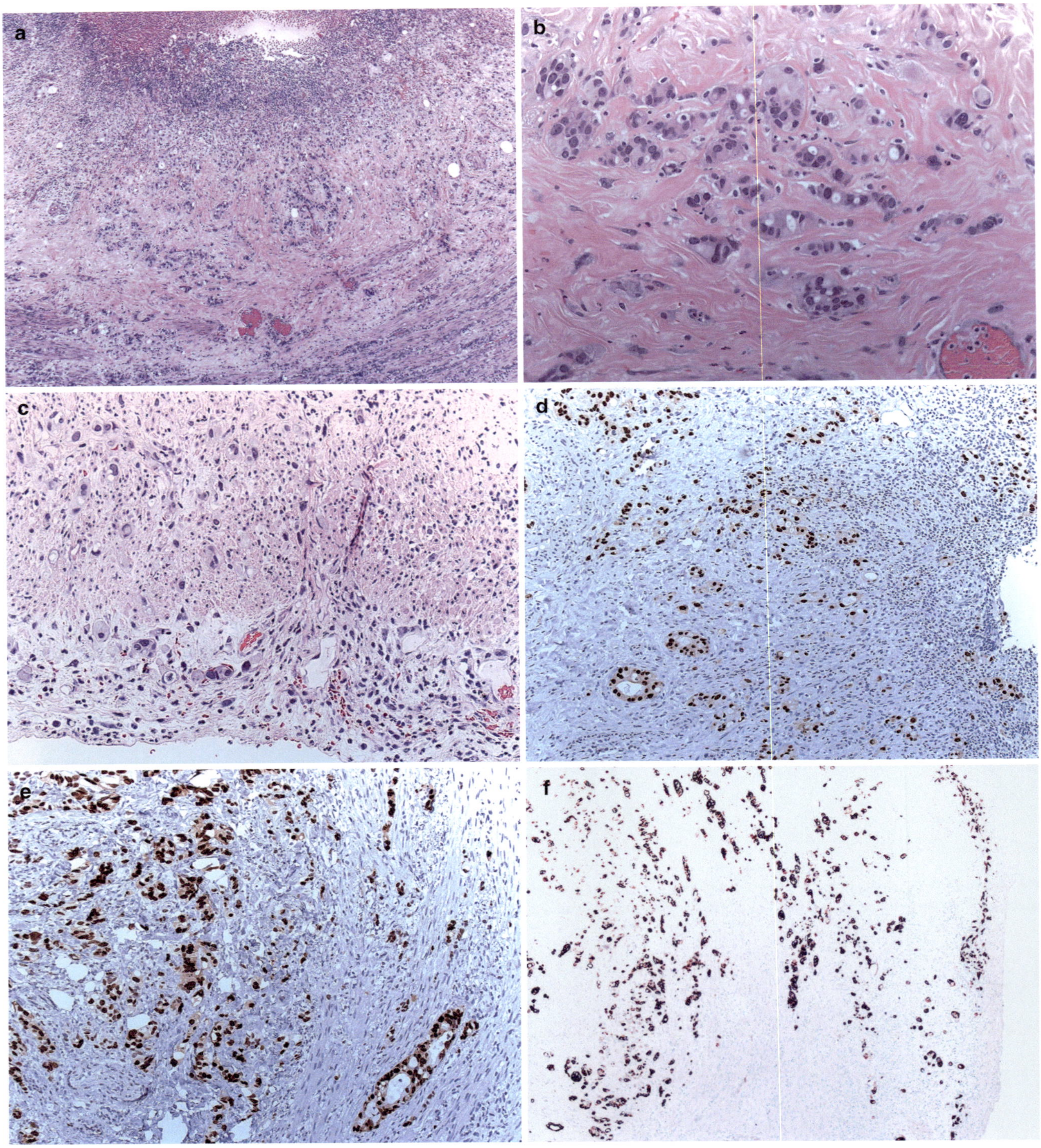

Fig. 4.60 Appendix with metastatic breast carcinoma. The patient had acute appendicitis, and this was initially referred in as a possible poorly differentiated variant of a goblet cell carcinoma, which is tenable given the pattern of distribution in (**a**), and the cell clusters with signet ring-like cells in (**b**). (**c**), The cells extending close to the serosa. (**d**), estrogen receptor (progestogen receptor had been lost since the patient's lumpectomy 4 years earlier). (**e**), GATA3 (BRST2 was similarly positive). (**f**), CK7 also showing both extension of cells to the serosa as well as the serosal mesothelial proliferation top right

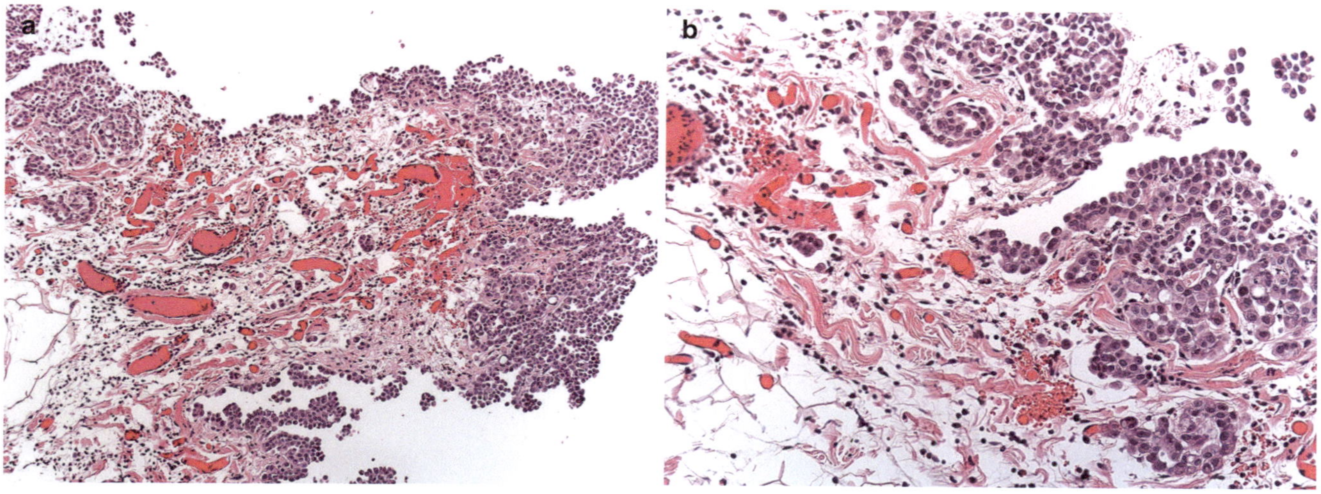

Fig. 4.61 Mesoappendix with involvement by an epithelioid mesothelioma that was widespread throughout the peritoneal cavity. (**a**), A papillary pattern is present with underlying tumor infiltrating down towards the fat. (**b**), Detail of top left of (**a**)

lesions and tumors associated with pregnancy (deciduosis) and gynecological diseases, but especially endometriosis. Secondary malignancies, usually carcinoma, can also invade the appendix. Sometimes this is a direct extension from contiguous organs, such as in cases of cecal carcinomas. The most common secondary tumors to involve the appendix are appendiceal involvement in other intra-abdominal malignancies, such as gastric or pancreatic carcinoma or gynecological malignancies. However, it can also be associated with disseminated malignancies, usually carcinomatosis from sites such as the breast.

References

1. Carr NJ, Bibeau F, Bradley RF, Dartigues P, Feakins RM, Geisinger KR, et al. The histopathological classification, diagnosis and differential diagnosis of mucinous appendiceal neoplasms, appendiceal adenocarcinomas and pseudomyxoma peritonei. Histopathology. 2017;71(6):847–58.
2. Umetsu SE, Shafizadeh N, Kakar S. Grading and staging mucinous neoplasms of the appendix: a case series and review of the literature. Hum Pathol. 2017;69:81–9.
3. Morano WF, Gleeson EM, Sullivan SH, Padmanaban V, Mapow BL, Shewokis PA, et al. Clinicopathological features and management of appendiceal mucoceles: a systematic review. Am Surg. 2018;84(2):273–81.
4. Misdraji J. Mucinous epithelial neoplasms of the appendix and pseudomyxoma peritonei. Mod Pathol. 2015;28(Suppl 1):S67–79.
5. Misdraji J, Yantiss RK, Graeme-Cook FM, Balis UJ, Young RH. Appendiceal mucinous neoplasms: a clinicopathologic analysis of 107 cases. Am J Surg Pathol. 2003;27(8):1089–103.
6. Yantiss RK, Shia J, Klimstra DS, Hahn HP, Odze RD, Misdraji J. Prognostic significance of localized extra-appendiceal mucin deposition in appendiceal mucinous neoplasms. Am J Surg Pathol. 2009;33(2):248–55.
7. Tang LH, Shia J, Soslow RA, Dhall D, Wong WD, O'Reilly E, et al. Pathologic classification and clinical behavior of the spectrum of goblet cell carcinoid tumors of the appendix. Am J Surg Pathol. 2008;32:1429–43.
8. Lee LH, McConnell YJ, Tsang E, Zerhouni S, Speers C, Kennecke H, et al. Simplified 2-tier histologic grading system accurately predicts outcomes in goblet cell carcinoid of the appendix. Hum Pathol. 2015;46(12):1881–9.
9. Maedler C, Arnason T, Dorreen A, Sapp H, Castonguay M, Murphy J, et al. Goblet cell carcinoid of the appendix. An interobserver variability study using two proposed classification systems. Ann Diagn Pathol. 2018;32:51–5.
10. Wang HL, Dhall D. Goblet or signet ring cells: that is the question. Adv Anat Pathol. 2009;16(4):247–54.

Neuroendocrine Tumors of the Gastrointestinal Tract

5

Hala El-Zimaity

The gut has been described as "the largest endocrine organ in the body" [1]. Intestinal endocrine cells are scattered in the mucosa between gut mucosal cells at the base of crypts, but they can be found higher in the crypt. The enterochromaffin (EC) cells, the prototype for this cell, are the largest endocrine cell population in the gastrointestinal (GI) tract and are characterized by fine red basal (subnuclear) granules. These cells were called EC cells because of their ability to bind chromium salts [1]; they also were called argentaffin cells [1] because of their capacity to bind and reduce silver ions [1]. The endocrine population of the large bowel is generally less diverse than that of the small intestine (Table 5.1). The EC cells are the most frequent endocrine cell subtype in the colon and rectum. Other cells, such as L-cells, occur from the duodenum to the rectum but are rarely found proximal to the terminal ileum. They secrete glucagon-like peptide 1 (GLP-1) that stimulates insulin and suppresses glucagon secretion, inhibits gastric emptying, and reduces appetite and food intake. Within the large bowel, their frequency increases from proximal to distal, being most concentrated in the rectum (a frequent site of large bowel L-cell neuroendocrine tumors [NETs]) [2]. Understanding the normal distribution of endocrine cells is helpful because it correlates with the preferred primary sites of specific NETs with some exceptions [3].

NETs are defined as epithelial neoplasms with a predominant neuroendocrine differentiation. Intestinal endocrine cells can be highlighted by neuroendocrine markers, which include synaptophysin, chromogranin A, CD56/NCAM1, protein gene product 9.5 (PGP9.5), and neuron-specific enolase. In clinical practice, only synaptophysin and chromogranin A and occasionally CD56 (which is more capricious) are used. Although the histologic features of these tumors depend on the site and cell of origin, many characteristics are shared regardless of site. Following the World Health Organization (WHO), NETs are classified as Grade 1 (G1-NET), G2-NET, neuroendocrine carcinoma (G3-NEC) large- or small-cell type, and mixed adenoneuroendocrine carcinoma (MANEC) (Table 5.2) [1]. Broadly, NETs fall into two main categories — well differentiated, Grade 1-G1 and Grade 2-G2 — while G3-NETs are included with carcinomas (NECs), along with large- and small-cell ("poorly differentiated") endocrine carcinomas, which behave aggressively, as in other organs. Grading is based on the mitotic

Table 5.1 The distribution of neuroendocrine cells in the gastrointestinal tract [52–54]

Distribution	Cell type	Hormone produced	Related NETs/syndromes
Small intestine	EC	Serotonin	EC-cell carcinoid (typical syndrome)
	L	Glucagon-like peptide 1, peptide YY	
	I	Cholecystokinin	There are no cholecystokinin-, gastric inhibitory polypeptide-, or motilin-producing tumors in the small intestine
	K	Gastric inhibitory peptide	
	M	Motilin	
	N	Neurotensin	
	PD1	Ghrelin	
Duodenum	G	Gastrin	Gastrinoma (ZES)
	δ (D)	Somatostatin	Somatostatinoma
Appendix	δ (D)	Somatostatin	Somatostatinoma
	EC	Serotonin	EC-cell carcinoid (typical syndrome)
	P/D1	Ghrelin	
Colorectum	δ (D)	Somatostatin	Somatostatinoma
	EC	Serotonin	EC-cell carcinoid (typical syndrome)
	P/D1	Ghrelin	
Rectum	L	Glucagon-like peptide 1, peptide YY	

EC enterochromaffin, *ZES* Zollinger–Ellison syndrome

H. H. Li-Chang et al., *Atlas of Intestinal Pathology*, Atlas of Anatomic Pathology,
https://doi.org/10.1007/978-3-030-12379-6_5

Table 5.2 World Health Organization 2010 classification of neuroendocrine tumors in the gastrointestinal tract

Grade	Mitotic count/10 HPFs	Ki-67 Labeling Index, %
NET, grade 1	<2	<3
NET, grade 2	2–20	3–20
NEC, grade 3	>20	>20

HPFs high-power fields, *NET* neuroendocrine tumor, *NEC* neuroendocrine carcinoma

count and proliferation rate (Table 5.2). Briefly, G1 tumors have a mitotic count of less than 2 per 10 high-power fields (HPFs) and/or less than 2% proliferation (ki27/Mib1) index. G2 tumors have a mitotic count of between 2 and 20 per 10 HPFs and/or 3 and 20% proliferation index. Last, G3 tumors have a mitotic count more than 20 per 10 HPFs and/or more than a 20% proliferative index [1].

Poorly differentiated NECs are often associated with a rapid clinical course, while well-differentiated NETs generally are indolent and have a much better prognosis; their overall five-year survival is approximately 67%. Occasionally, G3-NECs are ulcerated masses, as in conventional carcinomas. NET grade is highly dependent on the primary site. High-grade NETs/NECs) are more likely to arise from the rectum and the ampulla of Vater than from the appendix and small bowel [1]. Large- and small-cell NECs are frequently associated with and arise from conventional carcinomas and sometimes adenomas. The stomach and rarely the duodenum and the bowel in inflammatory bowel disease are the only organs in which there may be a hyperplasia/neoplasia sequence.

The most common locations of NETs in the GI tract are said to be the small intestine (38%), the rectum (34%), followed by the colon (16%), stomach (11%), and unknown sites (1%) [3]. However, since the implementation of screening colonoscopy, the proportion of rectal NETs has been higher than that of small intestinal NETs [4]. That distribution differs in Asian countries, where the rectum (48%) is the most frequent location, followed by the stomach (15%), colon (8%), small intestine (8%), and appendix (3%) [5]. This chapter covers the most frequently encountered NETs in the GI tract.

5.1 Well-Differentiated Endocrine Tumors

Well-differentiated NETs (G1 and G2, still often referred to as "carcinoid") have fairly uniform nuclei, coarsely stippled ("salt and pepper") chromatin, and finely granular cytoplasm. The tumor nests are arranged in trabecular, insular, or sheet-like patterns [1]. As the main lesions of G1- and G2-NETs are deep in the mucosa and submucosa, the overlying mucosa is generally intact or may show an erosion and occasionally an ulceration (Figs. 5.1 and 5.2).

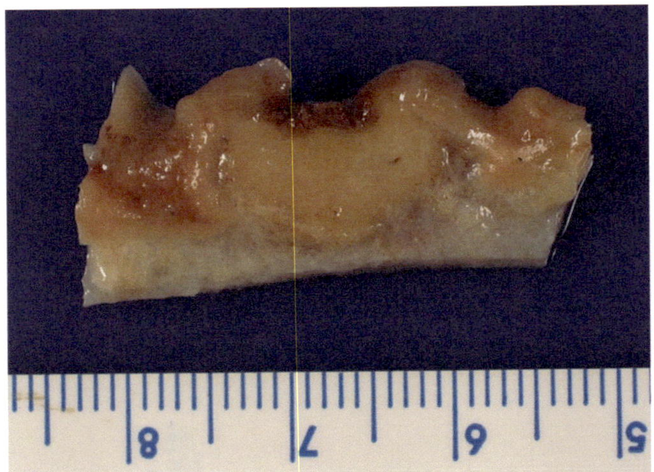

Fig. 5.1 Well-differentiated NETs are well-circumscribed tumors with a homogeneous cut surface

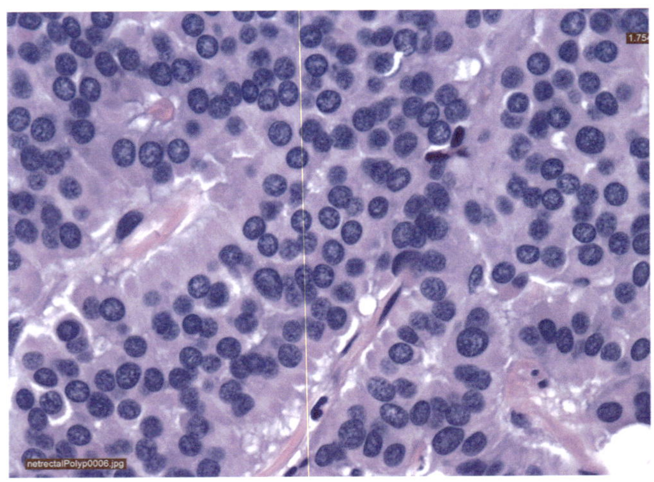

Fig. 5.2 The nuclei in well-differentiated NETs are relatively uniform and round. The nuclear chromatin is finely granular, with a salt and pepper appearance

5.2 Duodenum

Duodenal neuroendocrine tumors are uncommon [2, 3] but are sometimes biopsied at endoscopy when a duodenal nodule is encountered incidentally. Rarely, they are sought when Zollinger-Ellison syndrome is suspected. Some are functional, such as gastrin-producing "gastrinomas" and/somatostatin-producing "somatostatinomas," although signs and symptoms of the latter (diabetes, cholecystolithiasis, steatorrhea, hypochlorhydria [4]) may not be detected. Many duodenal NETs contain multiple substances, but most of these are nonfunctional. Gastrin-producing NETs are the most common duodenal NETs, followed by somatostatin-producing NETs and gangliocytic paragangliomas.

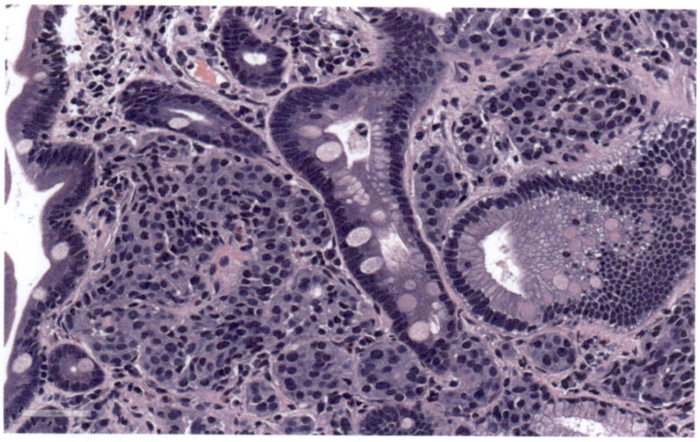

Fig. 5.3 Gastrin-producing endocrine tumor in the proximal duodenum, where the neoplastic cells infiltrate the mucosa as small nests and cords. The tumor cells have abundant eosinophilic cytoplasm with bland nuclei and rare, if any, mitotic figures

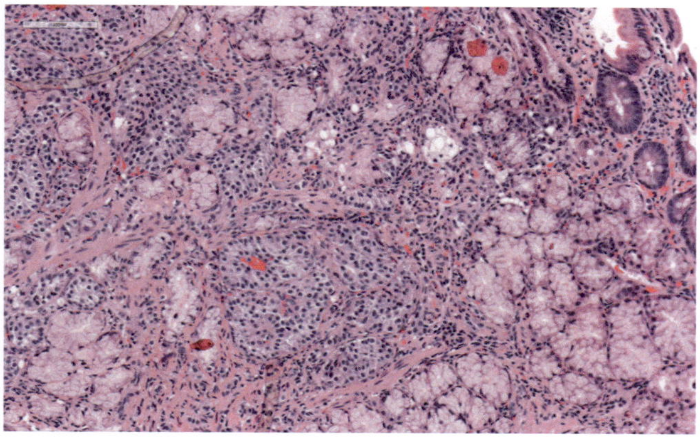

Fig. 5.4 Gastrin-producing endocrine tumor between Brunner glands. In contrast to the clear cytoplasm and basally located nuclei in Brunner glands, the tumor cells have eosinophilic cytoplasm and bland nuclei with smooth or stippled chromatin

5.2.1 Gastrin-Producing NETs

Duodenal gastrinomas occur sporadically or in association with multiple endocrine neoplasia, type 1 (MEN1) [2]. In MEN1, duodenal NETs including gastrinomas are often multiple and are associated with G-cell hyperplasia that is less common in sporadic gastrinomas. Gastrinomas associated with Zollinger-Ellison syndrome are frequently metastatic and are usually deeply infiltrating tumors with unfavorable clinical outcomes [2]. Case reports of G-cell hyperplasia with small NETs have been associated with long-term proton pump inhibitor (PPI) use and gastric *Helicobacter* [3]. It is interesting that gastric antral gastrinomas are vanishingly rare, whereas gastric antral G-cell hyperplasia is regularly seen in association with long-term PPI ingestion (Figs. 5.3, 5.4, and 5.5).

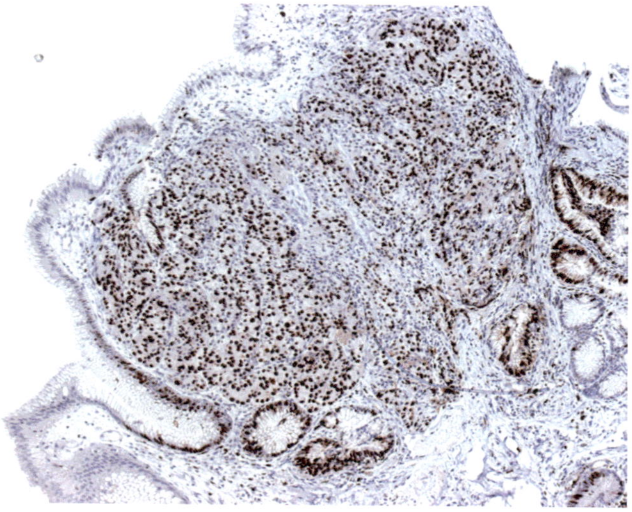

Fig. 5.5 Gastrin immunohistochemical stain highlights gastrin-producing tumor cell and G-cell hyperplasia

5.2.2 Somatostatin-Producing NETs

Somatostatin-producing NETs are usually found in the periampullary region [4]. Tumor cells frequently show a pseudo-glandular pattern in a solid or trabecular background of reasonably large cells with abundant granular eosinophilic cytoplasm [4, 5]. Psammoma bodies are occasionally present [4] but are more frequent in neurofibromatosis type 1 (NF1)-associated duodenal tumors (present in 60% of sporadic tumors versus all of NF1-associated tumors) [4]. In the duodenum, somatostatin-producing NETs have been reported in both MEN1 and NF1 [4]. In MEN1-associated somatostatin-producing NETs, somatostatin cell hyperplasia of the non-neoplastic mucosa is also seen [4]. Although the proliferative index is usually low, microinvasion (especially lymphatic invasion) and local lymph node metastases are frequently seen [6]. Although these show immunoreactivity for somatostatin, the somatostatin syndrome does not usually develop (Figs. 5.6, 5.7, 5.8, 5.9, 5.10, and 5.11) [4].

5.2.3 Gangliocytic Paraganglioma

Gangliocytic paragangliomas are rare tumors that occur predominantly in the second portion of the duodenum and ampulla. These tumors have a unique triphasic cellular component composed of an admixture of epithelioid endocrine (paraganglioid) cells, Schwann-like cells, and ganglion cells. The epithelial endocrine cells have an eosinophilic cytoplasm with ovoid nuclei arranged in a pseudoglandular pattern or in solid nests, often with psammomatous calcification, mimicking somatostatinoma.

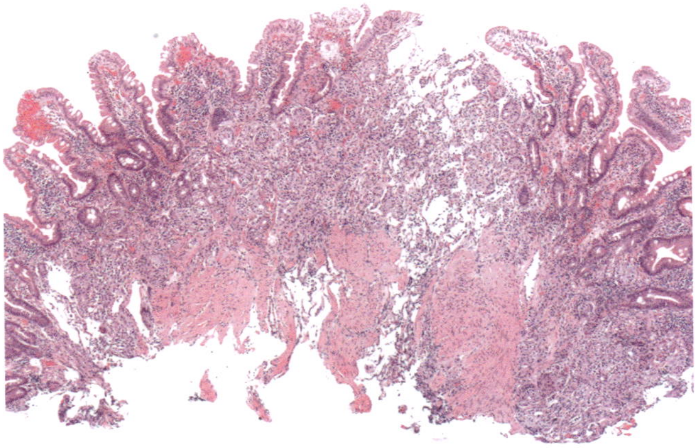

Fig. 5.6 A duodenal somatostatin-producing endocrine tumor. Tumor cells may be obscured by inflammation usually present in the mucosa

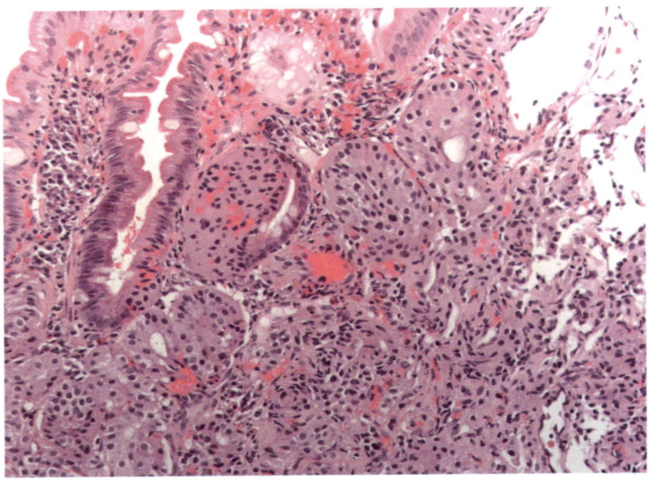

Fig. 5.7 Duodenal somatostatin-producing endocrine tumor. Tumor cells infiltrate the mucosa as small nests and cords. Tubular and glandular architectural patterns predominates

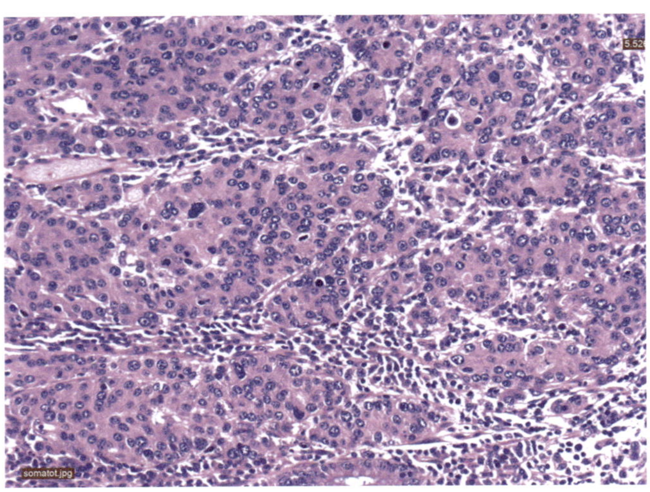

Fig. 5.8 High magnification of a duodenal somatostatin-producing tumor. Tumor cells have cytologic features typical of endocrine cells with slightly granular pale eosinophilic cytoplasm and monotonous nuclei with inconspicuous nucleoli

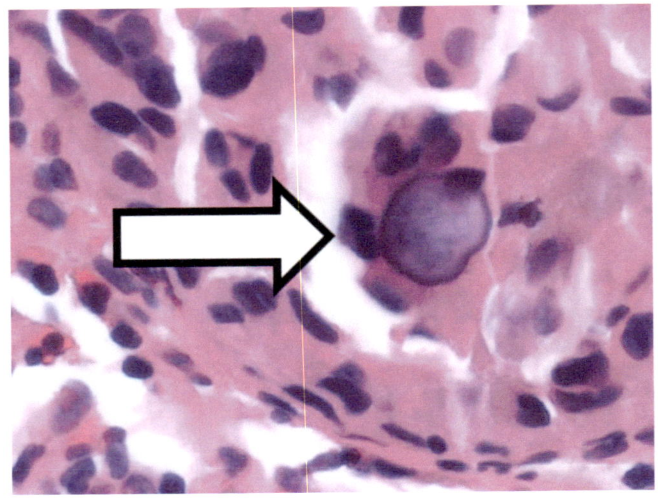

Fig. 5.9 High-power view of a psammoma body (*arrow*) present in approximately half of cases. (*Courtesy of* Dr. Olga Moshkin.)

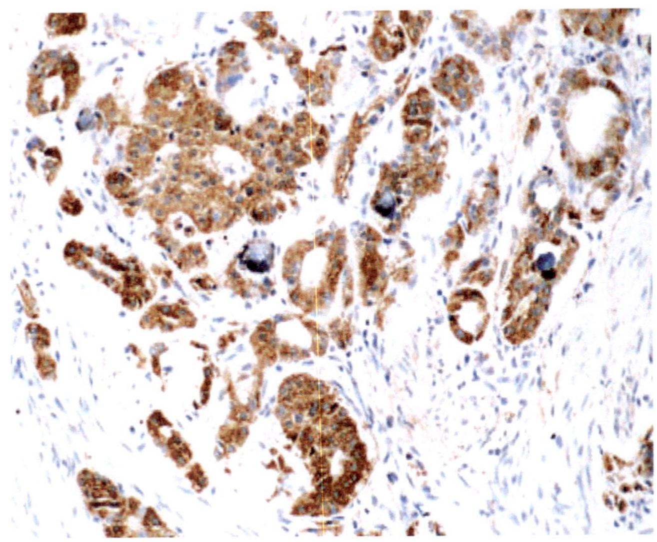

Fig. 5.10 Somatostatin stain is diffusely positive. Notice the psammoma bodies

These cells stain positive with pancreatic polypeptide and somatostatin. The Schwann-like cells stain positive for S100 protein, and the ganglion cells stain positive for synaptophysin [7, 8]. Most gangliocytic paragangliomas are confined to the mucosa and submucosa [9]. While most cases are benign, some cases with nodal metastases have been reported [10, 11]. These need to be differentiated from somatostatinomas and other nonfunctional neuroendocrine tumors of the duodenum with more aggressive behavior (Fig. 5.12).

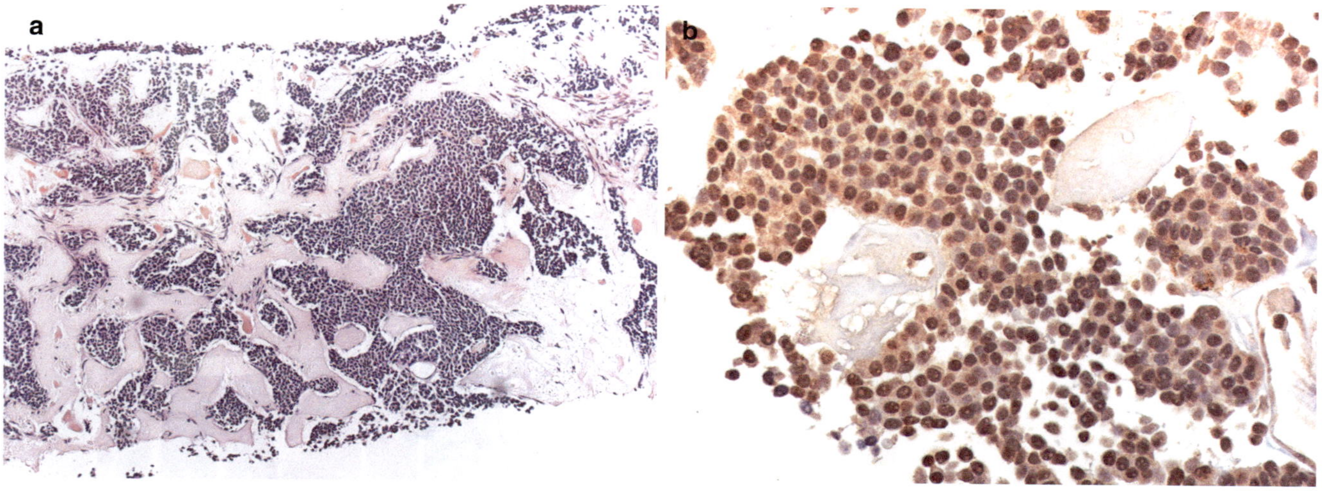

Fig. 5.11 Duodenal somatostatinoma, metastatic to the liver. (**a**) H&E. (**b**) Somatostain stain

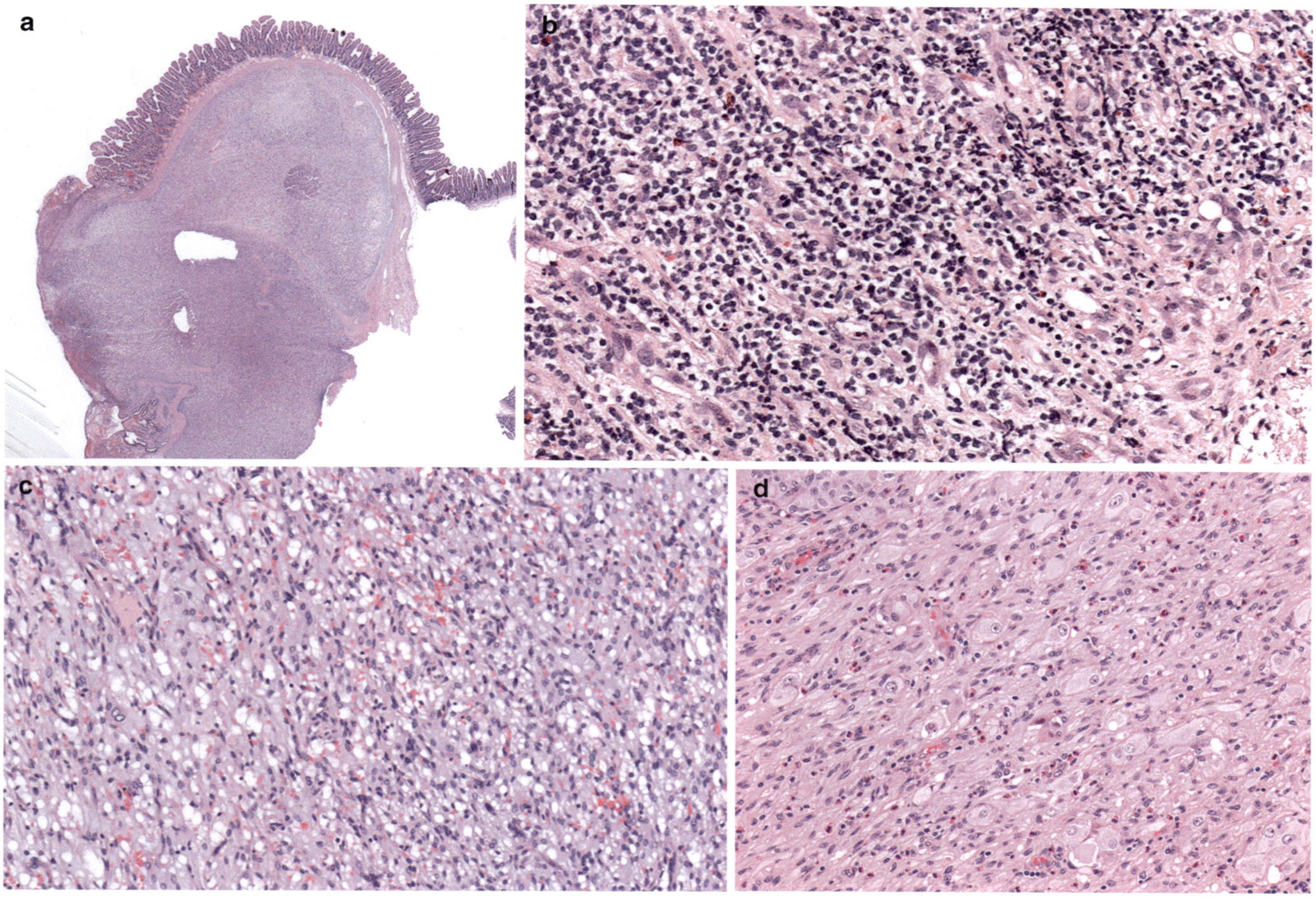

Fig. 5.12 (**a**) Low-power H&E image of a gangliocytic paraganglioma. The lesion is in the submucosa. Note the muscularis mucosae. High-magnification image shows the epithelioid component (appears similar to a well-differentiated neuroendocrine tumor) (**b**) as well as the other components (gangliocytic and schwannian) (**c**). This image shows mature ganglion cells, interspersed singly and in clusters within Schwannian stroma (**d**). The epithelioid endocrine tumor cells and the ganglion cells are positive with synaptophysin (**e**). S100 protein highlights Schwannian differentiation (**f**)

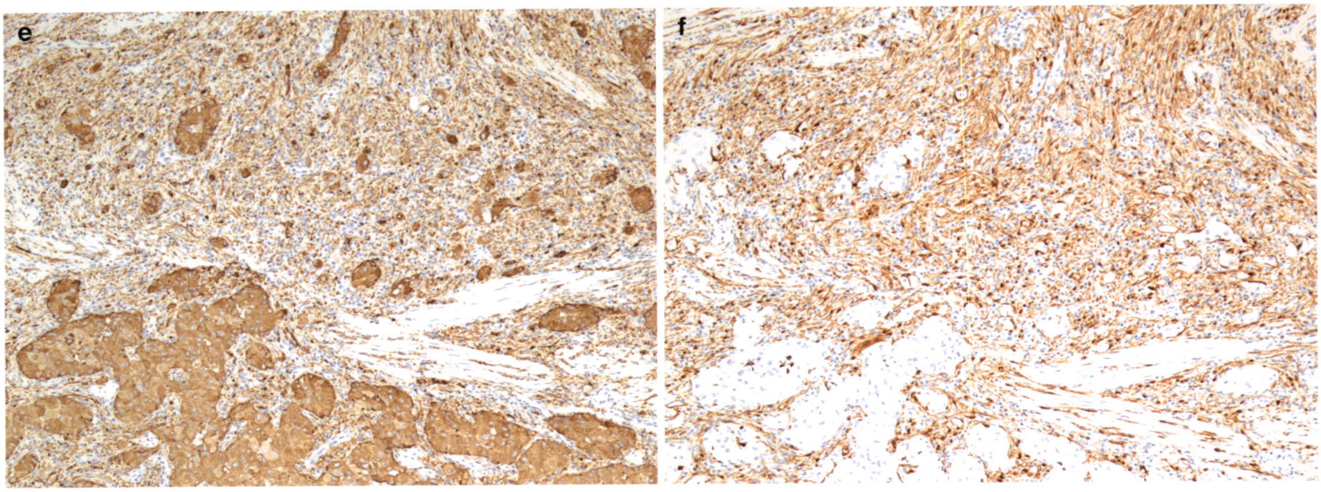

Fig. 5.12 (continued)

5.3 Jejunal and Terminal Ileum NETs

Small-bowel NETs have increased in frequency in the last decade, in part because of increased detection [12]. Interestingly, as the proportion of NETs has increased, the proportion of adenocarcinomas has decreased [13]. Little is known about jejunal NETs, since they are rare [14, 15] but mimic their ileal counterparts.

Endocrine tumors of the small intestine are mainly EC-cell, serotonin-producing NETs, and rarely L-cell, glucagon-like peptide and PP (pancreatic polypeptide)/PYY (pancreatic polypeptide PYY)-producing tumors [2].

Ileal NETs are EC-cell and mostly serotonin-producing, with a predominantly insular growth pattern forming small nests in the lamina propria with no intraepithelial component. The cells at the periphery of the nests are often palisaded with fine basal subnuclear red granules, while the cells deeper in the nests have less obvious granules [16]. These granules are readily appreciated in both primary tumors and metastases and are immunoreactive to serotonin antibodies, by far the best way of determining the small-bowel origin of tumors presenting with metastatic disease. The bulk of the tumor is typically in the submucosa, even with tumors with transmural invasion into the mesentery [16]. However, satellite tumors are common, and these tend to be mainly mucosal with focal submucosal invasion. They are invariably associated with lymphovascular channel permeation. Artifactual retraction spaces are commonly found between the nests and the thick collagen bundles mimicking lymphovascular spread. Tumors readily spread into the mesentery and also to the serosa, and once present peritoneal deposits can occur. Tumor deposits are associated with a more aggressive course.

These tumors can promote dense collagenous desmoplasia with fibrosis that stiffens the bowel, causing obstruction. A small subset causes peri- and intravascular elastosis in the mesenteric arterioles in particular, also known as mesenteric angiopathy; this can lead to ischemic necrosis and ulcers [17]. Polyps in the same segment as the tumor have been described as akin to prolapsed mucosa and others as consisting of granulation tissue [18, 19].

These tumors can present with metastases. Regional lymph nodes are the most common metastatic site, followed by the liver. Once metastatic to the liver, their active products can reach the systemic circulation, causing carcinoid syndrome [16]. The metastatic potential only partially correlates with proliferative indices or the mitotic count, and size is also important. Tumors of 1 cm or more are correlated with distant and nodal metastases [20, 21]. However, tumors less than 2 mm can metastasize; indeed, despite their slow clinical growth, these tumors can metastasize to nodes early. In general, the liver is the most common site of metastasis, and the small intestine is the most common source of NET metastases. The risk of metastasis is highest if the primary tumor was in the small intestine and lower with appendiceal and rectal NETs [22]. Multifocality is an issue with terminal ileum NETs and occurs in one third of cases (Figs. 5.13 and 5.14) [20, 23–25].

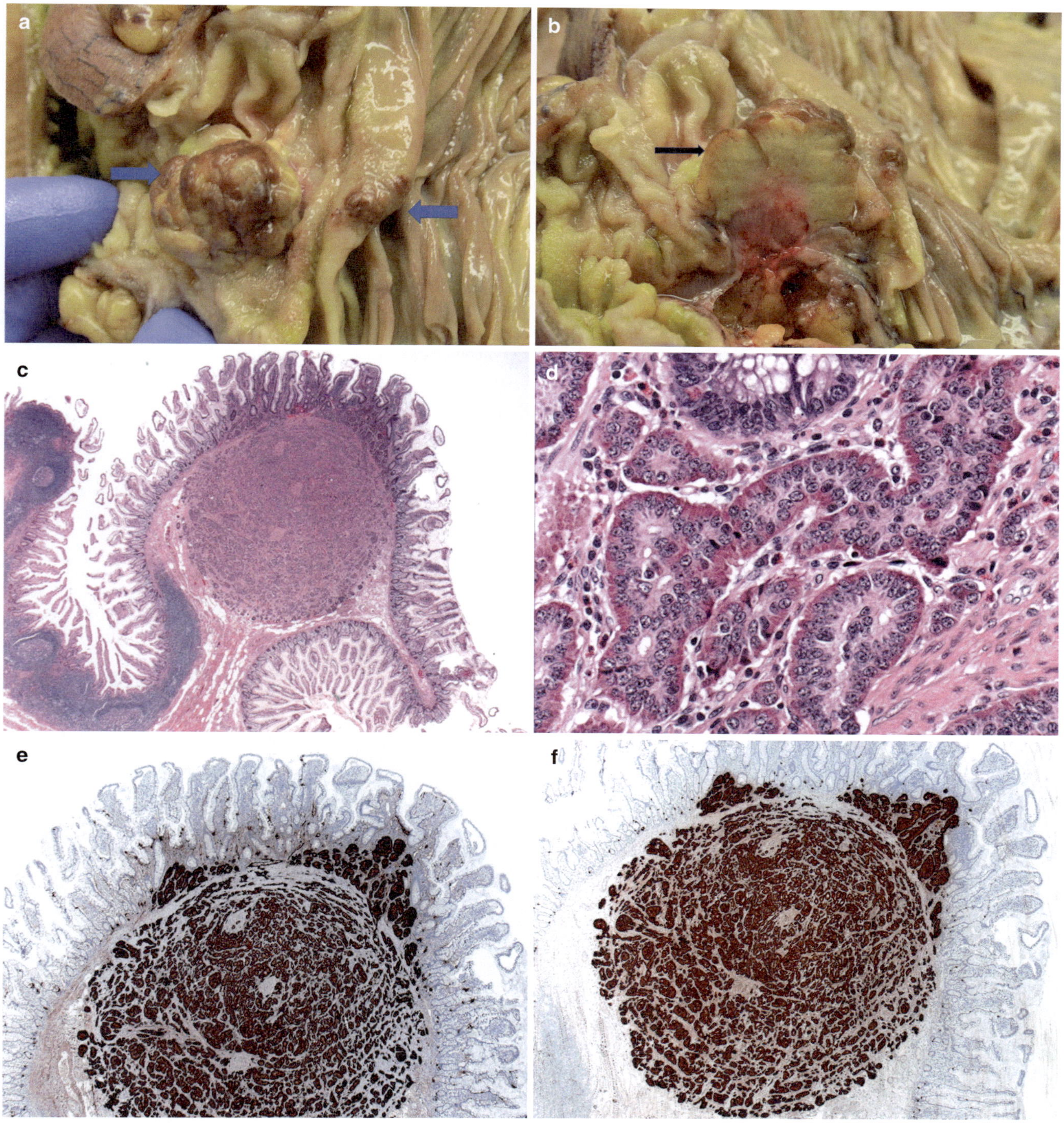

Fig. 5.13 (**a**) Endocrine tumor of the distal ileum with a satellite tumor to its right (*blue arrow*). The overlying mucosa is dark brown compared to the background mucosa. (**b**) A cross-section through the tumor reveals a pale yellowish nodule in the submucosa. The overlying mucosa (*solid black arrow*) is separate from and uninvolved by the tumor. (**c**) Low-power H&E view of a terminal ileum NET that presented as a polyp. The lesion was removed entirely by polypectomy. High-power view (**d**) with tumor cells displaying typical endocrine features with a predominantly insular growth pattern with small nests in the lamina propria. The tumor cells are positive for chromogranin A (**e**) and serotonin (**f**). Less than 5% of tumor cells are immunolabeled with MIB-1 (**g**)

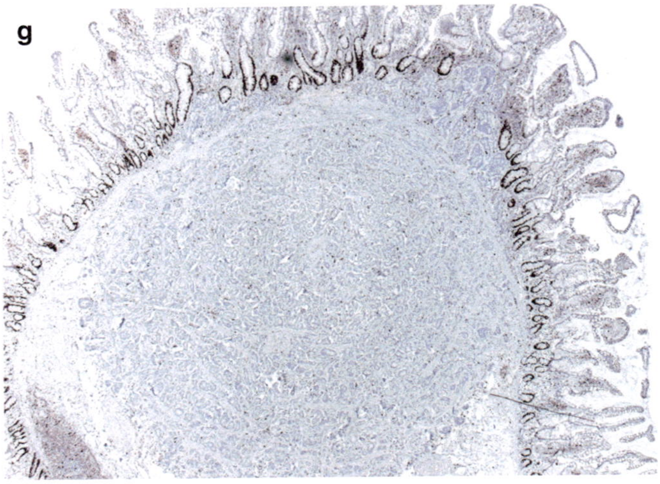

Fig. 5.13 (continued)

5.4 Appendix

NETs account for 50–77% of all appendiceal neoplasms and for 19% of all GI NETs [2]. There are two special types of appendiceal NETs: tubular carcinoid (TC) which has two main subcategories: EC-cell and L-cell variants, and so-called goblet cell carcinoid/carcinoma. According to the WHO classification, tubular carcinoids are classified as an NET, while goblet cell carcinoid is classified as a MANEC; these are discussed in the Appendix chapter (see Chap. 4) [2].

Well-differentiated NETs are the most common neoplasms in the appendix. Almost all are discovered incidentally in appendectomy specimens from acute appendicitis or incidental appendectomies performed during other abdominal surgical procedures. EC-cell NETs account for a sub-

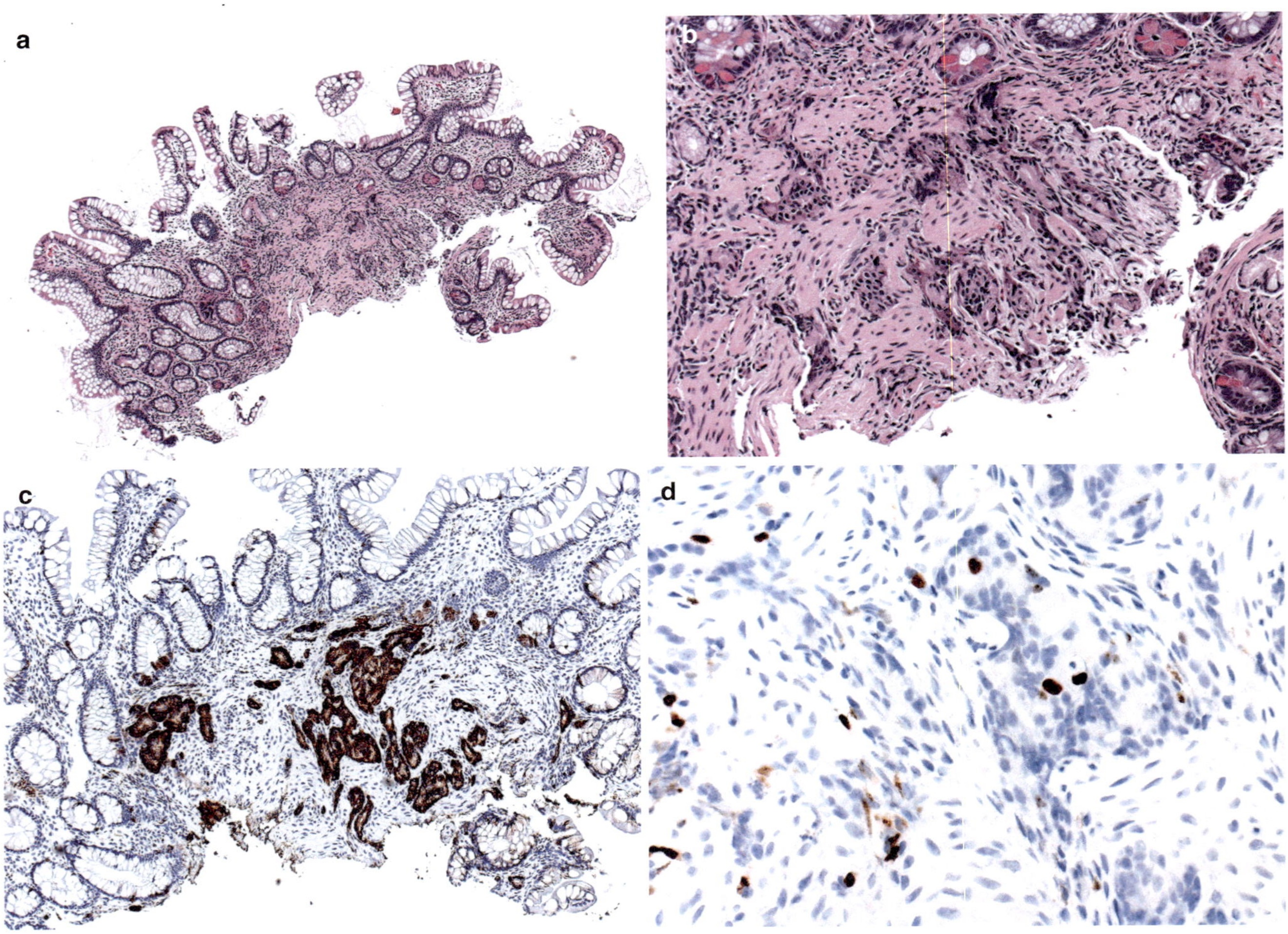

Fig. 5.14 Low-power (**a**) and high-power (**b**) H&E image of terminal ileum neuroendocrine with small tumor cell nests enmeshed in a collagenous stroma. Tumor cells display typical endocrine features. Peritumoral fibrosis results from serotonin secretion by tumor cells. Tumor cells stain positive for synaptophysin (**c**), with more than 50% immunolabeling with MIB-1 (**d**). An H&E image of a metastatic NET in a lymph node (**e**). Note the bland appearance of tumor cells, although this is a metastasis

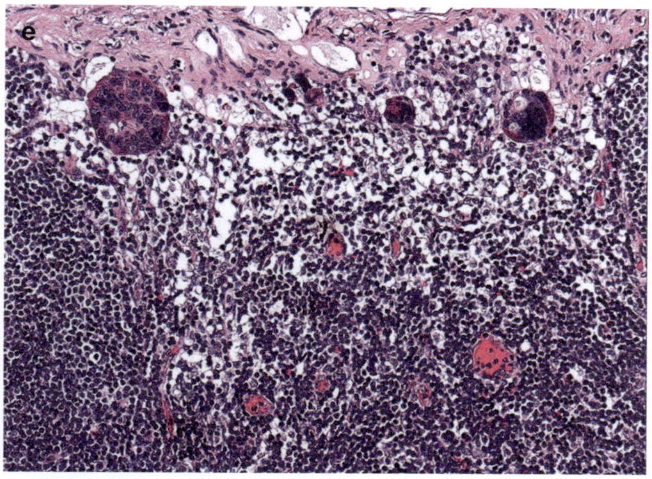

Fig. 5.14 (continued)

stantial portion of the appendiceal NETs and tend to occur at the tip of the appendix, while L-cell NETs tend to occur in the midpart of the appendix. They are readily distinguished on hematoxylin and eosin (H&E) stain by the subnuclear red granules at the periphery of tumor islands in EC-cell NETs [26]. The histologic features are comparable to those of ileal EC-cell NETs [27]. Appendiceal NETs form discrete tubules and short lines of cells within abundant stroma. Some contain mucus in the lumina [26]. Since they are often discovered in appendices removed for acute appendicitis, these tumors may be overlooked because of the intense inflammation present. Tubular NETs can be misdiagnosed as metastatic adenocarcinomas because they show little contact with the mucosa [2]. They have a trabecular pattern and are the appendiceal counterpart of L-cell NETs in the rectum [2]. Appendiceal NETs are the only GI tract carcinoid in which the nests of tumor cells are partly surrounded by S-100 spindle cells, presumably Schwann cells [16]. L-cell appendiceal NETs are PP/PYY-producing or L-cell NETs similar to those in the rectum. The cells produce enteroglucagons and peptide YY, and so they occasionally stain for glucagon [2]. Metastases are unusual for appendiceal carcinoids. In a large series from the Mayo Clinic, no tumor less than 2 cm in diameter metastasized [28], although occasional smaller NETs have metastasized.

Rare appendiceal NET cases have a clear cell change. It is characterized by foamy microvesicular cytoplasm in a nested or trabecular pattern. Cytoplasmic clearing has been attributed to glycogen, lipids, or mucin. Goblet cell carcinoid (GCC) and metastatic clear cell carcinoma of the kidney or ovary are the most important differentials. Although rare, it is helpful to recognize this variant, as it can be a close mimic to GCCs (Figs. 5.15 and 5.16).

GCC carcinomas of the appendix are covered in the Appendix chapter.

5.5 Large Intestine

Endocrine tumors of this segment are EC-cell, serotonin-producing NETs that end to be found in the proximal large bowel, L-cell, glucagon-like peptide, PP/PYY-producing tumors in the distal colon and rectum, and neuroendocrine carcinomas.

Endocrine tumors are more common in the rectum (54% of the cases), followed by the cecum (20%), sigmoid colon (7.5%), rectosigmoid colon (5.5%), and ascending colon (5%) [2]. The remaining abdominal colon is the least common site [16]. Most are located in the right colon, particularly in the cecum [29–31]. Most tumors are large when discovered, and about three fourths of those larger than 2 cm metastasize [29, 31]. However, the incidence of functioning tumors is very low [30]. NETs of the cecum and ascending colon are serotonin EC-cell type with the same histologic, cytologic, and cytochemical features as those of the jejuno-ileal EC-cell serotonin-producing NETs [2]. In contrast, the rectum is a relatively common site for NETs, and most are found incidentally on endoscopy performed for other reasons [32, 33].

Tumors from the distal colon and rectum are L-cell (glucagonlike-peptide-producing and PP/PYY-producing) NETs. A predominant trabecular pattern characterizes these, and they are often admixed with trabeculae with rosettes and occasionally with solid nests [2]. Contrary to EC-cell serotonin-producing NETs, the pattern in L-cell NETs shows a predominance of solid nests. The cytologic features resemble other GI NETs with the uniform round to oval nuclei with indistinct nucleoli and coarsely granular chromatin pattern. Most of these may not stain for chromogranin A but will stain for synaptophysin [16]. Interestingly, the tumor cells of some rectal carcinoids contain prostatic acid phosphatase, as do some in the small bowel [34, 35]. However, in a differential diagnosis with prostatic carcinoma with direct extension into the rectum, which can at times look like a well-differentiated endocrine tumor, one should run prostate-specific antigen, which is negative in carcinoid tumors.

As with other GI NETs, size correlates closely with the likelihood of metastases. Tumors smaller than 1 cm rarely metastasize [36, 37]. Approximately 6% of tumors between 1 and 1.9 cm and 24% of those over 2 cm metastasize to the liver [37–40]. Other poor prognostic features include deep invasion (into the muscularis propria or deeper), lymphovascular invasion, and a high mitotic rate (≥2 per 50 HPFs) [40, 41]. The main problem with these tumors is that the adequacy of excision can be difficult to assess, and the tumor site is challenging to find afterwards. It can be useful to rescope these patients and tattoo proximal and distal to the scar as soon as possible to allow the site to be observed again. L-cell tumors tend to be chromogranin A (CGA) –negative so that they cannot be followed with serial serum CGA levels (Fig. 5.17).

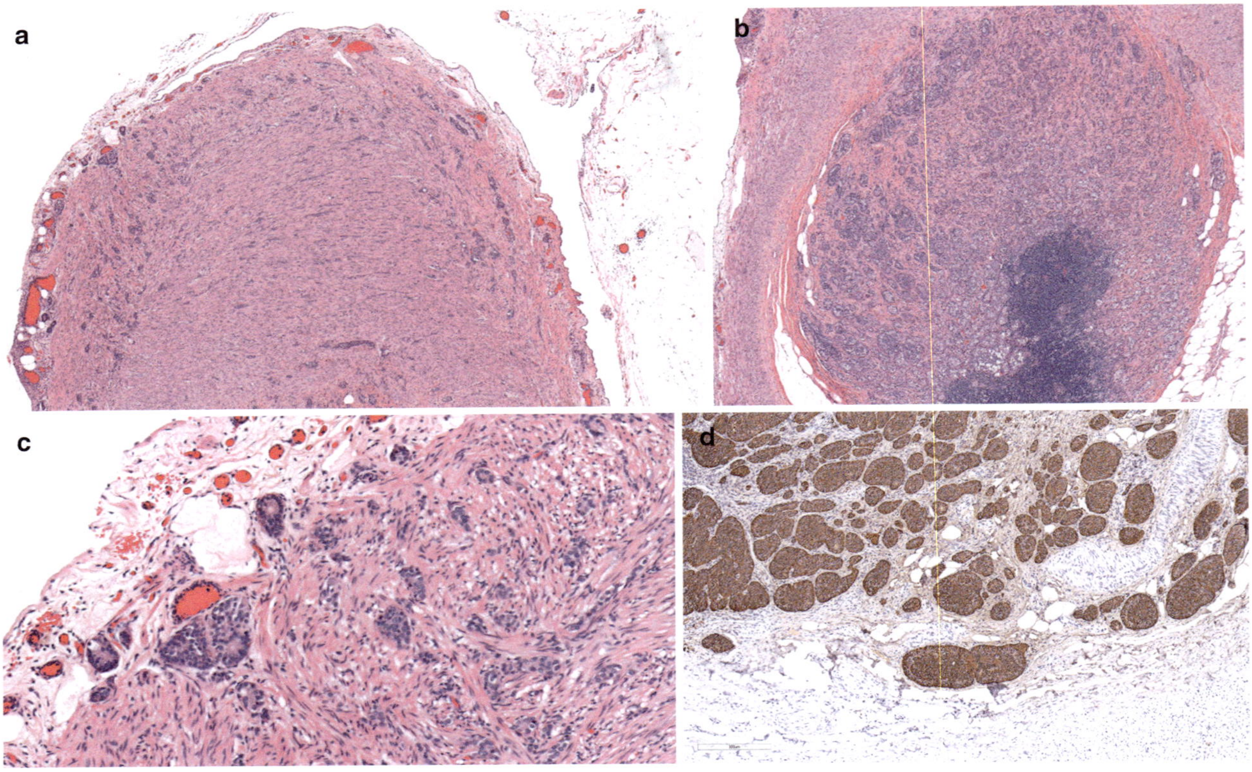

Fig. 5.15 Low-power (**a**) H&E image of an incidental NET seen in an appendix resected for acute appendicitis. Normal lymphoid follicles (lumen remnants) are found adjacent to the NET in the appendix tip (**b**). At high magnification (**c**), tumors cells showed eosinophilic cytoplasm and stippled or "salt and pepper" nuclear chromatin. Mitotic activity is absent. The tumor cells are positive for chromogranin (**d**)

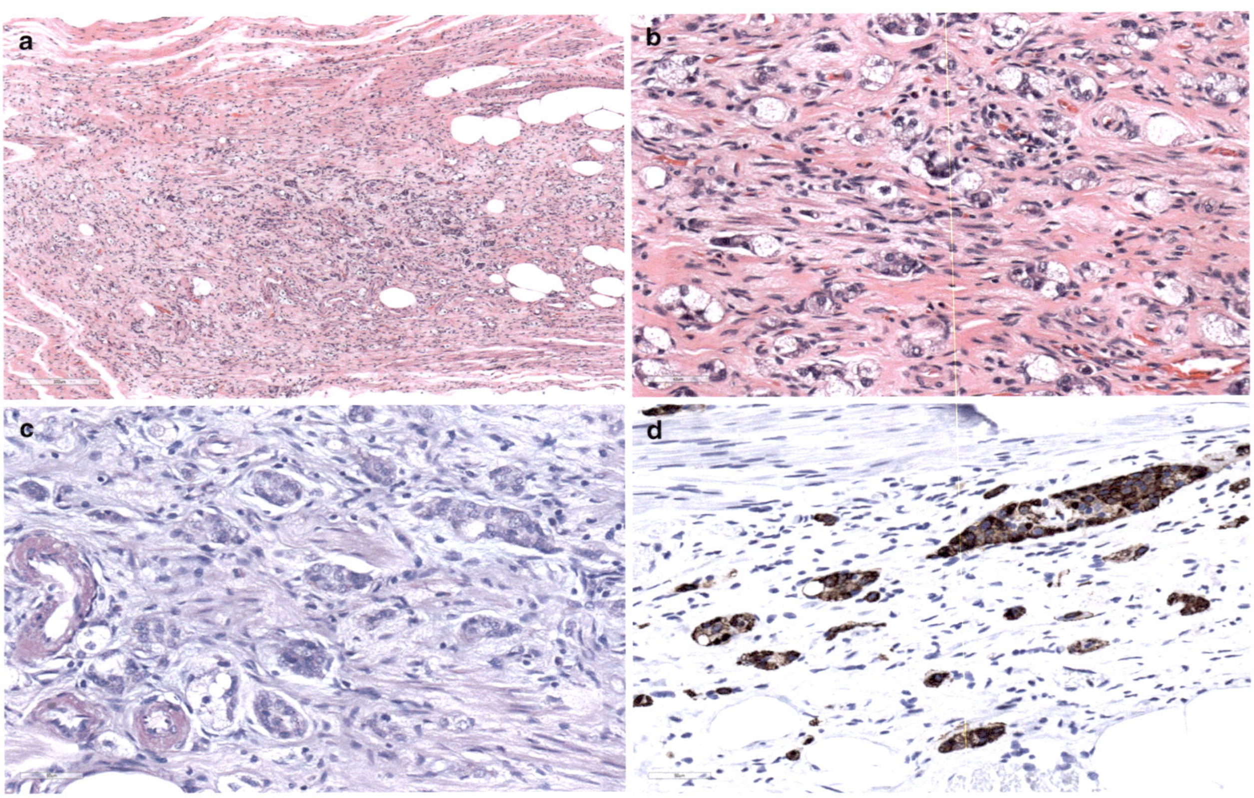

Fig. 5.16 Low-power (**a**) H&E image of clear cell carcinoid of the appendix. At high power (**b**) tumor cells are foamy with microvesicular clear cytoplasm. With a mucin stain, note the absence of the typical goblet cells of goblet cell carcinoids (**c**). Tumor cells are positive with a chromogranin stain (**d**)

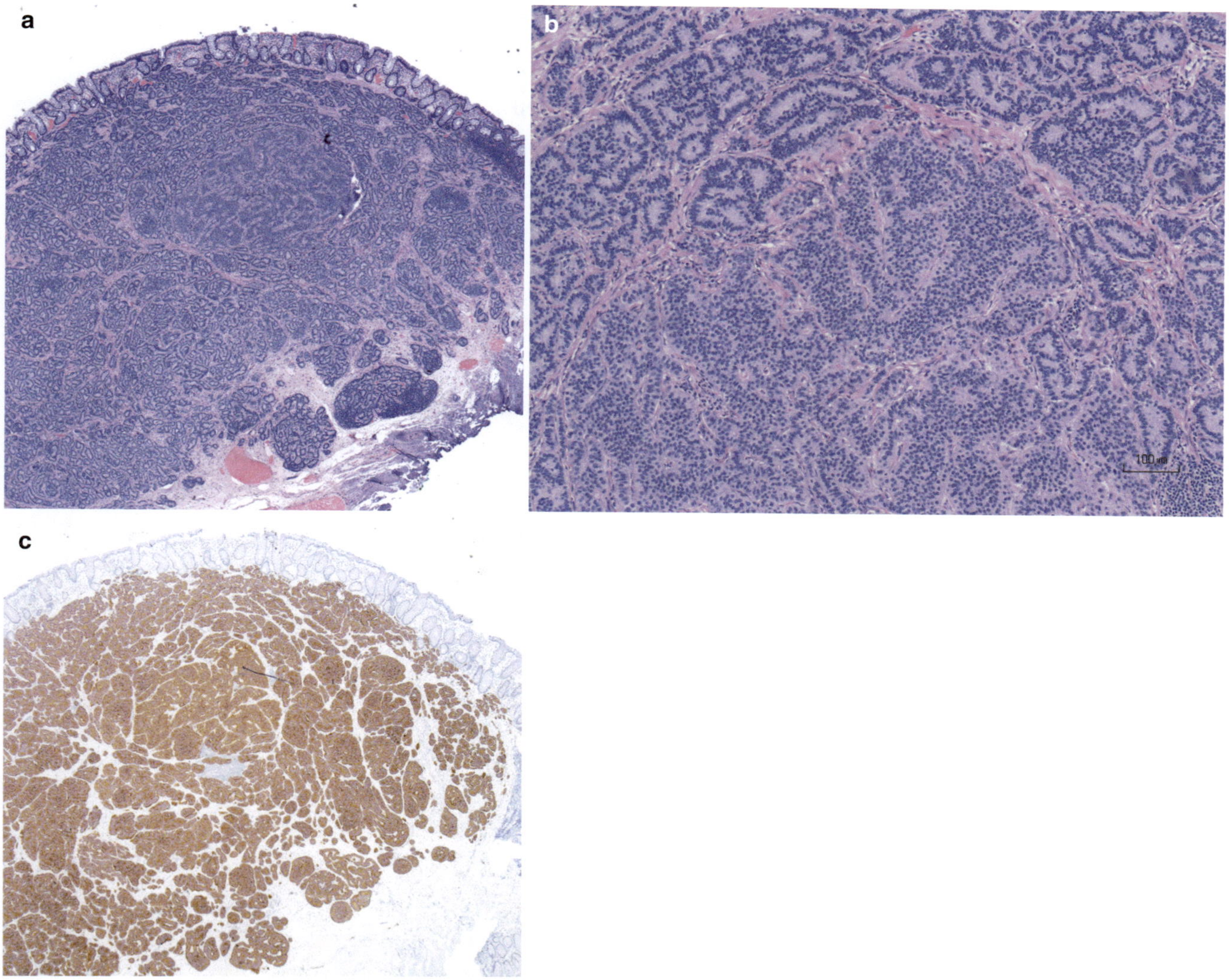

Fig. 5.17 Low-power view (**a**) of a well-differentiated neuroendocrine tumor in the mucosa and submucosa of a rectal "polyp" biopsied during routine endoscopy. This medium-power view (**b**) shows small tumor nests, cords/ribbons, and a few acinar structures. Tumor cells are positive for synaptophysin (**c**)

5.6 Neuroendocrine Carcinoma (NEC)

These are rare tumors with an aggressive clinical course and a poor prognosis [2, 42]. They are subclassified into three pathologic types: tumors that resemble other NETs but are G3 (proliferation induces >20%), small-cell carcinomas, and large-cell carcinomas. Many of the non-G3 tumors are MANECs [2]. Squamous cell carcinomas coexisting with NECs have also been reported in the esophagus and duodenum [43, 44]. These are grade 3 tumors that are morphologically identical to small-cell and large-cell NEC of the lung [9, 45]. Large-cell carcinoma is the most common colorectal NEC, followed by small-cell carcinoma and mixed carcinoma of small-cell and large-cell carcinoma [46]. NECs are more common in the colon, especially the right colon, than in the rectum [2, 47]. They are frequently associated with an overlying adenoma or adjacent adenocarcinoma [2], but they are not associated with NETs [2].

Small-cell carcinomas consist of small, round, ovoid, or spindle-shaped tumor cells with scant cytoplasm, arranged in a sheet-like pattern morphologically similar to their pulmonary counterparts. Nuclei of small-cell carcinomas show fine granular chromatin with absent or inconspicuous nucleoli. These typically express neuroendocrine markers (e.g., chromogranin, synaptophysin) by immunohistochemistry but can also express thyroid transcription factor 1 (TTF1), which does not immediately imply a bronchogenic metastasis. Patients usually have liver metastases at the time of original surgery [48], even when they are very small. Some tumors resemble intermediate bronchogenic NETs.

Large-cell carcinomas are composed of large-sized tumor cells with large vesicular nuclei with prominent nucleoli [49]. The nuclear-to-cytoplasmic ratio is lower than that of small-cell carcinomas [49–51]. These tumor cells have organoid, nesting, trabecular, rosette-like, and palisading patterns that suggest endocrine differentiation.

MANECs are composed of both adenocarcinoma and neuroendocrine carcinoma components, with each component accounting for more than 30% of the tumor [2]. Conversely, NETs arising in association with adenocarcinomas are exceedingly rare [2]. A neoplasm with morphologically recognizable glandular and neuroendocrine components is identified as a carcinoma, since both are malignant and need to be graded [2]. The identification of scattered neuroendocrine cells by immunohistochemistry in adenocarcinoma does not qualify as MANEC [2]. These tumors have not been well described in the GI tract because of their low frequency. Some otherwise typical carcinomas that have a large neuroendocrine component are best regarded as adenocarcinomas with a neuroendocrine component, as they tend to respond better to conventional therapy (Figs. 5.18, 5.19 and 5.20).

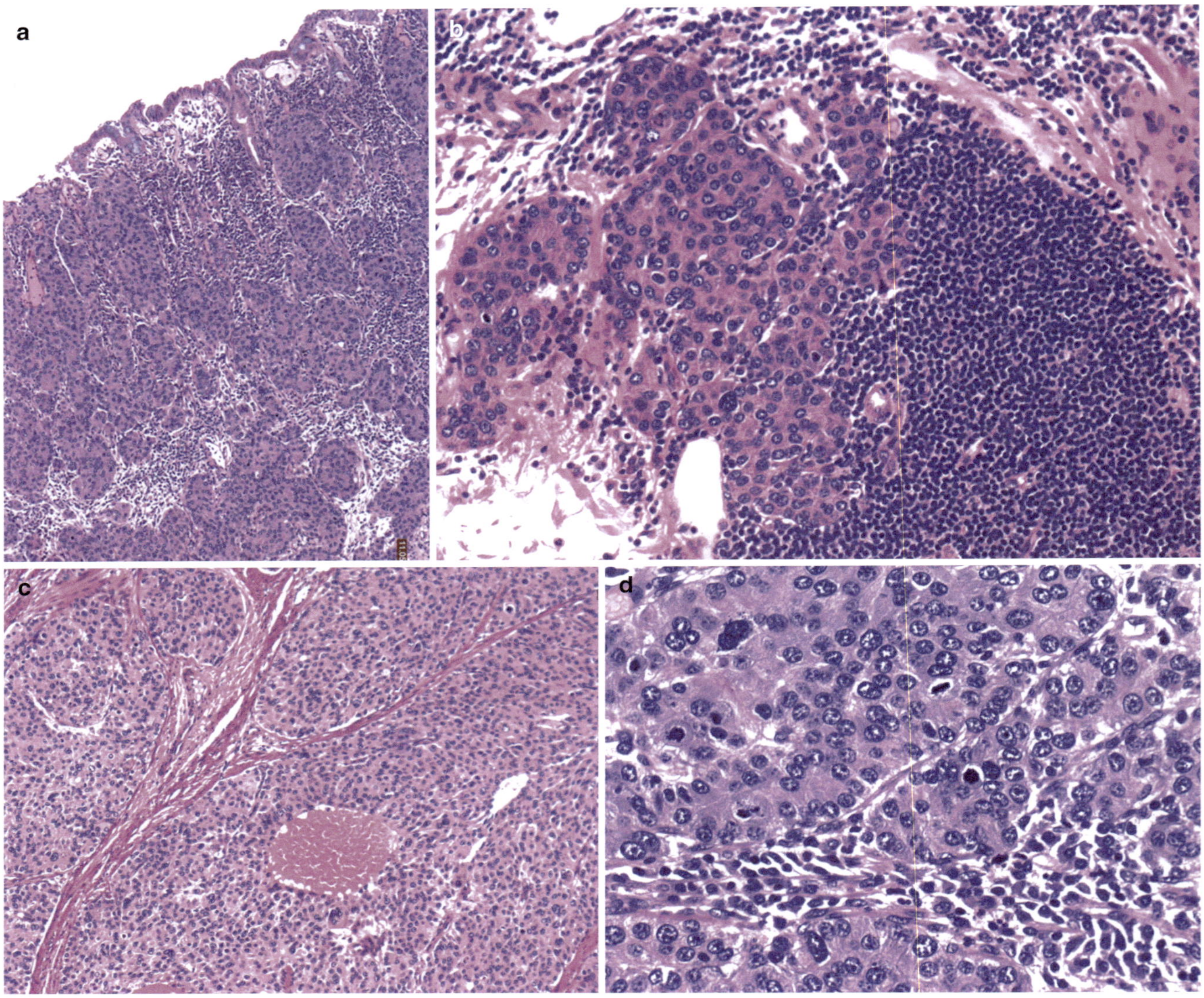

Fig. 5.18 Low-power H&E image of a large-cell NET (**a**) with lymph node metastases (**b**). Most have a brisk mitotic rate and show areas of necrosis (**c**). This high-power H&E image (**d**) shows typical features of large-cell neuroendocrine carcinoma (abundant cytoplasm, prominent nucleoli, and brisk mitoses (30 mitoses/10 HPFs). Tumor cells are positive for Cam 5.2 (**e**) and synaptophysin (**f**), with patchy staining for chromogranin (**g**); they are negative for CD56 (**h**). Chromogranin is specific but synaptophysin is more sensitive for demonstrating neuroendocrine differentiation. MIB-1 shows >50% positive (**i**)

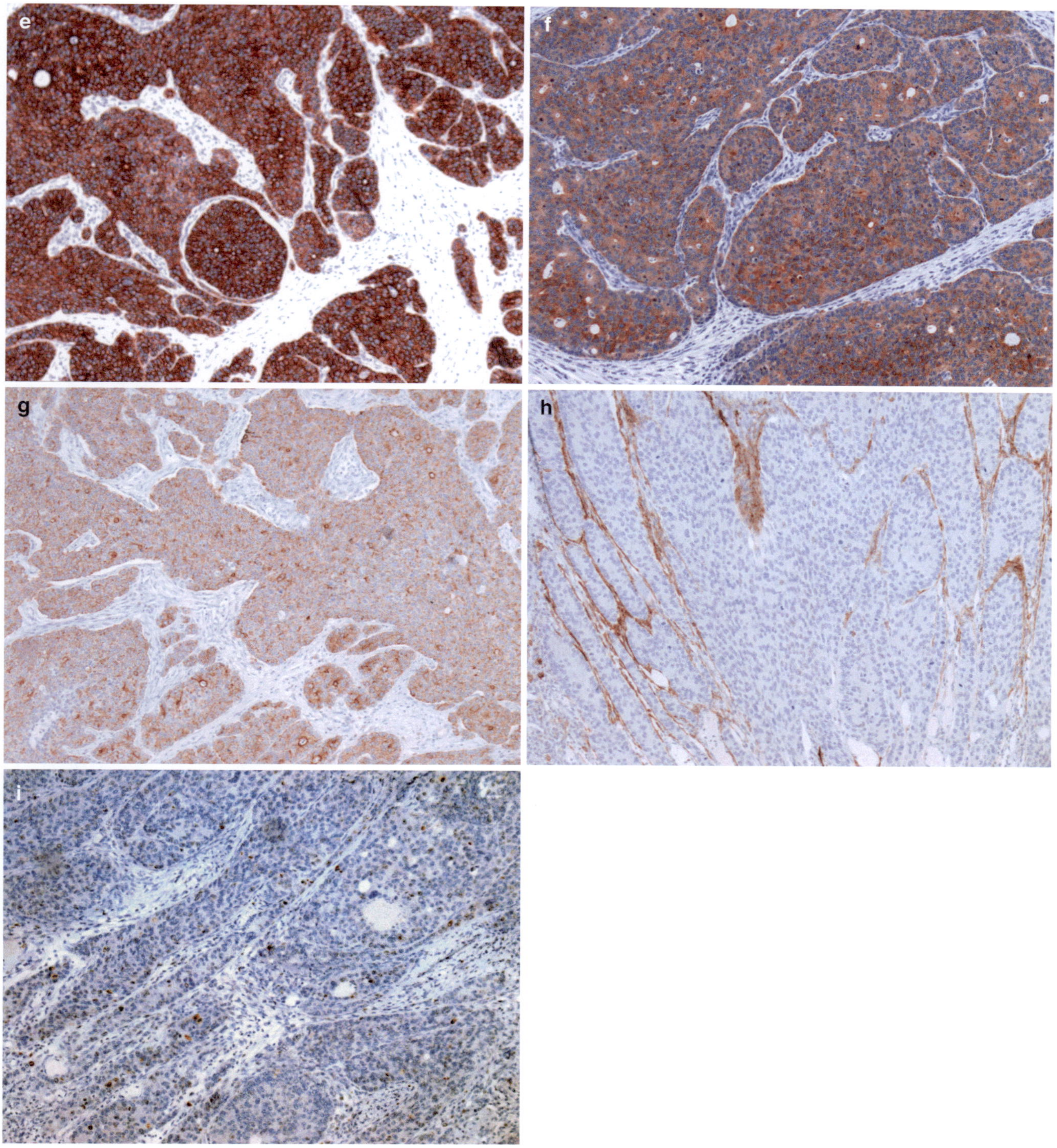

Fig. 5.18 (continued)

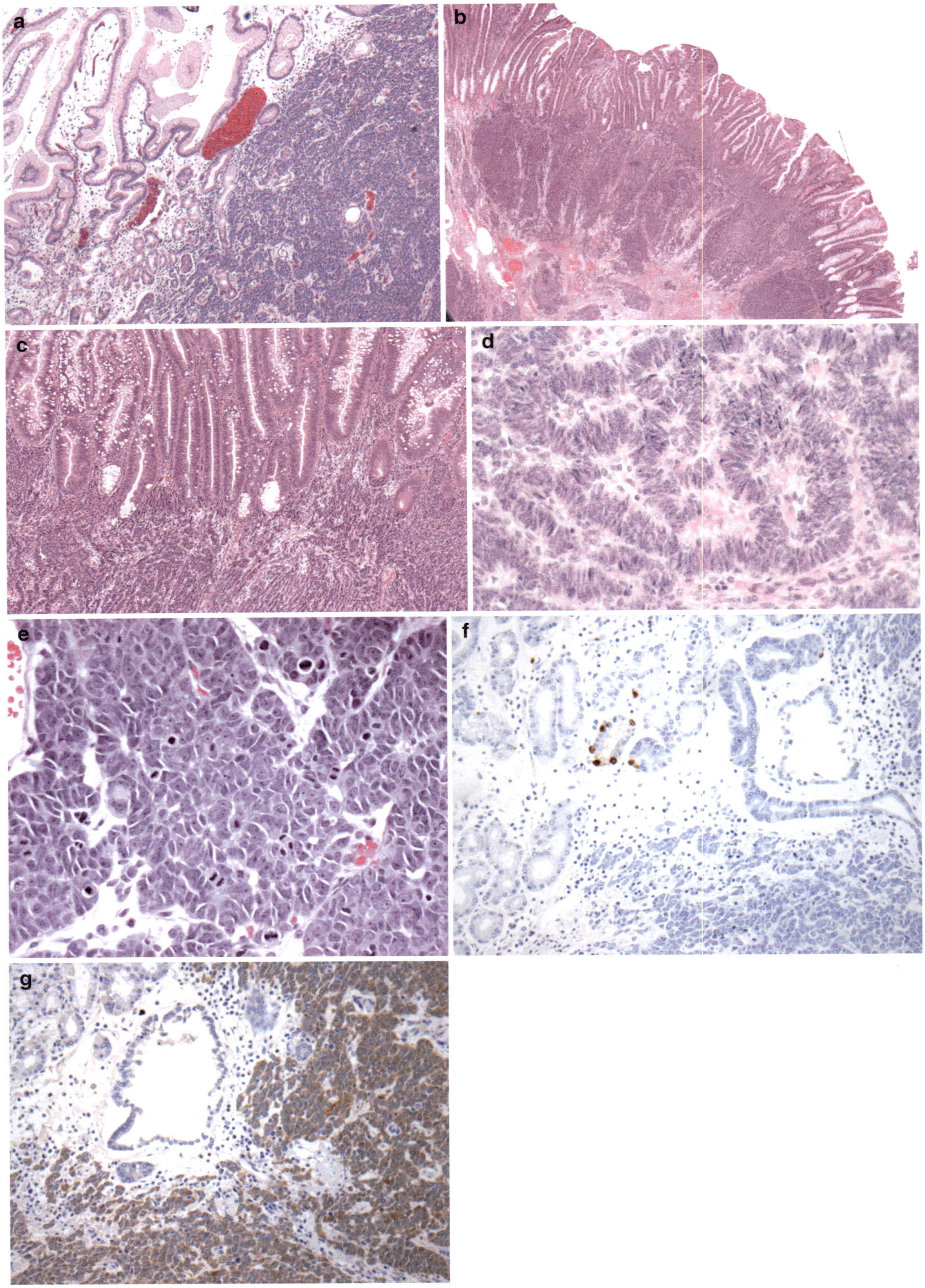

Fig. 5.19 Low-power H&E image of a small-cell carcinoma of the small bowel (**a**). (**b–d**) H&E images of a small-cell carcinoma arising from a tubular adenoma. This high-power image (**e**) shows the generic features seen in any small-cell carcinoma (salt and pepper chromatin, nuclear molding, karyorrhectic debris, prominent apoptosis, and high mitotic count). The absence of significant cytoplasm or prominent nucleoli distinguishes it from large-cell neuroendocrine carcinoma. This tumor was negative for chromogranin (**f**) but positive for PGP 9.5, which confirms its neuroendocrine differentiation (**g**)

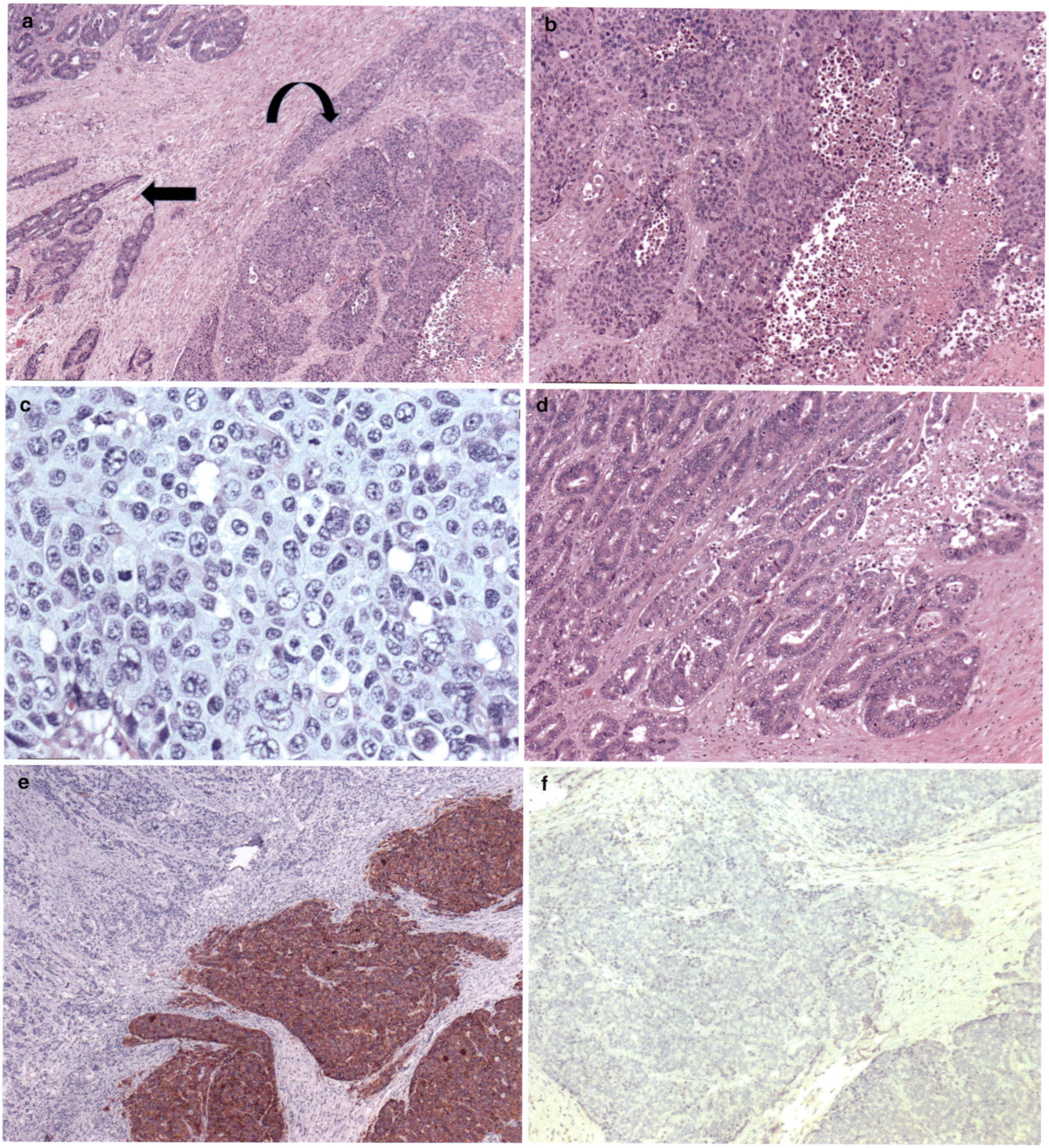

Fig. 5.20 The tumor shows features of small-cell NEC (*black curved arrow*) with foci of conventional adenocarcinoma (*solid black arrow*). These tumors are referred to as mixed adeno-neuroendocrine carcinomas as per the WHO 2010 nomenclature (**a**). High-power image of the focus with small-cell neuroendocrine carcinoma (**b** and **c**); note the generic features of any small-cell carcinoma (salt and pepper chromatin, nuclear molding, high mitotic count). High-power image of the focus with conventional adenocarcinoma (**d**). Synaptophysin stain highlights focus with small-cell neuroendocrine carcinoma only (**e**). Chromogranin stain is negative (**f**)

References

1. Fitzgerald TL, Mosquera C, Lea CS, McMullen M. Primary site predicts grade for gastroenteropancreatic neuroendocrine tumors. Am Surg. 2017;83:799–803.
2. Bosman FT, Carneiro F, Hruban RH, Theise ND. WHO classification of tumours of the digestive system. Geneva: WHO Press; 2010.
3. Merchant SH, VanderJagt T, Lathrop S, Amin MB. Sporadic duodenal bulb gastrin-cell tumors: association with helicobacter pylori gastritis and long-term use of proton pump inhibitors. Am J Surg Pathol. 2006;30:1581–7.
4. Garbrecht N, Anlauf M, Schmitt A, Henopp T, Sipos B, Raffel A, et al. Somatostatin-producing neuroendocrine tumors of the duodenum and pancreas: incidence, types, biological behavior, association with inherited syndromes, and functional activity. Endocr Relat Cancer. 2008;15:229–41.
5. Hartel M, Wente MN, Sido B, Friess H, Buchler MW. Carcinoid of the ampulla of Vater. J Gastroenterol Hepatol. 2005;20:676–81.
6. Vanoli A, La Rosa S, Klersy C, Grillo F, Albarello L, Inzani F, et al. Four neuroendocrine tumor types and neuroendocrine carcinoma of the duodenum: analysis of 203 cases. Neuroendocrinology. 2017;104:112–25.
7. Perrone T, Sibley RK, Rosai J. Duodenal gangliocytic paraganglioma. An immunohistochemical and ultrastructural study and a hypothesis concerning its origin. Am J Surg Pathol. 1985;9:31–41.
8. Okubo Y, Wakayama M, Nemoto T, Kitahara K, Nakayama H, Shibuya K, et al. Literature survey on epidemiology and pathology of gangliocytic paraganglioma. BMC Cancer. 2011;11:187.
9. Delle Fave G, Kwekkeboom DJ, Van Cutsem E, Rindi G, Kos-Kudla B, Knigge U, et al. ENETS consensus guidelines for the management of patients with gastroduodenal neoplasms. Neuroendocrinology. 2012;95:74–87.
10. Buchler M, Malfertheiner P, Baczako K, Krautzberger W, Beger HG. A metastatic endocrine-neurogenic tumor of the ampulla of Vater with multiple endocrine immunoreaction--malignant paraganglioma? Digestion. 1985;31:54–9.
11. Inai K, Kobuke T, Yonehara S, Tokuoka S. Duodenal gangliocytic paraganglioma with lymph node metastasis in a 17-year-old boy. Cancer. 1989;63:2540–5.
12. Modlin IM, Champaneria MC, Chan AK, Kidd M. A three-decade analysis of 3,911 small intestinal neuroendocrine tumors: the rapid pace of no progress. Am J Gastroenterol. 2007;102:1464–73.
13. Bilimoria KY, Bentrem DJ, Wayne JD, Ko CY, Bennett CL, Talamonti MS. Small bowel cancer in the United States: changes in epidemiology, treatment, and survival over the last 20 years. Ann Surg. 2009;249:63–71.
14. Godwin JD. Carcinoid tumors. An analysis of 2,837 cases. Cancer. 1975;36:560–9.
15. Vinik AI, McLeod MK, Fig LM, Shapiro B, Lloyd RV, Cho K. Clinical features, diagnosis, and localization of carcinoid tumors and their management. Gastroenterol Clin N Am. 1989;18: 865–96.
16. Lewin. Weinstein and Riddell's gastrointestinal pathology and its clinical implications. In: Riddell R, Jain D, editors. 2e. Philadelphia: Wolters Kluwer; 2014.
17. Eckhauser FE, Argenta LC, Strodel WE, Wheeler RH, Bull FE, Appelman HD, et al. Mesenteric angiopathy, intestinal gangrene, and midgut carcinoids. Surgery. 1981;90:720–8.
18. Allibone RO, Hoffman J, Gosney JR, Helliwell TR. Granulation tissue polyposis associated with carcinoid tumours of the small intestine. Histopathology. 1993;22:475–80.
19. Abrahams NA, Vesoulis Z, Petras RE. Angiogenic polypoid proliferation adjacent to ileal carcinoid tumors: a nonspecific finding related to mucosal prolapse. Mod Pathol. 2001;14: 821–7.
20. Burke AP, Thomas RM, Elsayed AM, Sobin LH. Carcinoids of the jejunum and ileum: an immunohistochemical and clinicopathologic study of 167 cases. Cancer. 1997;79:1086–93.
21. Yarze JC, Herlihy KJ, Coombes JM, Bauer WM, Fritz HP, D'Agostino JA. Detection of asymptomatic ileal carcinoid tumors during ileal intubation at screening colonoscopy: a case series. Am J Gastroenterol. 2009;104:3114–5.
22. Riihimaki M, Hemminki A, Sundquist K, Sundquist J, Hemminki K. The epidemiology of metastases in neuroendocrine tumors. Int J Cancer. 2016;139:2679–86.
23. Moertel CG, Sauer WG, Dockerty MB, Baggenstoss AH. Life history of the carcinoid tumor of the small intestine. Cancer. 1961;14:901–12.
24. Strodel WE, Talpos G, Eckhauser F, Thompson N. Surgical therapy for small-bowel carcinoid tumors. Arch Surg. 1983;118:391–7.
25. Yantiss RK, Odze RD, Farraye FA, Rosenberg AE. Solitary versus multiple carcinoid tumors of the ileum: a clinical and pathologic review of 68 cases. Am J Surg Pathol. 2003;27:811–7.
26. Carr NJ, Sobin LH. Neuroendocrine tumors of the appendix. Semin Diagn Pathol. 2004;21:108–19.
27. Kloppel G, Perren A, Heitz PU. The gastroenteropancreatic neuroendocrine cell system and its tumors: the WHO classification. Ann N Y Acad Sci. 2004;1014:13–27.
28. Moertel CG, Weiland LH, Nagorney DM, Dockerty MB. Carcinoid tumor of the appendix: treatment and prognosis. N Engl J Med. 1987;317:1699–701.
29. Rosenberg JM, Welch JP. Carcinoid tumors of the colon. A study of 72 patients. Am J Surg. 1985;149:775–9.
30. Spread C, Berkel H, Jewell L, Jenkins H, Yakimets W. Colon carcinoid tumors. A population-based study. Dis Colon Rectum. 1994;37:482–91.
31. Ballantyne GH, Savoca PE, Flannery JT, Ahlman MH, Modlin IM. Incidence and mortality of carcinoids of the colon. Data from the Connecticut tumor registry. Cancer. 1992;69:2400–5.
32. Caplin M, Sundin A, Nillson O, Baum RP, Klose KJ, Kelestimur F, et al. ENETS consensus guidelines for the management of patients with digestive neuroendocrine neoplasms: colorectal neuroendocrine neoplasms. Neuroendocrinology. 2012;95:88–97.
33. Jetmore AB, Ray JE, Gathright JB, McMullen KM, Hicks TC, Timmcke AE. Rectal carcinoids: the most frequent carcinoid tumor. Dis Colon Rectum. 1992;35:717–25.
34. Azumi N, Traweek ST, Battifora H. Prostatic acid phosphatase in carcinoid tumors. Immunohistochemical and immunoblot studies. Am J Surg Pathol. 1991;15:785–90.
35. Kimura N, Sasano N. Prostate-specific acid phosphatase in carcinoid tumors. Virchows Arch A Pathol Anat Histopathol. 1986;410:247–51.
36. Soga J. Early-stage carcinoids of the gastrointestinal tract: an analysis of 1914 reported cases. Cancer. 2005;103:1587–95.
37. Koura AN, Giacco GG, Curley SA, Skibber JM, Feig BW, Ellis LM. Carcinoid tumors of the rectum: effect of size, histopathology, and surgical treatment on metastasis free survival. Cancer. 1997;79:1294–8.
38. Capella C, Heitz PU, Hofler H, Solcia E, Kloppel G. Revised classification of neuroendocrine tumours of the lung, pancreas and gut. Virchows Arch. 1995;425:547–60.
39. Mani S, Modlin IM, Ballantyne G, Ahlman H, West B. Carcinoids of the rectum. J Am Coll Surg. 1994;179:231–48.
40. Shields CJ, Tiret E, Winter DC, International Rectal Carcinoid Study Group. Carcinoid tumors of the rectum: a multi-institutional international collaboration. Ann Surg. 2010;252:750–5.
41. Fahy BN, Tang LH, Klimstra D, Wong WD, Guillem JG, Paty PB, et al. Carcinoid of the rectum risk stratification (CaRRs): a strategy for preoperative outcome assessment. Ann Surg Oncol. 2007;14:1735–43.

42. Cai W, Tan Y, Ge W, Ding K, Hu H. Pattern and risk factors for distant metastases in gastrointestinal neuroendocrine neoplasms: a population-based study. Cancer Med. 2018;7:2699–709.
43. Yamamoto J, Ohshima K, Ikeda S, Iwashita A, Kikuchi M. Primary esophageal small cell carcinoma with concomitant invasive squamous cell carcinoma or carcinoma in situ. Hum Pathol. 2003;34:1108–15.
44. Nassar H, Albores-Saavedra J, Klimstra DS. High-grade neuroendocrine carcinoma of the ampulla of vater: a clinicopathologic and immunohistochemical analysis of 14 cases. Am J Surg Pathol. 2005;29:588–94.
45. Rindi G, Kloppel G, Couvelard A, Komminoth P, Korner M, Lopes JM, et al. TNM staging of midgut and hindgut (neuro) endocrine tumors: a consensus proposal including a grading system. Virchows Arch. 2007;451:757–62.
46. Shia J, Tang LH, Weiser MR, Brenner B, Adsay NV, Stelow EB, et al. Is nonsmall cell type high-grade neuroendocrine carcinoma of the tubular gastrointestinal tract a distinct disease entity? Am J Surg Pathol. 2008;32:719–31.
47. Kloppel G, Rindi G, Anlauf M, Perren A, Komminoth P. Site-specific biology and pathology of gastroenteropancreatic neuroendocrine tumors. Virchows Arch. 2007;451(Suppl 1):S9–27.
48. Burke AB, Shekitka KM, Sobin LH. Small cell carcinomas of the large intestine. Am J Clin Pathol. 1991;95:315–21.
49. Travis WD, Linnoila RI, Tsokos MG, Hitchcock CL, Cutler GB, Nieman L, et al. Neuroendocrine tumors of the lung with proposed criteria for large-cell neuroendocrine carcinoma. An ultrastructural, immunohistochemical, and flow cytometric study of 35 cases. Am J Surg Pathol. 1991;15:529–53.
50. Kajiwara H, Hirabayashi K, Miyazawa M, Nakamura N, Hirasawa T, Muramatsu T, et al. Immunohistochemical expression of somatostatin type 2A receptor in neuroendocrine carcinoma of uterine cervix. Arch Gynecol Obstet. 2009;279:521–5.
51. Stojsic Z, Brasanac D, Bilanovic D, Mitrovic O, Stevanovic R, Boricic I. Large-cell neuroendocrine carcinoma of the ampulla of Vater. Med Oncol. 2010;27:1144–8.
52. Ahlman H, Nilsson. The gut as the largest endocrine organ in the body. Ann Oncol. 2001;12 Suppl 2:S63–8.
53. Gunawardene AR, Corfe BM, Staton CA. Classification and functions of enteroendocrine cells of the lower gastrointestinal tract. Int J Exp Pathol. 2011;92:219–31.
54. Solcia E, Vanoli A. Histogenesis and natural history of gut neuroendocrine tumors: present status. Endocr Pathol. 2014;25:165–70.

6 Lymphoproliferative Disorders of the Small and Large Intestine

Romulo Celli and Dhanpat Jain

The gastrointestinal (GI) tract by its nature is continuously exposed to the outside world and plays a central role in our immunological response to a number of potential microbial pathogens and other antigens. Gut-associated lymphoid tissue (GALT) is a cardinal element of the normal GI cellular environment. Lymphocyte immunomodulation is a source of protection (providing pathogen-specific reactions), but it also can act as the substrate for clonal proliferation and disease (lymphoproliferative disorders). It is no surprise, then, that the GI tract is the most common extranodal site of lymphoma—accounting for roughly 10–20% of total cases [1]. Approximately 50% of extranodal lymphomas occur in the stomach, and the remaining cases are distributed about evenly between the small and large intestines [2]. Overall, the most common diagnosis is of diffuse large B-cell lymphoma (DLBCL), followed by low-grade marginal zone lymphoma. The most impressive aspect of these tumors is their remarkable heterogeneity in gross and histologic patterns. Diagnosis of these conditions requires recognition of both the classic and not-so-classic phenotypes of disease. Ancillary diagnostic methods, such as B-cell and T-cell receptor gene rearrangement by polymerase chain reaction or specific translocations are often needed to clarify complex cases, but may be redundant in certain scenarios. In the setting of a complex case, effective communication amongst laboratories is imperative when performing immunophenotyping and/or molecular assays to subtype lymphomas, or when distinguishing neoplastic from reactive processes. The following images are a sampling of the diverse disease phenotypes (gross and histologic) seen in the small and large intestines (Figs. 6.1, 6.2, 6.3, 6.4, 6.5, 6.6, 6.7, 6.8, 6.9, 6.10, 6.11, 6.12, 6.13, 6.14, 6.15, 6.16, 6.17, 6.18, 6.19, 6.20, 6.21, 6.22, 6.23, 6.24, 6.25, 6.26, 6.27, 6.28, 6.29, 6.30, 6.31, 6.32, 6.33, 6.34, 6.35, 6.36, 6.37, 6.38, 6.39, 6.40, 6.41, 6.42, 6.43, 6.44, 6.45, 6.46 and 6.47).

H. H. Li-Chang et al., *Atlas of Intestinal Pathology*, Atlas of Anatomic Pathology,
https://doi.org/10.1007/978-3-030-12379-6_6

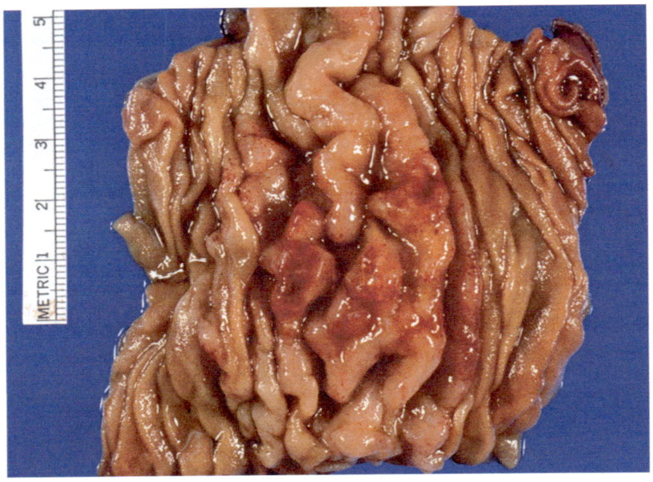

Fig. 6.1 Gross appearance of lymphomas in the GI tract is highly varied and may closely mimic an inflammatory process or epithelial neoplasms. The following photographs illustrate the spectrum of gross findings of lymphomas involving the small and large bowel. This image depicts diffuse thickening of the mucosal folds without a distinct mass lesion. This is a nonspecific finding that can be seen early in the disease process and tends to mimic an inflammatory disorder rather than a neoplasm. This was an example of immunoproliferative small intestinal disease (IPSID), but the appearance is not specific to any particular lymphoproliferative disease

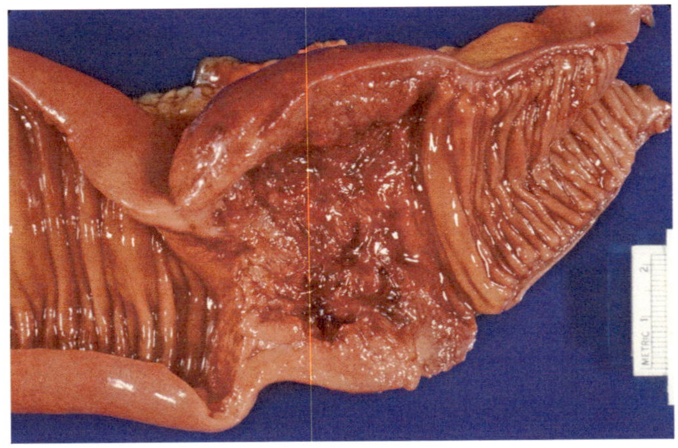

Fig. 6.2 Many advanced lymphomas often present with symptomatic disease and show discrete mass lesions that may take the form of a large polyp, a fungating ulcer or ulceroproliferative lesion, or mural thickening. This lesion is a large ulcer with diffuse mural thickening of the small intestine. (Approximately 30% of intestinal lymphomas present in this fashion [3].) The borders of this lesion are very indistinct, and the texture is soft and "fish flesh" in appearance—all features that are in contrast to most epithelial malignancies. Symptomatic obstruction is less often seen than in adenocarcinoma because of the lack of a desmoplastic response. The most common lymphoma of intestines is diffuse large B-cell lymphoma (DLBCL), as in this case of a small bowel resection

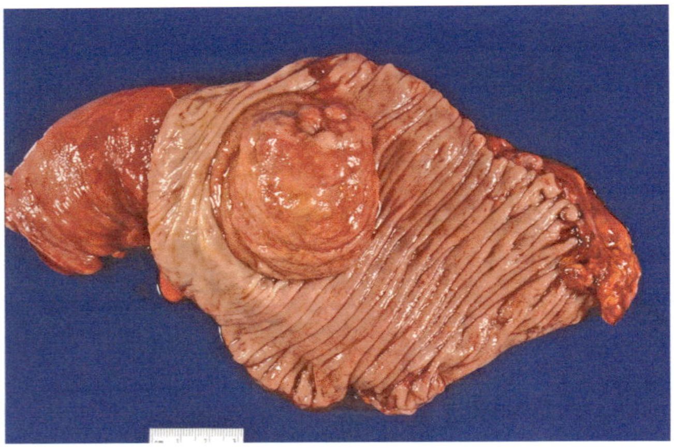

Fig. 6.3 Lymphoma presenting as a fungating polypoid mass, which was seen protruding into the small bowel lumen. This turned out to be a follicular lymphoma, but this gross appearance is not specific for any subtype

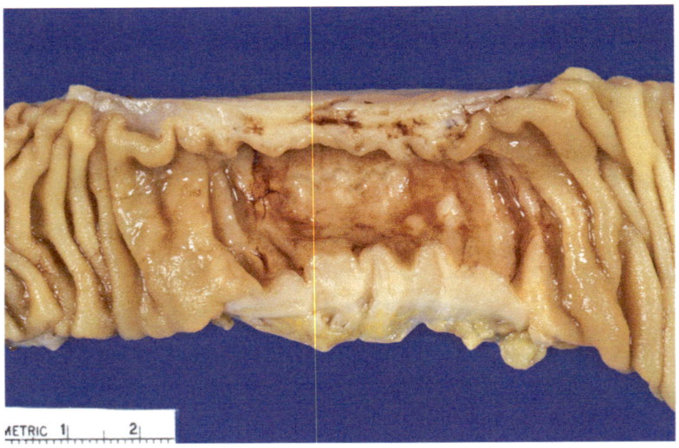

Fig. 6.4 An example of small bowel lymphoma presenting as an ulcer. The underlying wall is slightly thickened, but no distinct mass is seen, and the adjacent folds appear only minimally thickened

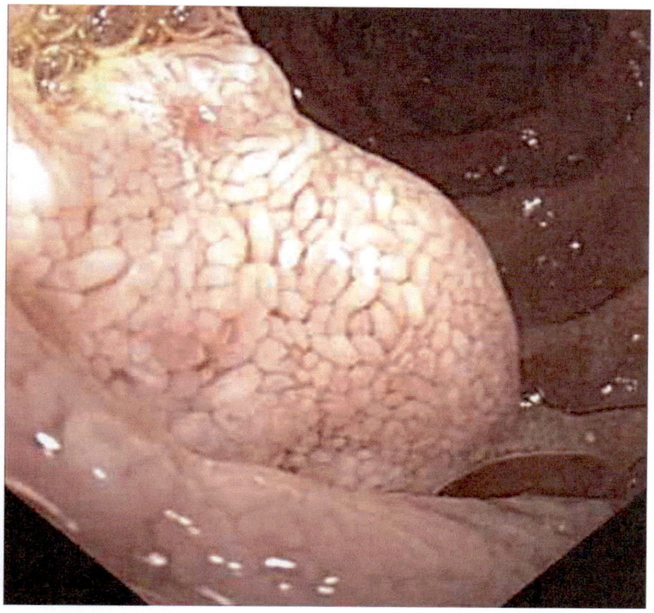

Fig. 6.5 Endoscopic appearance of the duodenum involved by follicular lymphoma, showing multiple tiny nodules instead of a single discrete mass. Most cases of follicular lymphoma in the intestines present in this manner [4]

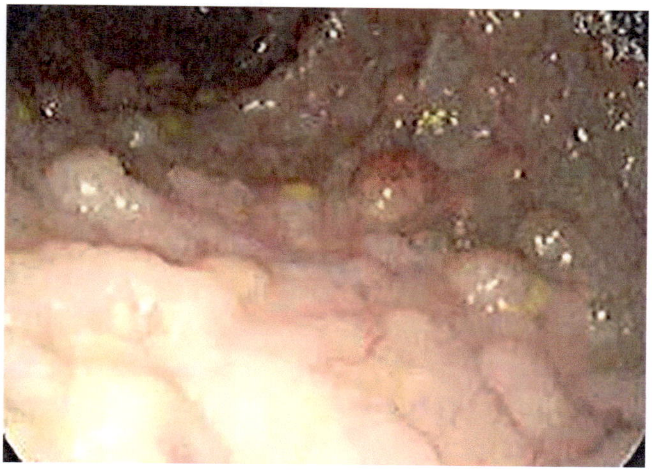

Fig. 6.6 Endoscopic appearance of the ascending colon showing numerous broad-based sessile polyps diffusely carpeting the entire large bowel (lymphomatoid polyposis), which turned out to be mantle cell lymphoma. Presentation with this appearance is most often seen with mantle cell lymphoma, but it is not specific; sometimes marginal zone and follicular lymphomas may present similarly

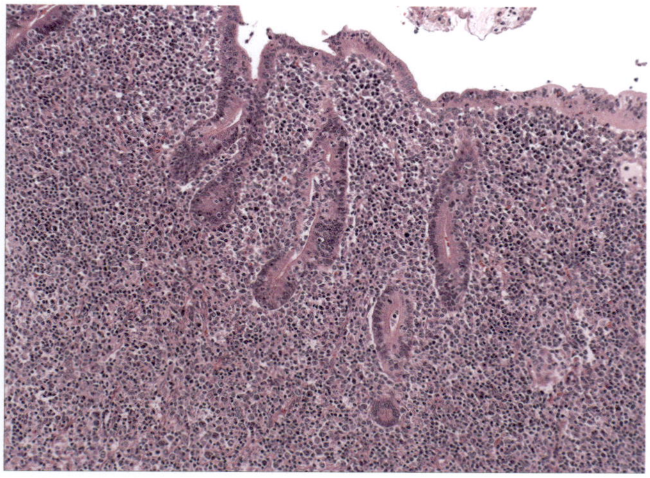

Fig. 6.7 Extranodal marginal zone lymphoma or lymphoma of mucosa-associated lymphoid tissue (MALT) of the small bowel. This medium-magnification view of the tumor shows infiltration of the lamina propria by a diffuse, polymorphic cell population composed of small lymphocytes, plasma cells, monocytoid B cells, and sparse eosinophils. Although the majority of the cells are B cells, there is often a population of admixed T cells that can be easily highlighted with immunostains. Note that the crypts are few, indicative of the expansile and destructive nature of the infiltrate. A cluster of monocytoid B-cells is seen infiltrating a crypt with reactive epithelial changes and forming a "lymphoepithelial lesion". These lesions are the characteristic histologic finding of MALT lymphomas ("MALTomas") of the GI tract, but are often sparse or absent in the small bowel and colonic lesions. IPSID is a variant of extranodal MALT lymphoma of the small bowel that is characterized by defective immunoglobulin formation, whereby the plasma cells secrete only the heavy alpha chains without the light chains (so it is also called *alpha heavy chain disease*). IPSID has been primarily described in young adults from the Middle East and has been attributed to an abnormal response to intestinal infection with *Campylobacter* species. It typically affects the proximal small bowel [5]. There has been a steady decline in its incidence, even in the Middle East

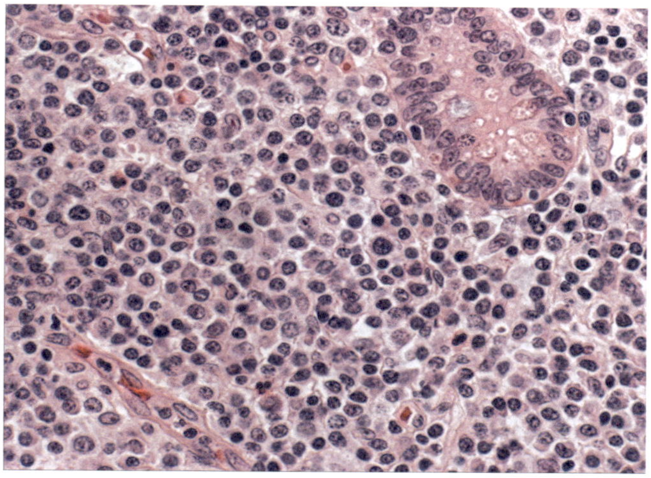

Fig. 6.8 Higher-magnification picture of a MALT lymphoma in the small intestine. Note the polymorphous appearance of the infiltrate with many lymphocytes and plasma cells. The immunophenotype of the tumor cells is a nonspecific B-cell phenotype with expression of CD20 and other pan-B-cell markers, and negativity for CD5, CD10, cyclin D1, and CD23. Neoplastic lymphocytes show surface clonal immunoglobulin, often but not exclusively surface immunoglobin M (sIgM)

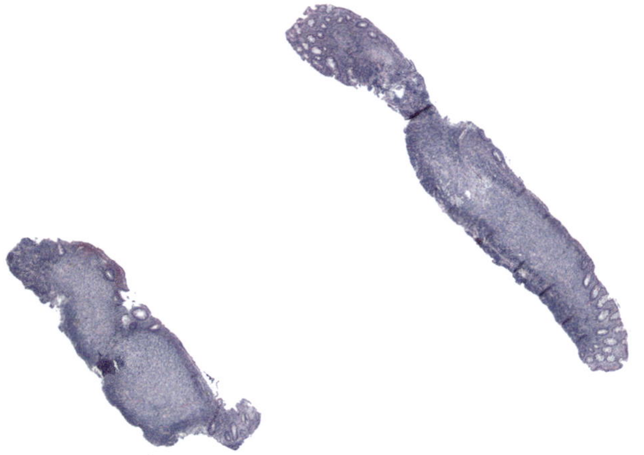

Fig. 6.9 Example of a colonic MALT lymphoma, which was identified during a screening colonoscopy as a small mucosal bump. Many such lesions are small and incidentally identified, and pose a diagnostic challenge. The lesion is characterized by infiltration of the lamina propria by a mixed population of small and medium-sized lymphocytes, some of which appear as monocytoid B cells. The infiltrate is often polymorphous and lacks a true germinal center, which can be appreciated at low power in this biopsy specimen. Sometimes residual germinal centers can be seen that have been overrun or infiltrated by neoplastic B cells. A few lymphoepithelial lesions are also seen, but these should not be taken as diagnostic of a lymphoma. The immunophenotype of these B cells is similar to their gastric and small-bowel counterparts, and is not specific. The diagnosis of such incidentally identified small lesions often requires incorporation of histology, immunophenotype, and molecular data

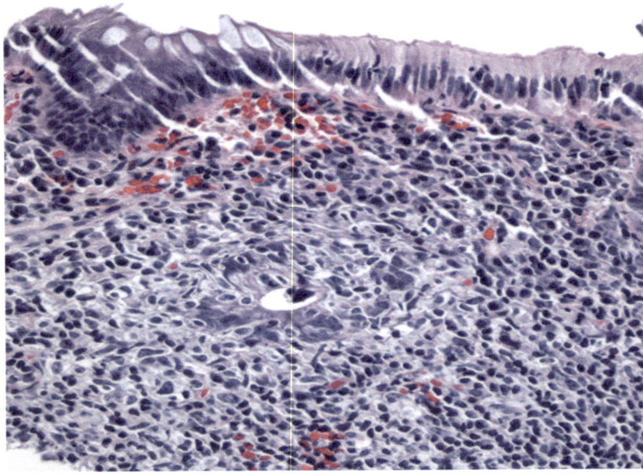

Fig. 6.10 Higher magnification of the same lesion as in Fig. 6.9, showing the monocytoid B cells and a few lymphoepithelial lesions. Note the intimate relationship of small lymphocytes traversing the columnar, reactive-appearing epithelial cells. The classic molecular alteration of t(11;18)(q21;21) *API2-MALT1*, encountered in a subset of gastric MALT lymphomas, is encountered infrequently in the intestinal variant [6]. The underlying etiology of most cases of intestinal MALT is still unknown, although some hypothesize that an as-yet-undiscovered infectious organism may be the culprit—similar to the role of *H. pylori* in gastric MALT or *C. jejuni* in IPSID. There are no standardized treatment guidelines, but intestinal MALT lymphomas are generally indolent [7]

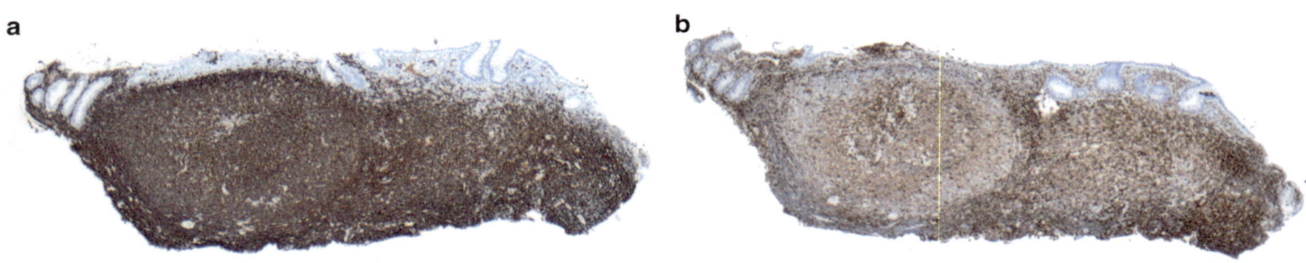

Fig. 6.11 Colonic MALT lymphoma showing the infiltrate to be positive for B-cell markers CD20 (**a**) and CD43 (**b**). A sprinkling of T cells is often present, as highlighted with CD3 and CD5. The neoplastic B cells are negative for BCL-2, CD10 and CD5

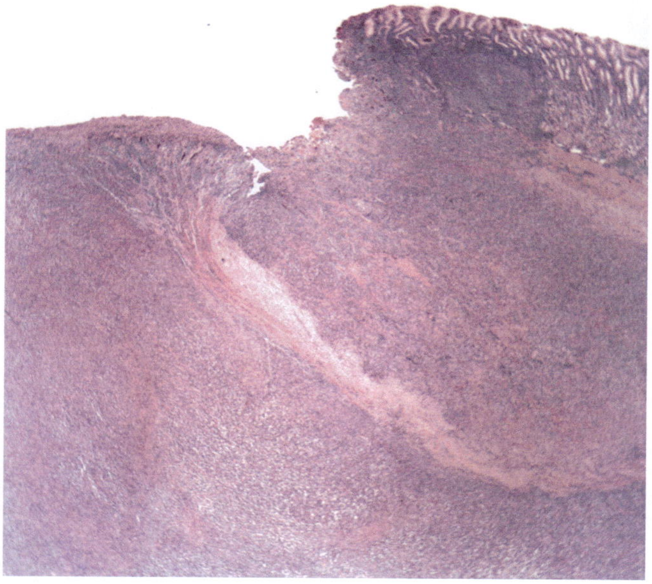

Fig. 6.12 Example of a DLBCL involving the small bowel, showing diffuse involvement of all layers of the intestinal wall (mucosa, submucosa, and circular and longitudinal muscle) by a monomorphic lymphocytic population. This is the same lesion shown in Fig. 6.2

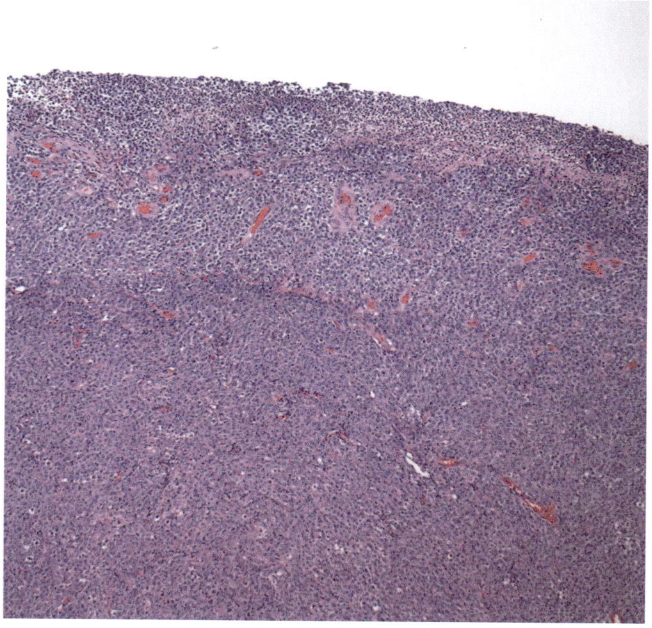

Fig. 6.13 Higher magnification of the same tumor, showing large lymphocytes with high nucleus-to-cytoplasm (N:C) ratio and prominent nucleoli. These cells intersect muscular fibers with scant desmoplastic response. DLBCL of intestines tends to express a germinal center–like immunophenotype (CD10+, BCL6+, MUM1-) [8]. These lymphomas are more likely than their gastric counterparts to develop several adverse prognostic events [9]

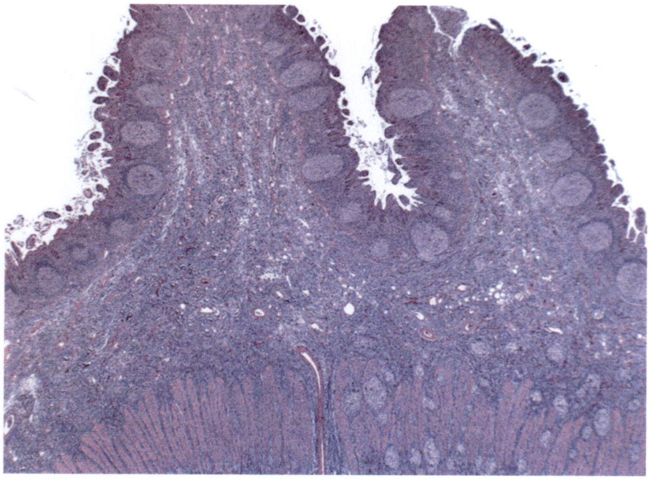

Fig. 6.14 Follicular lymphomas in the intestine can present as multiple nodular lesions or a single mass lesion. These are quite rare in the intestines (representing about 3% of intestinal lymphoma cases). In the intestines, they most commonly occur in the duodenum, especially in the periampullary region [10, 11]. Follicular lymphoma involving small intestine with a transmural lymphoid infiltrate is shown. The formation of follicles is obvious even at this low magnification. Once the lymphomas transform or become diffuse, the follicular architecture may be lost

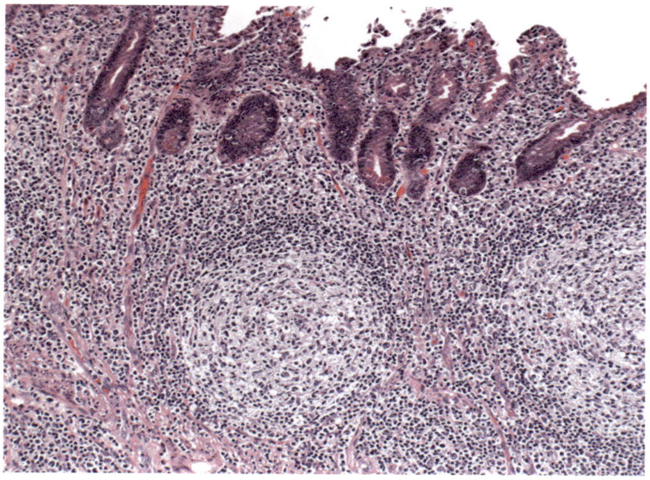

Fig. 6.15 Higher magnification of the neoplastic follicles in the follicular lymphoma, showing lack of a well-formed mantle zone and absence of tingible body macrophages in the germinal center. Tumor cells are monomorphic and disrupt the normal polarized histology of the germinal centers. Most are centrocytes, with a few admixed centroblasts. Most intestinal follicular lymphomas are of low grade, with a higher proportion of centrocytes

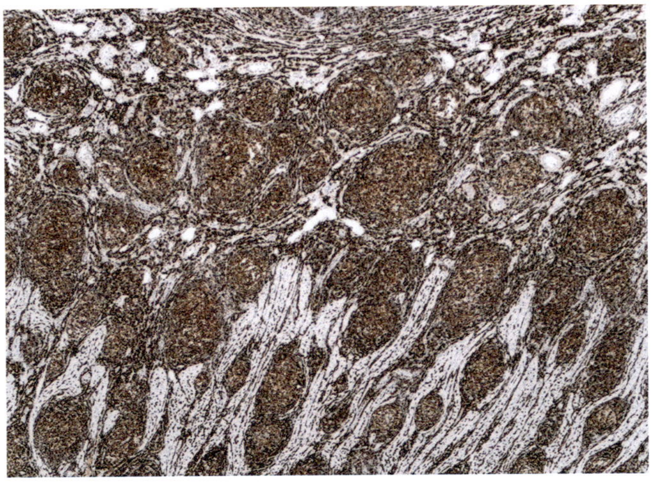

Fig. 6.16 Neoplastic follicles of the tumor shown in Fig. 6.15 diffusely express BCL-2, as shown here

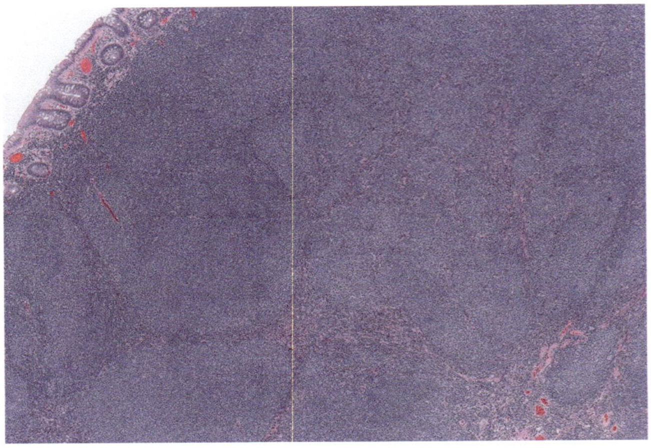

Fig. 6.18 Colonic follicular lymphoma. This higher-power examination of Fig. 6.17 shows diffuse infiltration of the colonic muscular wall by the infiltrating neoplastic lymphocytes, forming vague follicles

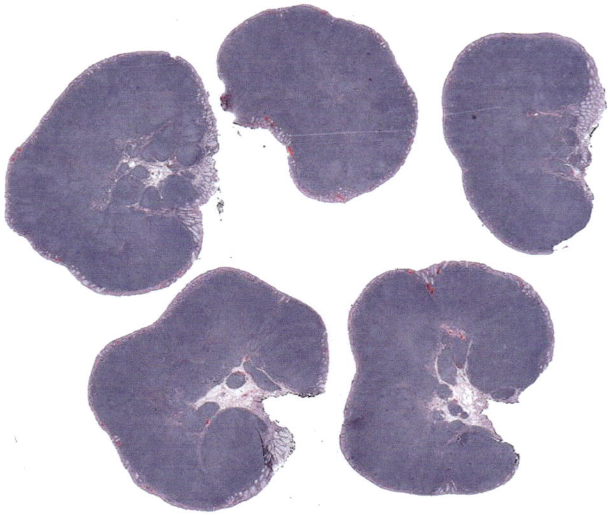

Fig. 6.17 Colonic follicular lymphoma. Follicular lymphoma rarely arises in the colon; when it does, it demonstrates an indolent clinical phenotype [12]. Low-power examination again shows a diffusely nodular appearance of the "small blue" lymphocytes, here below relatively preserved colonic mucosa. The follicles are less conspicuous than in the small-intestinal case illustrated in Fig. 6.14

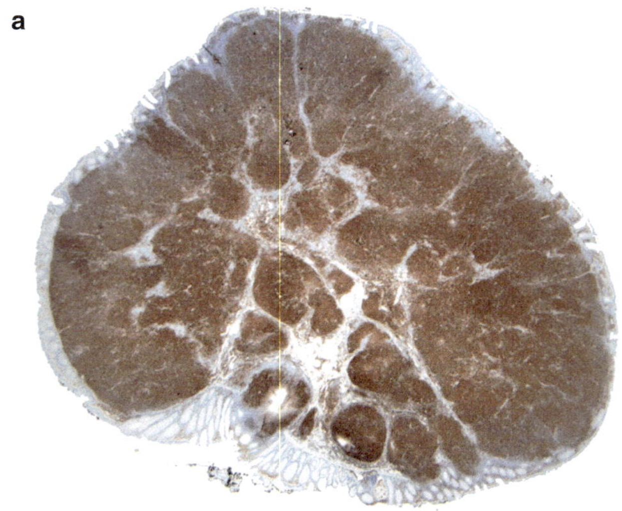

Fig. 6.19 The immunophenotype of colonic follicular lymphomas is similar to its small-intestinal and nodal counterparts, with CD20, CD10 (**a**) and BCL-2 (**b**) positivity, including the cells in the center of the follicles, and lack of expression of CD3 (**c**) and CD5. Similar to the nodal type, the t(14;18) (q32;q21) *IgH/bcl2* is highly prevalent by molecular analysis [4, 12]

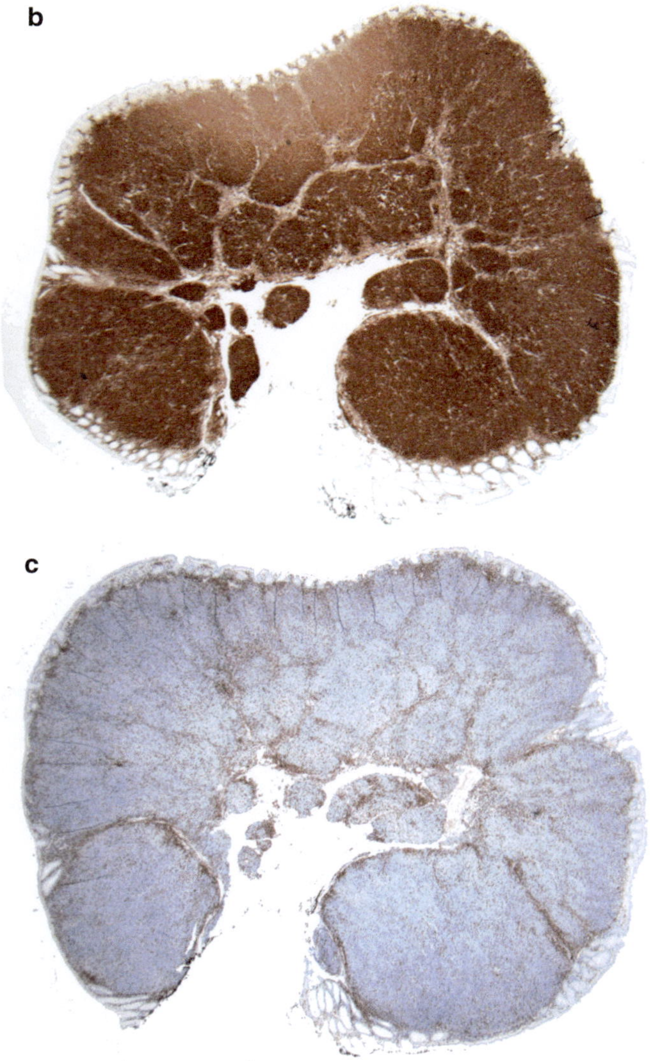

Fig. 6.19 (continued)

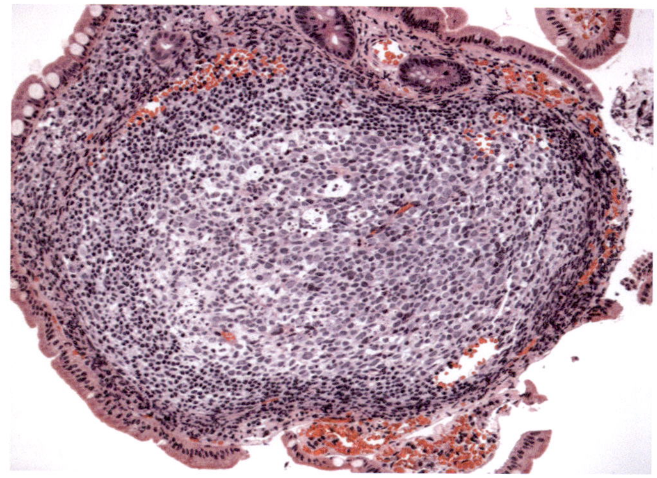

Fig. 6.20 A reactive follicle in a small-bowel biopsy is shown here for comparison. In contrast to the morphology of follicular lymphoma, there is a well-formed mantle and a marginal zone. In addition, numerous tingible-body macrophages are seen in the reactive germinal center, imparting a "starry-sky" appearance. Compared with Fig. 1.15, the cells in this germinal center are polymorphic. Immunohistochemistry (IHC) shows expression of BCL-2 in the marginal zone and lack of expression in the center of the follicles

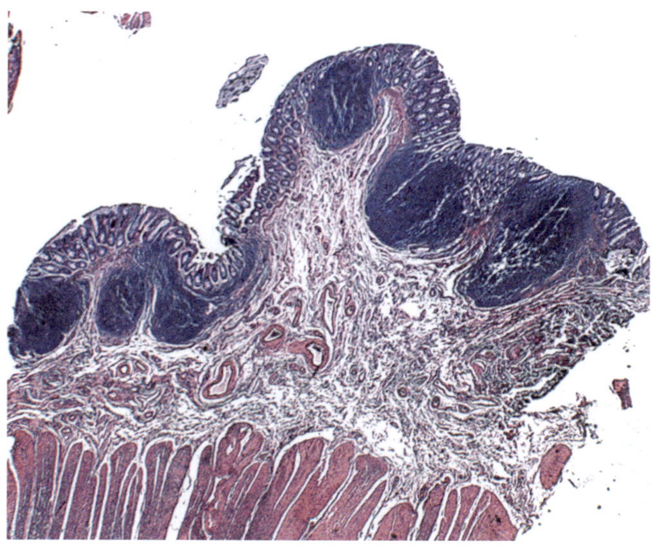

Fig. 6.21 Mantle cell lymphoma (MCL) of the colon presenting as polyposis. Numerous small lymphoid nodules as seen here can be grossly mistaken for sessile polyps and an epithelial polyposis syndrome (*see* Fig. 6.6). This is the classic, albeit not exclusive, appearance of intestinal mantle cell lymphoma [13]

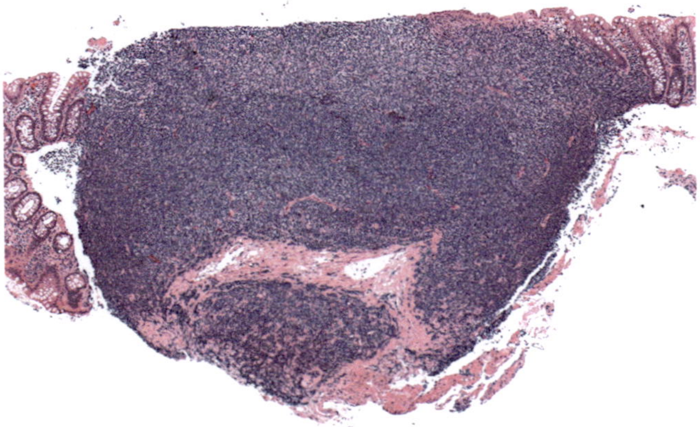

Fig. 6.22 The "polyps" consist of focal areas of lamina propria expanded by aggregates of neoplastic lymphocytes, which often also extend into the submucosa

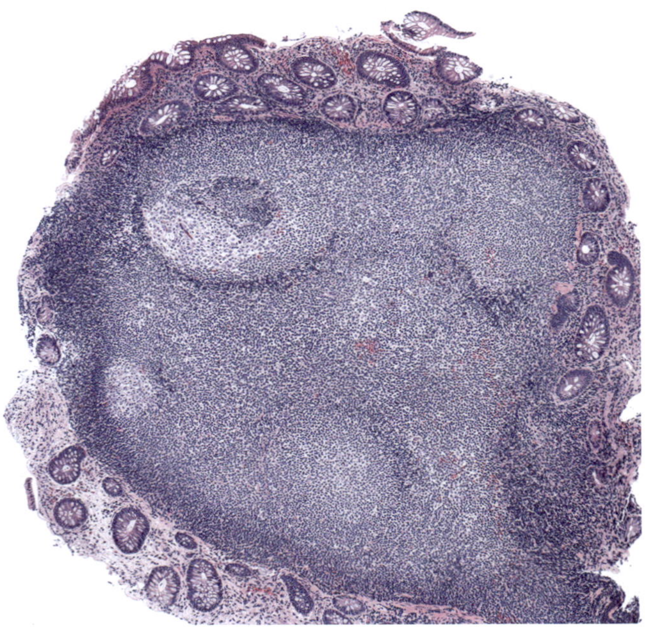

Fig. 6.23 On hematoxylin and eosin (H&E) stain, a classic appearance of expanded, confluent mantle zones is sometimes seen, as shown here

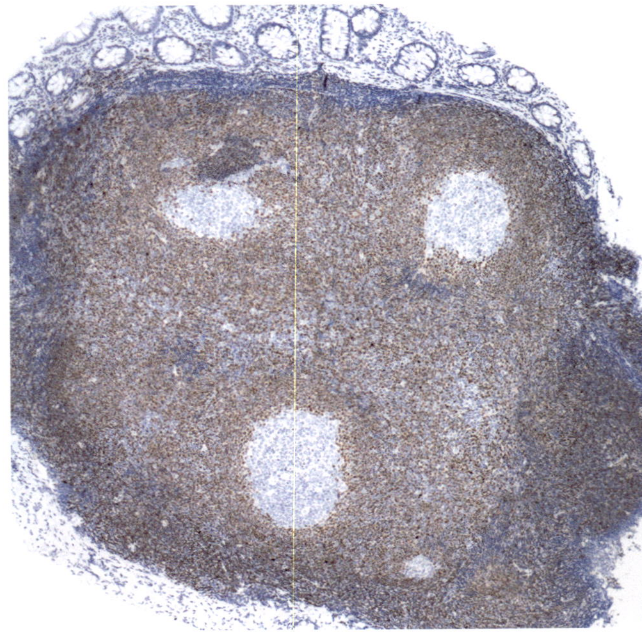

Fig. 6.24 Tumor cells of MCL express CD20 and CD5 and overexpress cyclin D1 as a result of t(11;14)(q13;q32) *CCND1:IgH*. Shown here is a cyclin D1 immunostain, with positivity in the expanded, submucosal neoplastic mantle zone. Distinction from small lymphocytic lymphoma (also CD5-positive) is important, as MCL portends a much worse prognosis

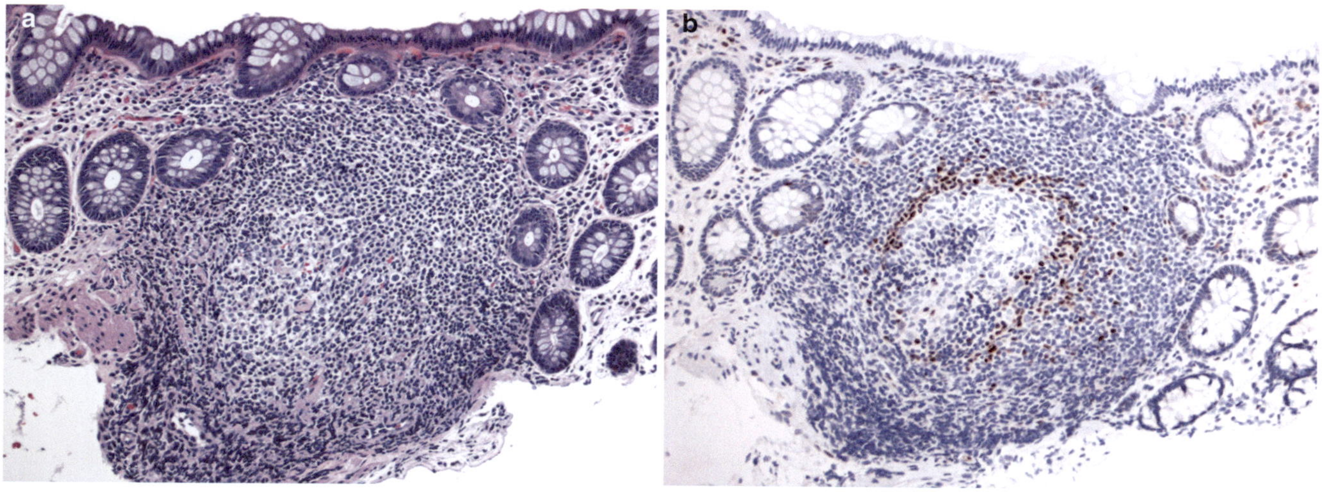

Fig. 6.25 MCL in situ. In occasional cases with prominent mantle zones (**a**), cyclin D1 IHC (**b**) will highlight clusters of B cells in the reactive follicle. Studies show that patients with these findings generally follow a benign clinical course not requiring treatment, but they must be followed carefully for possible development of lymphoma in the future [14, 15]. This finding can also be seen in some patients with systemic or nodal MCL, suggesting subtle GI tract involvement, though it is still called "MCL in situ"

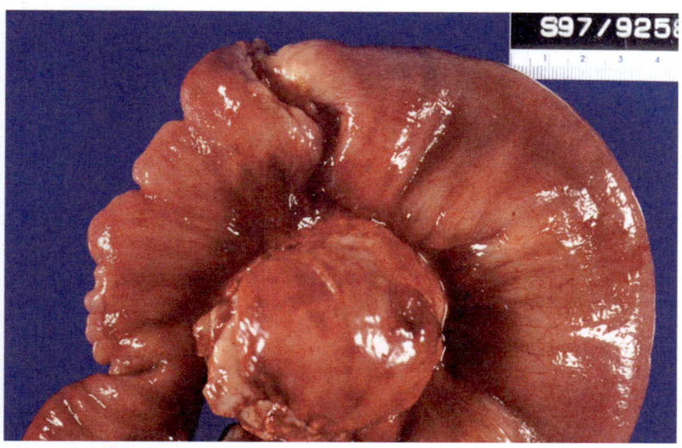

Fig. 6.26 Gross image of a case of Burkitt lymphoma that presented with intussusception. The second most common site of presentation of Burkitt lymphoma is the GI tract. Severe abdominal pain, bleeding, or acute abdomen are classic presentations of this aggressive neoplasm, particularly in children [16]. Intussusception, as shown in this image, can occur because of projection of the tumor mass into the gut lumen

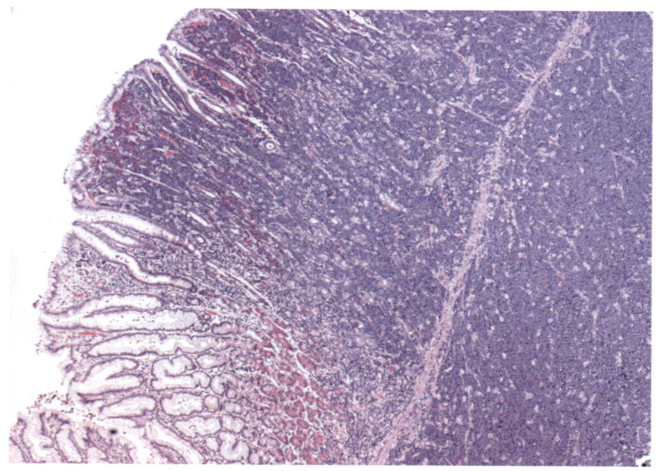

Fig. 6.27 Low magnification of a Burkitt lymphoma, showing a tight aggregate of medium-sized lymphocytes with numerous mitoses, apoptotic cells, and tingible-body macrophages (giving the "starry-sky" appearance). This entity is the most common pediatric intestinal non-Hodgkin lymphoma and can be split epidemiologically into endemic and sporadic cases, and cases in immunodeficient patients

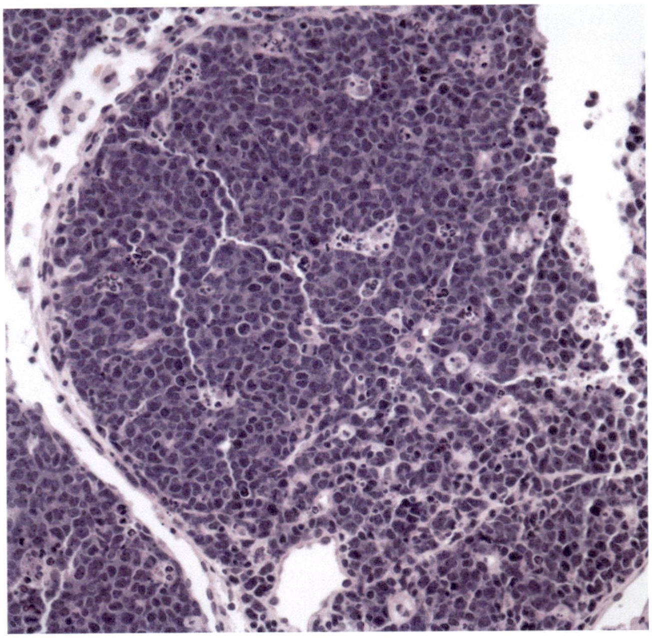

Fig. 6.28 High-power view of Burkitt lymphoma. Tumor cells are medium-sized and demonstrate a high N:C ratio with occasional nucleoli. Individual mitoses and tingible-body macrophages can be appreciated at this power. Although the tumors are very biologically aggressive, the rapidly dividing cells of Burkitt lymphoma are typically quite sensitive to chemotherapy, and high 5-year survival rates have been achieved. Care must be taken to avoid the tumor lysis syndrome [17]

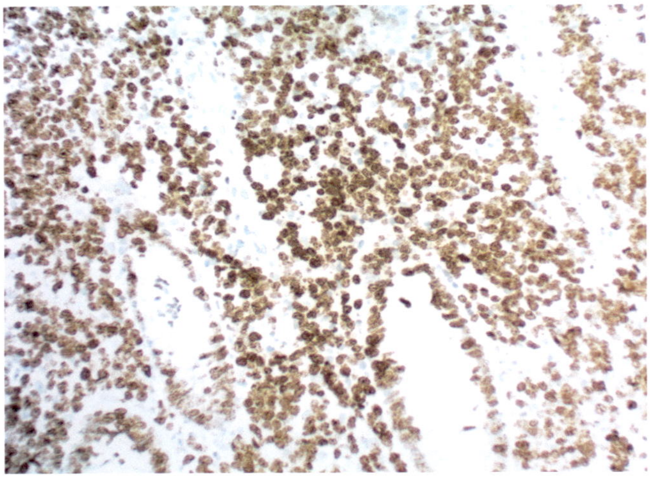

Fig. 6.29 Burkitt lymphoma typically shows a very high Ki-67 index (90–100%), indicative of very rapidly dividing tumor cells. Molecular confirmation can be performed with polymerase chain reaction (PCR) for t(8;14)

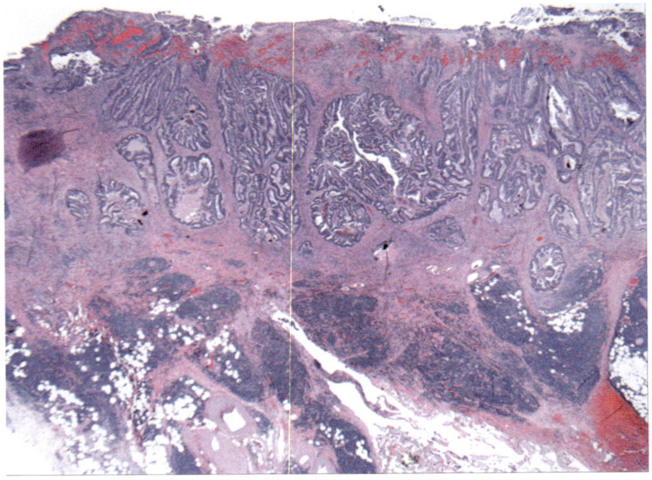

Fig. 6.30 The intestines are rarely involved by small lymphocytic lymphoma (SLL)/chronic lymphocytic leukemia (CLL), which sometimes is detected incidentally in resections performed for other reasons, such as diverticular disease or carcinoma. This image shows a proliferation of small monomorphic lymphocytes in the muscular portion of the bowel wall, subjacent to an adenocarcinoma. The disease can sometimes also be encountered incidentally in an adjacent lymph node in such resection specimens. SLL typically occurs in middle-aged to older adults

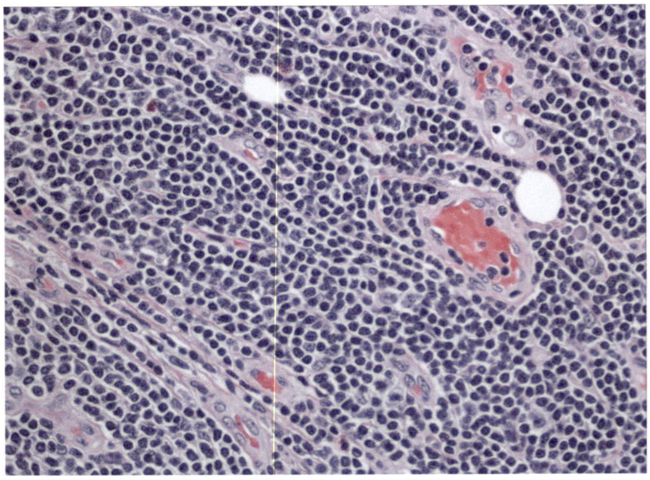

Fig. 6.31 Higher magnification of an SLL showing small, monomorphic lymphocytes with hyperchromatic nuclei with coarsely clumped chromatin. When it is the cause of presentation, SLL has usually undergone high-grade transformation to DLBCL or MCL

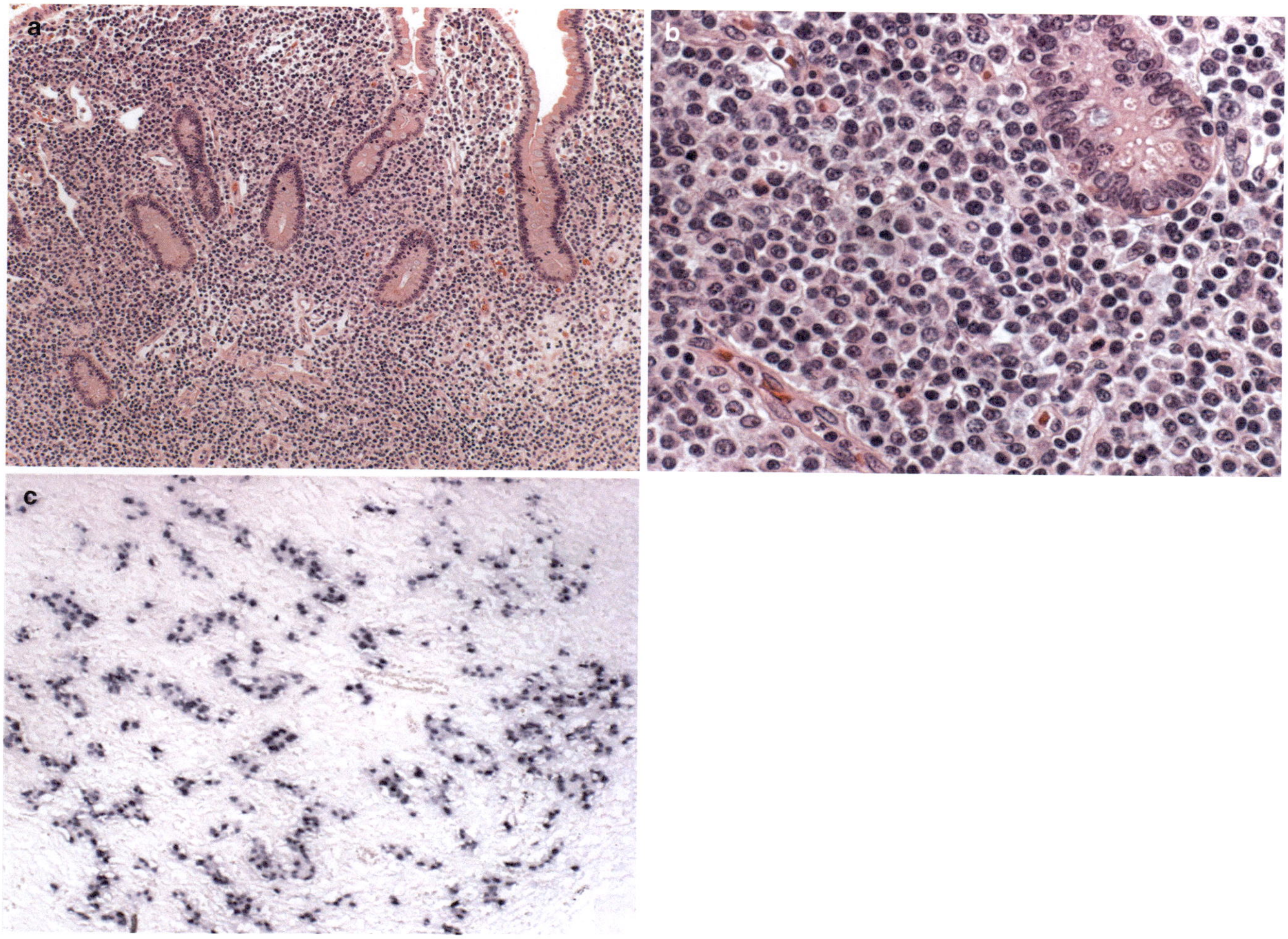

Fig. 6.32 Post-transplant lymphoproliferative disorder (PTLD). PTLD can be divided among monomorphic and polymorphic microscopic phenotypes. These images show a polymorphic type. Often the infiltrate is dense and expansile (**a**), a finding that should raise concern in the post-transplantation setting. The infiltrate is an admixture of small lymphocytes, plasma cells, immunoblasts, and eosinophils, and tends to mimic an inflammatory process (**b**). Most PTLD cases are associated with reactivation of the Epstein-Barr virus (EBV) in carriers [18]. This fact is important because detecting EBV, either by Epstein-Barr encoded RNA (EBER) on tissue (**c**) or by PCR in blood, can have treatment implications. EBV-positive tumors may be treated with a reduction in immunosuppression, allowing for an adequate T-cytotoxic response against infected B cells [19]

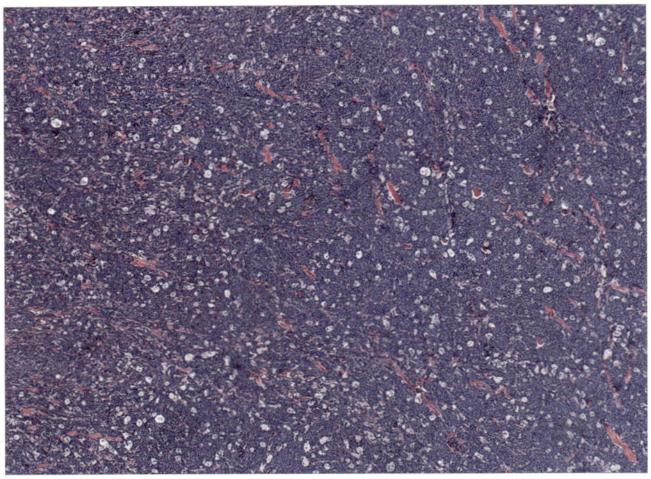

Fig. 6.33 Post-transplant lymphoproliferative disorder (PTLD), monomorphic type. This type of PTLD can take the form of any other lymphoma comprising monomorphic cells, most often DLBCL. This case of monomorphic lymphoma demonstrates the phenotype of a Burkitt lymphoma, with a very high mitotic count and numerous apoptotic bodies

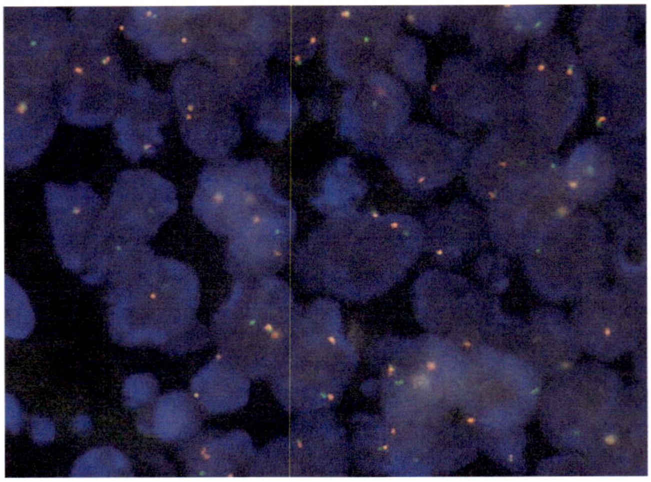

Fig. 6.34 Monomorphic PTLD of the Burkitt type, showing C-Myc rearrangement on fluorescence in situ hybridization (FISH) that is similar to sporadic Burkitt lymphoma with t(8;14). Other types of monomorphic lymphomas may also show immunophenotype and molecular abnormalities typical of the variant in a non-transplant setting. This case was also positive for EBER

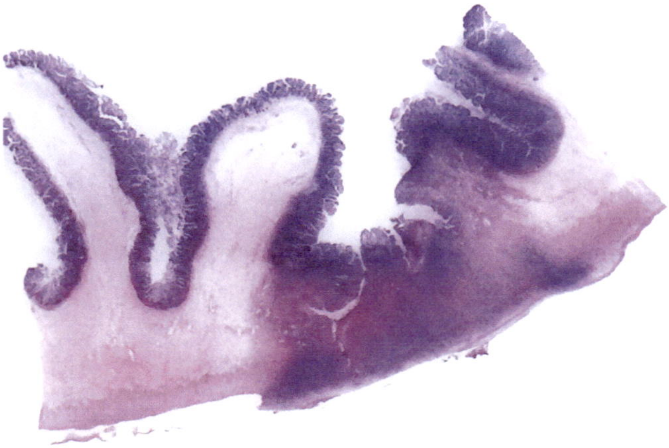

Fig. 6.35 Low magnification of enteropathy-associated T-cell lymphoma (EATL), showing a diffuse, polymorphous lymphocytic transmural infiltrate with ulceration that led to perforation. Note that the adjacent uninvolved mucosa shows changes of celiac disease (enteropathy). This is a highly aggressive tumor, with multifocality and dissemination being common features at presentation [20]. (*Courtesy of* Dr. Harold Sanchez; Bridgeport Hospital, Bridgeport, CT, USA.)

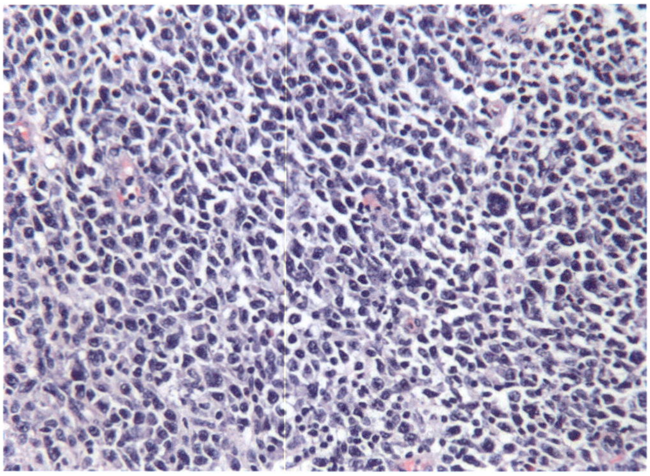

Fig. 6.36 Higher magnification of the same case, showing the diffuse, polymorphous lymphocytic infiltrate in the lamina propria, consisting of small lymphocytes, large immunoblast-like cells, plasma cells, and a few eosinophils. The immunophenotype typical of EATL is CD3+, CD7+, CD5-, CD8- (abnormal T-cell phenotype). Cases are almost always negative for EBER, a feature that can be used to distinguish EATL (types I or II) from disseminated extranodal NK/T-cell lymphoma. (*Courtesy of* Dr. Harold Sanchez.)

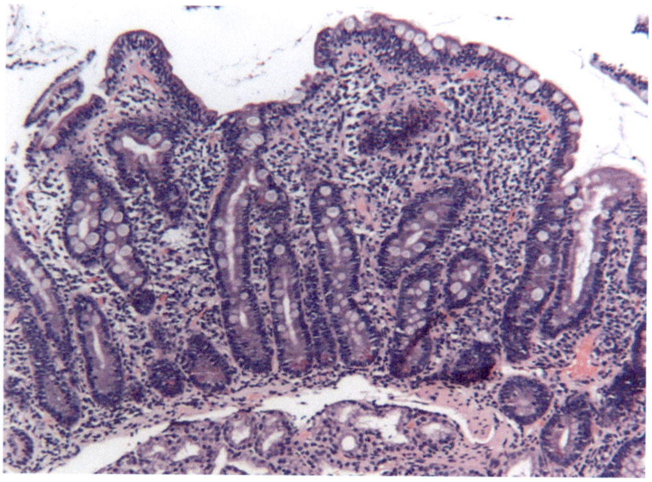

Fig. 6.37 Higher magnification of the adjacent mucosa, showing histologic changes associated with celiac disease, with villous blunting, crypt hyperplasia, increased intraepithelial lymphocytes (IELs), and lamina propria lymphoplasmacytic infiltrate. Celiac disease precedes the diagnosis of lymphoma by many years in most cases. In some patients, the diagnosis of celiac disease is made at the same time as the lymphoma, whereas others have only celiac-associated HLA phenotype or dermatitis herpetiformis [20]. (*Courtesy of* Dr. Harold Sanchez.)

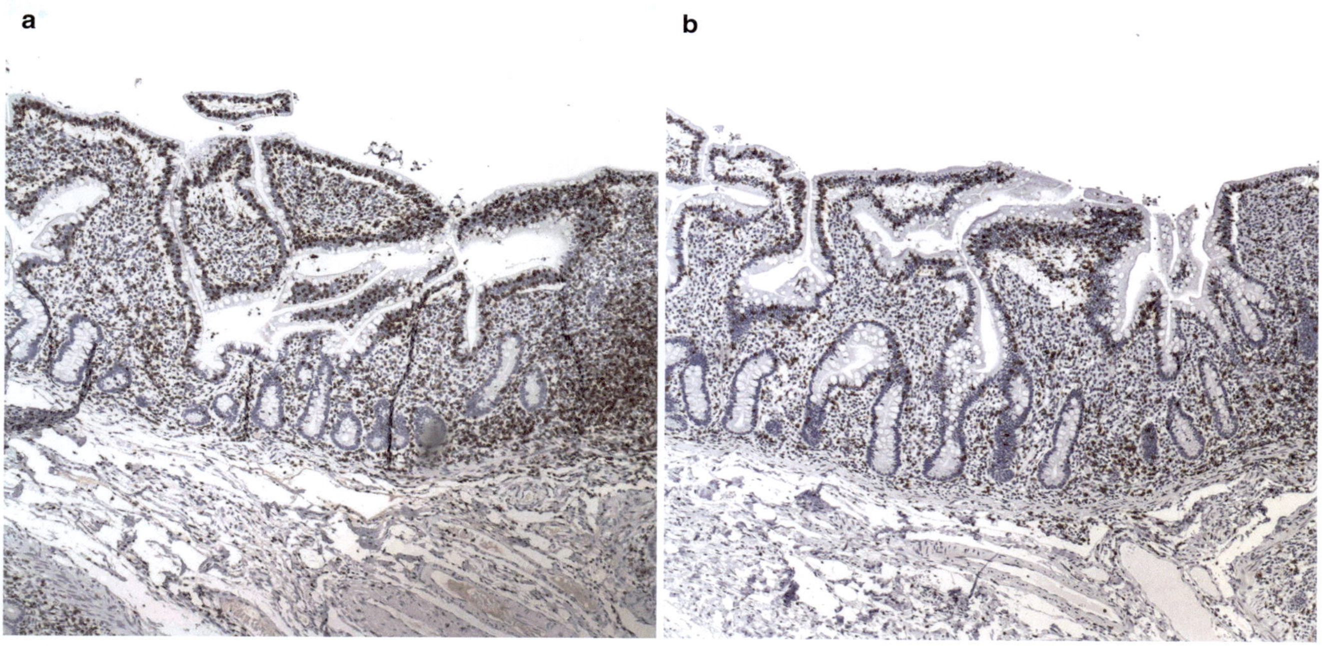

Fig. 6.38 The adjacent mucosa with enteropathy-type changes may show IELs that share the same phenotype as the EATL cells, with positivity for CD3+ (**a**) and loss of CD8 expression (**b**). (*See also* Fig. 6.39.) In contrast to type I EATL, type II is characterized by a proliferation of small monomorphic lymphocytes, is not associated with celiac disease, and is seen primarily in Asians. Type II EATL has recently been reclassified as monomorphic T-cell lymphoma. (*Courtesy of* Dr. Harold Sanchez.)

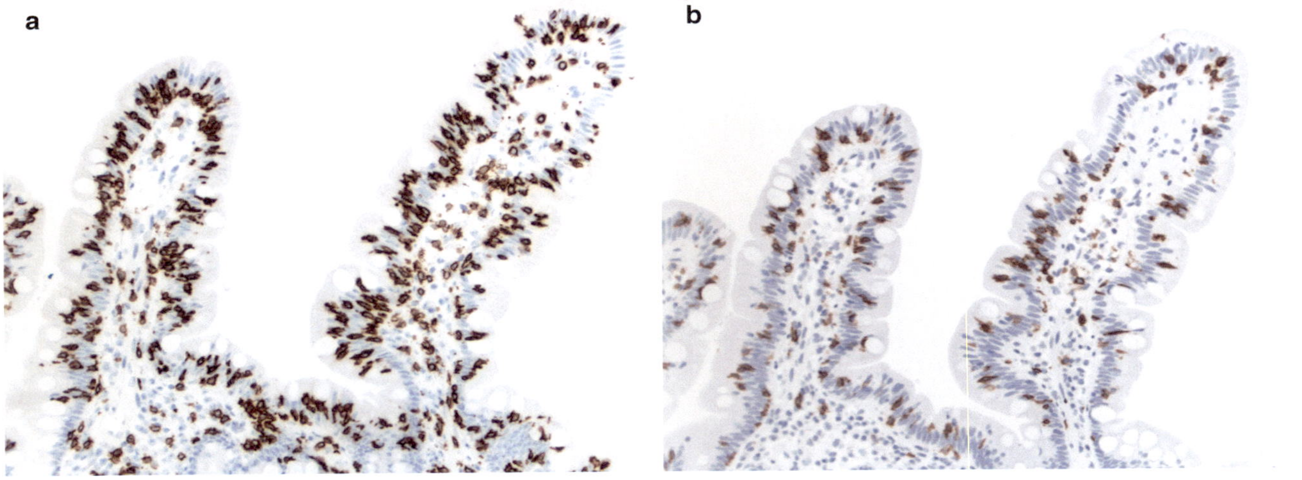

Fig. 6.39 Development of refractory celiac disease (RCD), which is resistant to a gluten-free diet, may precede progression to EATL in some cases. These images show examples of RCD. This entity is divided into two types. Type I is characterized by continued symptoms despite a gluten-free diet, with enteropathy and intra-epithelial lymphocytes (IELs) demonstrating a normal T-cell immunophenotype. Type II exhibits aberrant T-cell immunophenotyping of the IELs. The distinction between these two is prognostically important, as Type II is more likely to progress to EATL [21]. IHC shows IELs that express CD3 (**a**) but have lost CD8 expression (**b**)

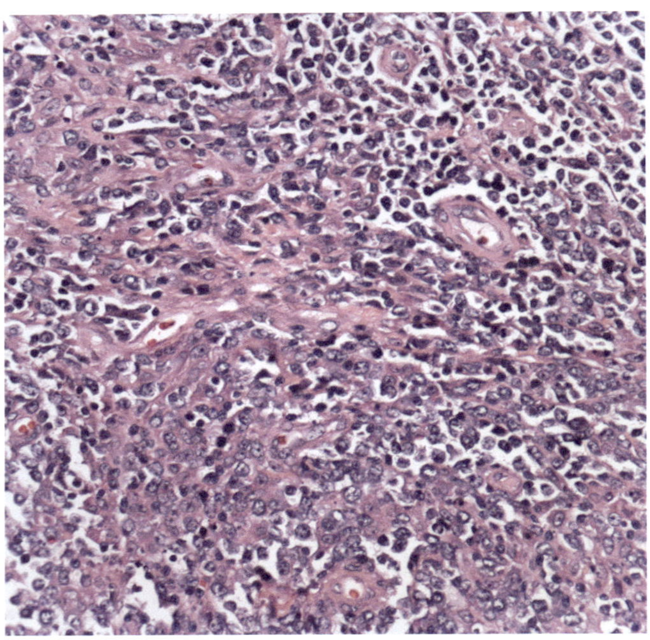

Fig. 6.40 Some enteropathy-associated lymphomas are B-cell lymphomas, as shown here. High magnification shows features that are compatible with a diffuse large B-cell lymphoma (DLBCL), with large cells demonstrating high N:C ratios. The cells were positive for CD20, with an otherwise nonspecific immunophenotype. Indeed, celiac disease has been linked to increased rates of numerous B-cell non-Hodgkin lymphomas (both GI and extraintestinal) [22]

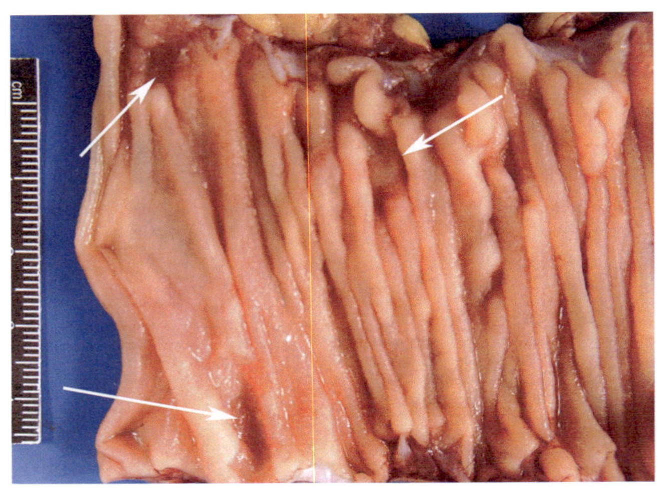

Fig. 6.41 Ulcerative jejunitis. Another complication of celiac disease, ulcerative jejunitis presents with small ulcers in the jejunum/ileum. This gross photograph of a small bowel resection shows a few bland ulcers (*arrows*) without any discrete mass or wall thickening. The gross appearance is deceptively benign, but has been shown to be a manifestation of EATL [23]

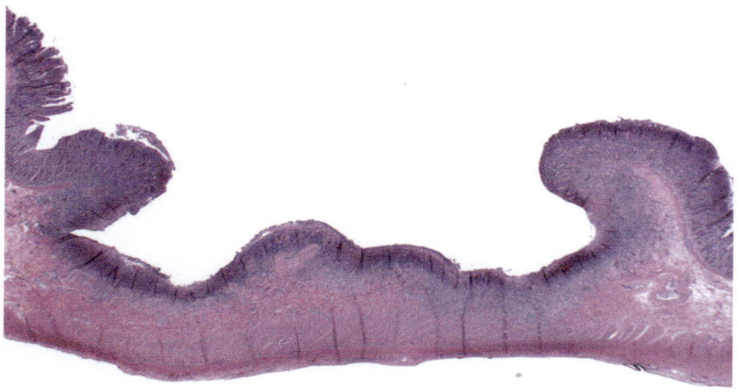

Fig. 6.42 Histology of ulcerative jejunitis, showing a deep ulcer with a dense, polymorphic cell population at the ulcer base at low magnification

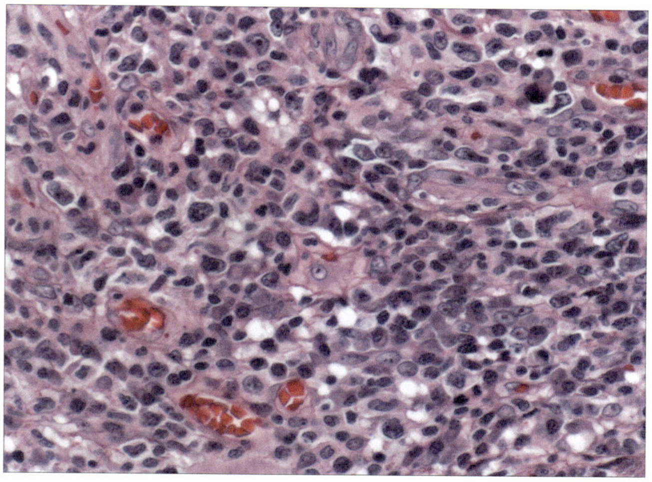

Fig. 6.43 Higher magnification shows a polymorphic lymphoid population with small cells admixed with larger cells and rare bizarre lymphoid cells in the background

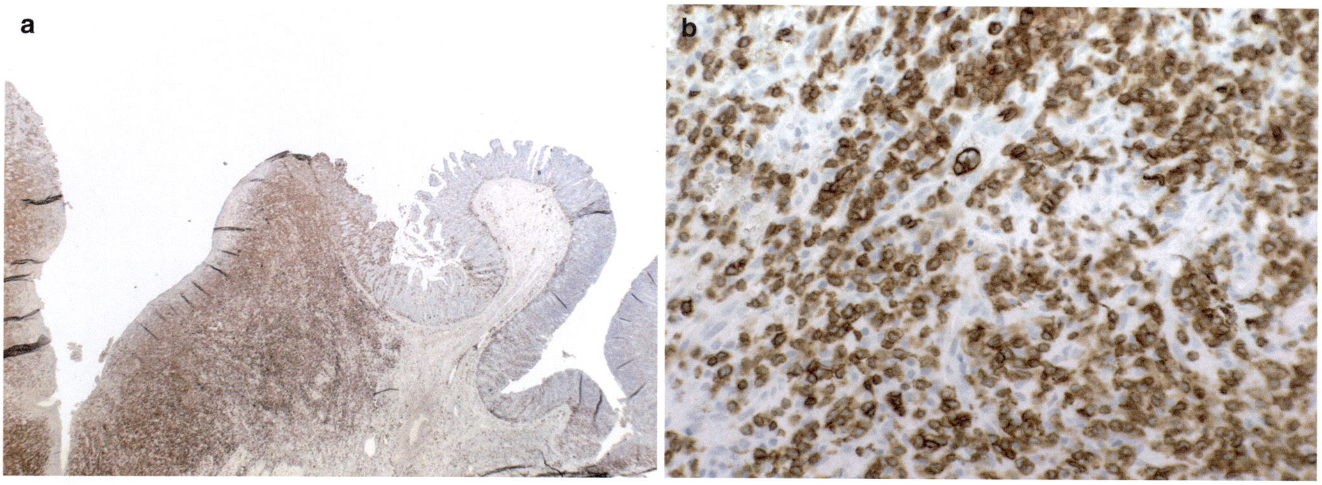

Fig. 6.44 Immunostain (CD3) reveals almost the entire infiltrate to be T cells (**a**). Higher magnification of CD3 immunostain shows that the larger cells are also CD3+ T cells (**b**). The mucosa adjacent to the ulcer shows features of enteropathy, although in this case the patient had no evidence of celiac disease. The monoclonal nature of the T cell can invariably be demonstrated with T-cell receptor (TCR) gene rearrangement, as in this case

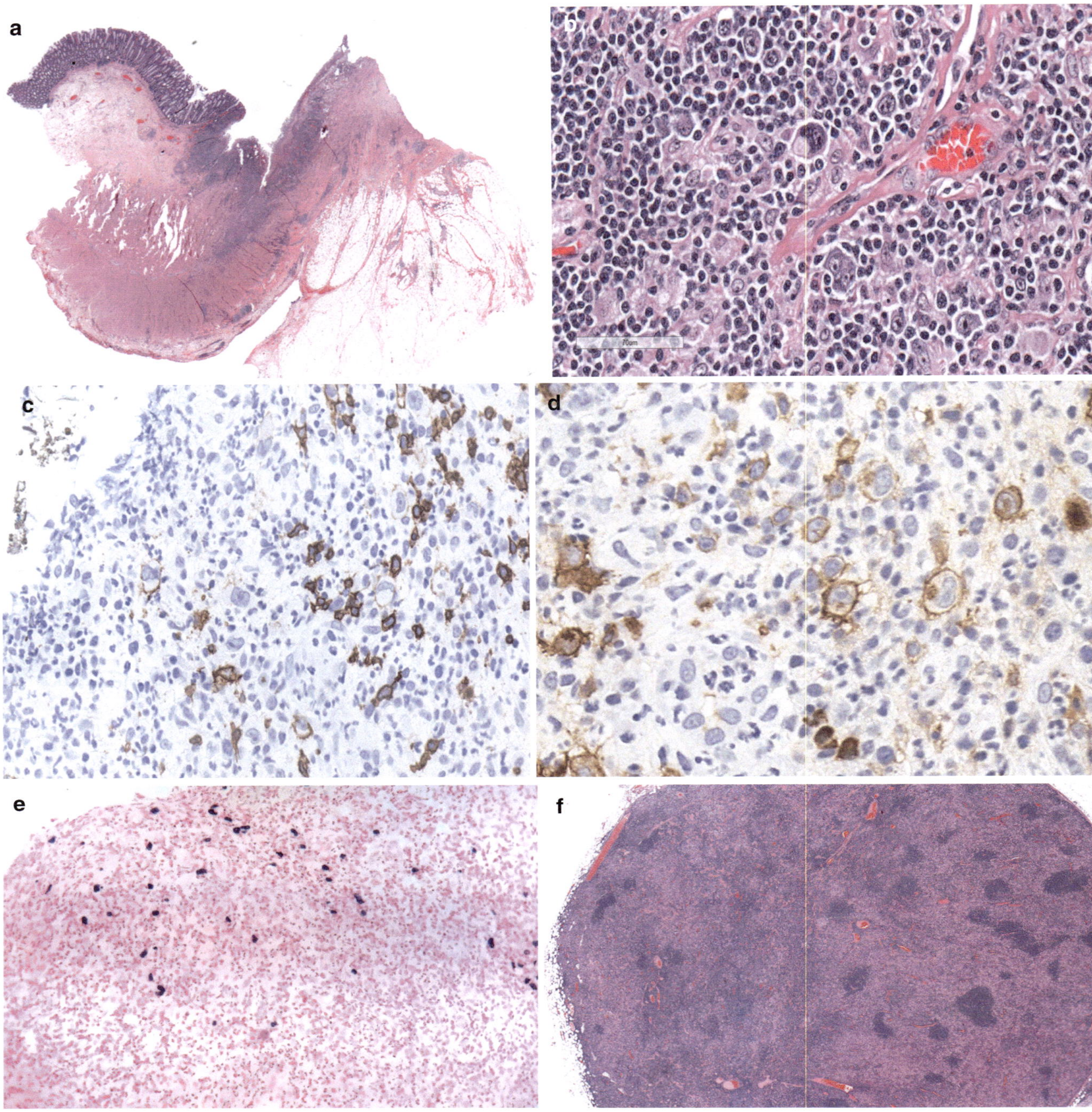

Fig. 6.45 EBV-associated B-cell lymphoproliferative disease with Hodgkin's-like features. (**a**) Low magnification shows a diffuse transmural infiltrate in this rectal resection from a 78-year-old man. (**b**) On higher magnification, the infiltrate is polymorphous and comprises mixed inflammatory infiltrate consisting of scattered large cells resembling Reed-Sternberg (RS) cells, as well as histiocytes, lymphocytes, plasma cells, and eosinophils. (**c**) and (**d**) The large RS-like cells are positive for CD20 (**c**), CD15, CD30 (**d**), and Mum1. (**e**) There is EBER positivity in scattered cells, including the large B cells and RS-like cells. (**f**) The lymph nodes were involved in this case and showed similar findings. The differential diagnosis includes Hodgkin disease and EBV-associated mucocutaneous ulcer of the elderly. The mimicry with Hodgkin disease is obvious with the presence of RS-like cells, although with recognition of Hodgkin disease as mostly B-cell lymphomas, this separation seems like another "grey zone" in the field of lymphomas. These typically occur in the elderly and in some cases the morphology is of a DLBCL with EBV positivity. The proper classification and nomenclature of these lymphomas is still evolving. The overlap with PTLD is also obvious. The possibility of an underlying immunodeficiency should always be excluded [24]

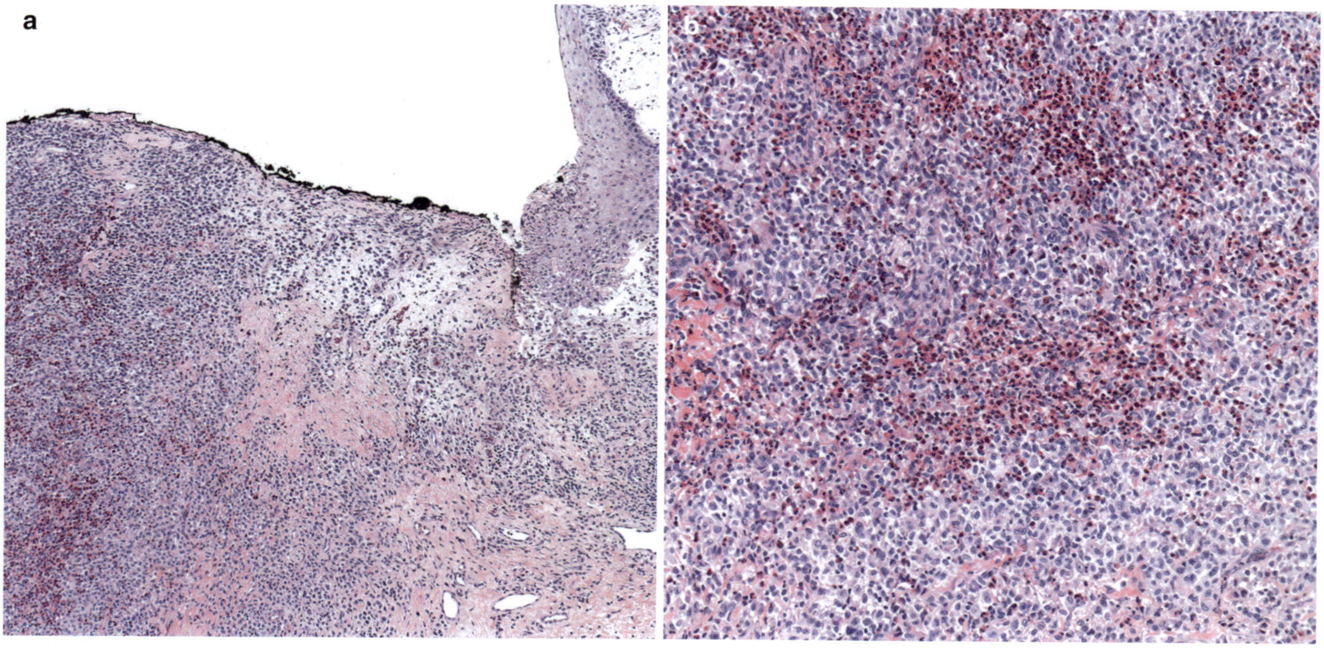

Fig. 6.46 Peri-anal Langerhans cell histiocytosis. This rare entity involves multiple tissues and organ types. Recently, it has been reported as a potential cause of peri-anal fistulas [25]. This case shows surface anal ulceration (**a**) and underlying mixed inflammatory infiltrate characterized (on higher power, **b**) by a proliferation of Langerhans cells demonstrating nuclear grooves and a moderate amount of amphophilic cytoplasm, as well as abundant accompanying eosinophils ("eosinophilic granuloma"). The neoplastic cells can be highlighted with a CD1a stain. The classic finding is of so-called Birbeck granules in the cytoplasm, seen by electron microscopy

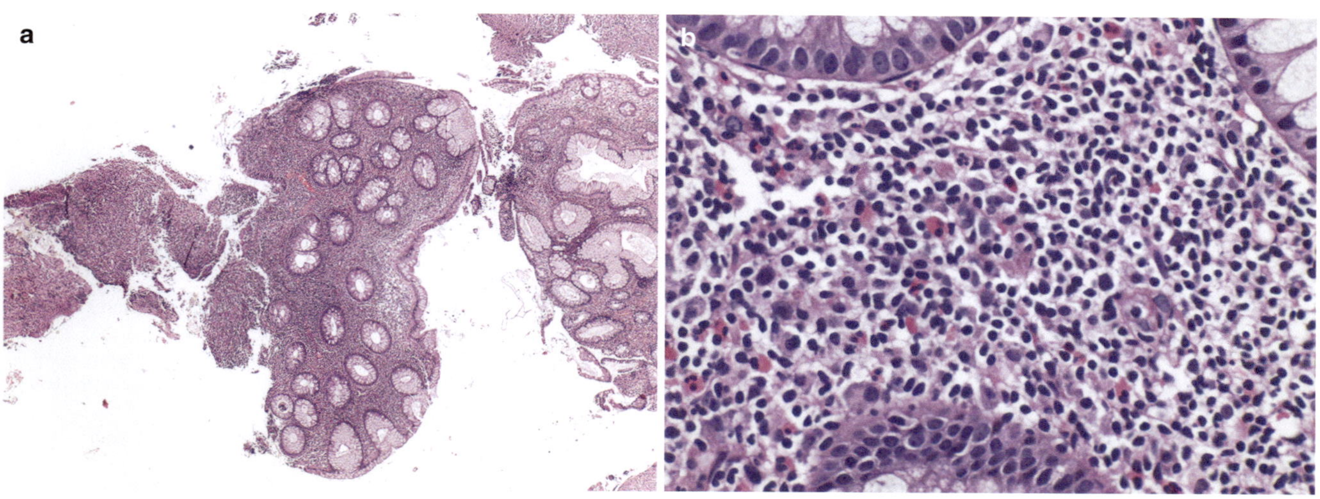

Fig. 6.47 Indolent T-cell lymphoproliferative disease of the GI tract. This 71-year-old man carried a diagnosis of ulcerative colitis and was found to have multiple raised mucosal lesions; biopsies were performed. (**a**) Low magnification shows expansion of the lamina propria by a dense lymphocytic population. (**b**) Lesional cells characteristically demonstrate eosinophilic cytoplasmic granules on higher power. (**c**) By immunophenotyping, cells were CD3+. They were also CD5-, CD7-, CD4-/CD8-, and showed rearranged T-cell receptor (TCR) gene. (**d**) The proliferative activity as shown with MIB stain was low. This patient showed persistence of the lesions (limited to the colon) over the course of 10 years despite no treatment for lymphoma. The cell of origin remains unidentified but is likely related to mucosa-associated γδT-cells. This rare disorder shows overlap with NK-cell enteropathy; both are indolent lymphoproliferative disorders of unclear nature. NK-cell enteropathy may involve multiple sites in the GI tract and may present similarly with ulceration, polyps, or mucosal thickening. The infiltrate has a phenotype consistent with NK cells (CD3+, CD5-, CD7+, CD4-, CD8-, CD56+, cytotoxic granules+) and possibly represent γδT cells. The TCR is not rearranged and EBV is negative. The infiltrate may persist despite chemotherapy and sometimes regresses spontaneously [26–28]. (*Courtesy of* Dr. Jay Mehta; Mumbai, India.)

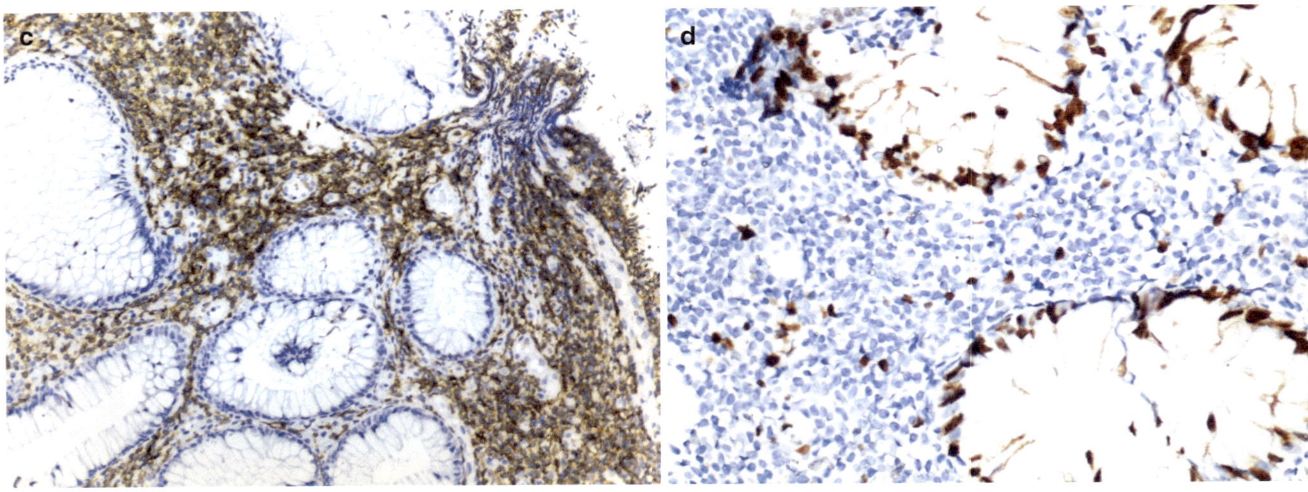

Fig. 6.47 (continued)

References

1. Arora N, Manipadam MT, Pulimood A, Ramakrishna BS, Chacko A, Kurian SS, Nair S. Gastrointestinal lymphomas: pattern of distribution and histological subtypes: 10 years experience in a tertiary centre in South India. Indian J Pathol Microbiol. 2011;54:712–9.
2. Freeman C, Berg JW, Cutler SJ. Occurrence and prognosis of extranodal lymphomas. Cancer. 1972;29:252–60.
3. Ghimire P, Wu GY, Zhu L. Primary gastrointestinal lymphoma. World J Gastroenterol. 2011;17:697–707.
4. Shia J, Teruya-Feldstein J, Pan D, Hegde A, Klimstra DS, Chaganti RSK, et al. Primary follicular lymphoma of the gastrointestinal tract: a clinical and pathologic study of 26 cases. Am J Surg Pathol. 2002;26:216–24.
5. Fine KD, Stone MJ. Alpha-heavy chain disease, Mediterranean lymphoma, and immunoproliferative small intestinal disease: a review of clinicopathological features, pathogenesis, and differential diagnosis. Am J Gastroenterol. 1999;94:1139–52.
6. Ye H, Liu H, Attygalle A, Wotherspoon AC, Nicholson AG, Charlotte F, et al. Variable frequencies of t(11;18)(q21;q21) in MALT lymphomas of different sites: significant association with CagA strains of *H pylori* in gastric MALT lymphoma. Blood. 2003;102:1012–8.
7. Akasaka R, Chiba T, Dutta AK, Toya Y, Mizutani T, Shozushima T, et al. Colonic mucosa-associated lymphoid tissue lymphoma. Case Rep Gastroenterol. 2012;6:569–75.
8. Connor J, Ashton-Key M. Gastric and intestinal diffuse large B-cell lymphomas are clinically and immunophenotypically different. An immunohistochemical and clinical study. Histopathology. 2007;51:697–703.
9. Ibrahim EM, Ezzat AA, El-Weshi AN, Martin JM, Khafaga YM, Rabih WA, et al. Primary intestinal diffuse large B-cell non-Hodgkin's lymphoma clinical features, management, and prognosis of 66 patients. Ann Oncol. 2001;12:53–8.
10. LeBrun DP, Kamel OW, Cleary ML, Dorfman RF, Warnke R. Follicular lymphomas of the gastrointestinal tract. Pathologic features in 31 cases and bcl-2 oncogenic protein expression. Am J Pathol. 1992;140:1327–35.
11. Yoshino T, Miyake K, Ichimura K, Mannami T, Ohara N, Hamazaki S, Akagi T. Increased incidence of follicular lymphoma in the duodenum. Am J Surg Pathol. 2000;24:688–93.
12. Damaj G, Verkarre V, Delmer A, Solal-Celigny P, Yakoub-Agha I, Cellier C, et al. Primary follicular lymphoma of the gastrointestinal tract: a study of 25 cases and a literature review. Ann Oncol. 2003;14:623–9.
13. Salar A, Juanpere N, Bellosillo B, Domingo-Domenech E, Espinet B, Seoane A, et al. Gastrointestinal involvement in mantle cell lymphoma: a prospective clinic, endoscopic, and pathologic study. Am J Surg Pathol. 2006;30:1274–80.
14. Hsu P, Yang T, Sheikh-Fayyaz S, Brody J, Bandovic J, Roy S, et al. Mantle cell lymphoma with in situ or mantle zone growth pattern: a study of five cases and review of literature. Int J Clin Exp Pathol. 2014;7:1042–50.
15. Carvajal-Cuenca A, Sua LF, Silva NM, Pittaluga S, Royo C, Song JY, et al. In situ mantle cell lymphoma: clinical implications of an incidental finding with indolent clinical behavior. Haematologica. 2012;97:270–8.
16. Gupta V, Sangwaiya A, Sharma J, Kaira V, Ratan K, Sen R. Burkitt's lymphoma masquerading as intestinal obstruction: an uncommon entity with variable clinical presentation. Clin Cancer Investig J. 2014;3:441–3.
17. Ferry JA. Burkitt's lymphoma: clinicopathologic features and differential diagnosis. Oncologist. 2006;11:375–83.
18. O'Malley DP, Goldstein NS, Banks PM. The recognition and classification of lymphoproliferative disorders of the gut. Hum Pathol. 2014;45:899–916.
19. Heslop HE. How I treat EBV lymphoproliferation. Blood. 2009;114:4002–8.
20. Arps DP, Smith LB. Classic versus type II enteropathy-associated T-cell lymphoma: diagnostic considerations. Arch Pathol Lab Med. 2013;137:1227–31.
21. Rubio-Tapia A, Murray JA. Classification and management of refractory coeliac disease. Gut. 2010;59:547–57.
22. Smedby KE, Akerman M, Hildebrand H, Glimelius B, Ekbom A, Askling J. Malignant lymphomas in coeliac disease: evidence of increased risks for lymphoma types other than enteropathy-type T cell lymphoma. Gut. 2005;54:54–9.
23. Elsing C, Placke J, Gross-Weege W. Ulcerative jejunoileitis and enteropathy-associated T-cell lymphoma. Eur J Gastroenterol Hepatol. 2005;17:1401–5.
24. Dojcinov SD, Venkataraman G, Pittaluga S, Wlodarska I, Schrager JA, Raffeld M, et al. Age-related EBV-associated lymphoprolif-

erative disorders in the Western population: a spectrum of reactive lymphoid hyperplasia and lymphoma. Blood. 2011;117:4726–35.
25. Akbayram S, Akgun C, Ozen S, Kaya A, Tuncer O, Yuca SA, et al. A case of langerhans cell histiocytosis with anal fistula. Kurume Med J. 2009;56:79–83.
26. Perry AM, Warnke RA, Hu Q, Gaulard P, Copie-Bergman C, Alkan S, et al. Indolent T-cell lymphoproliferative disease of the gastrointestinal tract. Blood. 2013;122:3599–606.
27. McElroy MK, Read WL, Harmon GS, Weidner N. A unique case of an indolent CD56-positive T-cell lymphoproliferative disorder of the gastrointestinal tract: a lesion potentially misdiagnosed as natural killer/T-cell lymphoma. Ann Diagn Pathol. 2011;15:370–5.
28. Mansoor A, Pittaluga S, Beck PL, Wilson WH, Ferry JA, Jaffe ES. NK-cell enteropathy: a benign NK-cell lymphoproliferative disease mimicking intestinal lymphoma: clinicopathologic features and follow-up in a unique case series. Blood. 2011;117:1447–52.

Anal Neoplasms

7

Hector H. Li-Chang

Though definitions of the anal canal vary, it is commonly understood that this site variably comprises (1) a proximal segment lined by colonic mucosa, (2) a middle segment lined by metaplastic or specialized epithelium known as the anal transition zone (ATZ), and (3) a distal segment lined by non-keratinizing squamous epithelium that lacks skin adnexal structures (in contrast to the perianal skin, which has keratinizing epithelium as well as skin adnexal structures). The anal canal can thus be involved by neoplasms from the distal rectum, such as colorectal adenocarcinomas and neuroendocrine tumors, as well as lesions arising from the ATZ and squamous mucosa. Malignancies of the anus comprise 2.5% of all cancers of the digestive system, and although they are rarer than malignancies in other sites, they remain of diagnostic importance to the practicing pathologist. Furthermore, human papillomavirus (HPV)–associated preneoplastic lesions are also commonly biopsied and are important for screening and management. This chapter also details both some rare malignancies and some benign neoplasms.

7.1 HPV-Associated Squamous Intraepithelial Lesions

The Lower Anogenital Squamous Terminology (LAST) standardization project recommends that for HPV-associated lesions, the term "low-grade squamous intraepithelial lesion" (LSIL) should be used instead of the former terminology of "anal intraepithelial neoplasia 1" [1]. With the appropriate exophytic architectural background, the term "condyloma acuminatum" is appropriate. These lesions show mitotic activity and mild atypia in the basal third of the epithelium. Atypia consists of mildly increased nuclear size and increased nuclear-to-cytoplasmic ratios. Maturation begins in the middle third and is relatively normal in the upper third. Koilocytosis can be more subtle than that observed in other sites such as the cervix. In Fig. 7.1, koilocytosis is present only as rare nuclei in the stratum corneum. Some cases traditionally classified as anal intraepithelial neoplasia 2 (AIN 2) are classified as LSIL following immunohistochemical examination (p16/Ki-67) [2, 3].

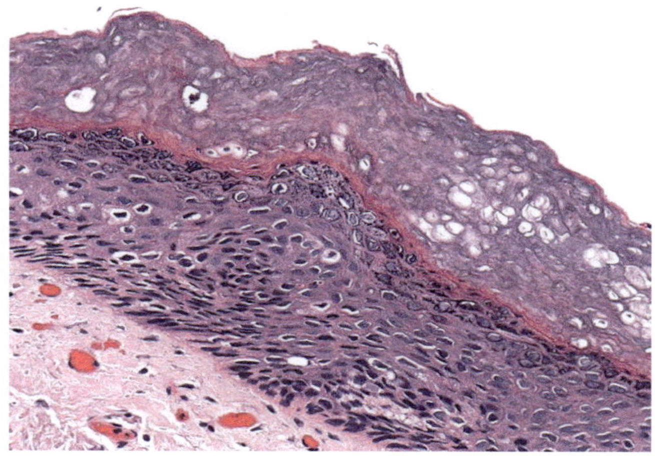

Fig. 7.1 Low-grade squamous intraepithelial lesion ((LSIL)

Under the LAST classification, both AIN 2 and AIN 3/carcinoma in situ are diagnosed as "high-grade intraepithelial lesion" (HSIL), as there is no biologic distinction between the two categories, and interobserver agreement is poor, but an additional qualifier denoting the lesion as either AIN 2 or AIN 3 is optional. In HSIL/AIN 2, mitotic figures and moderate to severe atypia are limited to the basal two thirds of the epithelium. Atypia consists of increased nuclear size, irregular nuclear membranes, and increased nuclear-to-cytoplasmic ratios [1]. There is little to no cytoplasmic

H. H. Li-Chang et al., *Atlas of Intestinal Pathology*, Atlas of Anatomic Pathology,
https://doi.org/10.1007/978-3-030-12379-6_7

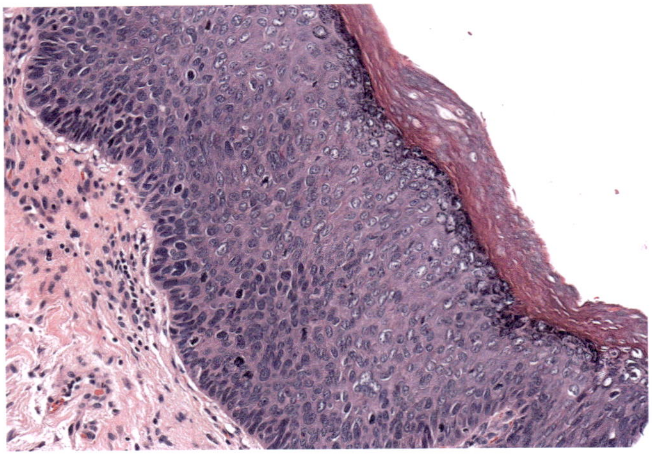

Fig. 7.2 High-grade squamous intraepithelial lesion (HSIL)

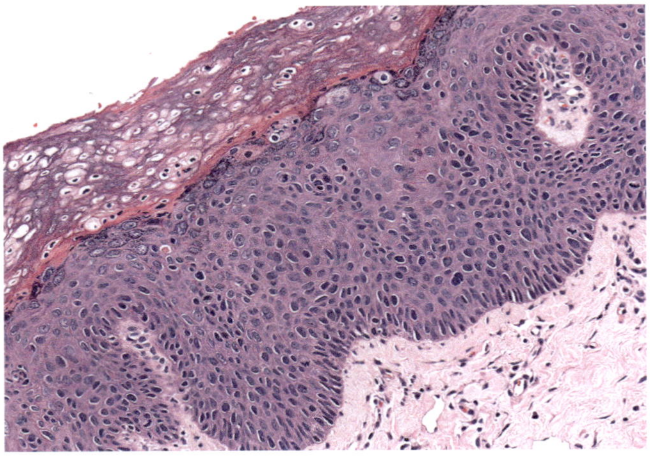

Fig. 7.3 High-grade squamous intraepithelial lesion (HSIL)

maturation in the middle third of the epithelium (Fig. 7.2). Occasionally, p16 and Ki-67 serve to adjudicate between diagnoses of LSIL and HSIL.

Distinguishing between LSIL and HSIL can at times be difficult and may be subject to interobserver variability. When entertaining a diagnosis of AIN 2, p16 immunohistochemistry is recommended, showing diffuse "block" expression of p16. Full-thickness expression of Ki-67 (MIB-1) can also assist in diagnosing HSIL in equivocal cases. Some authorities diagnose HSIL if atypia is of sufficient severity but is confined to basal third of the epithelium. In Fig. 7.3, there is sufficient hyperchromasia and nuclear irregularity to qualify as HSIL, and more convincing HSIL was present nearby. Koilocytes may still be present and do not necessarily suggest a diagnosis of LSIL or preclude a diagnosis of HSIL [4].

In severe dysplasia (AIN 3), there is moderate to severe atypia and mitotic activity that extends to the superficial third of the epithelium, with minimal to absent cytoplasmic differentiation at the most superficial third (Fig. 7.4). The

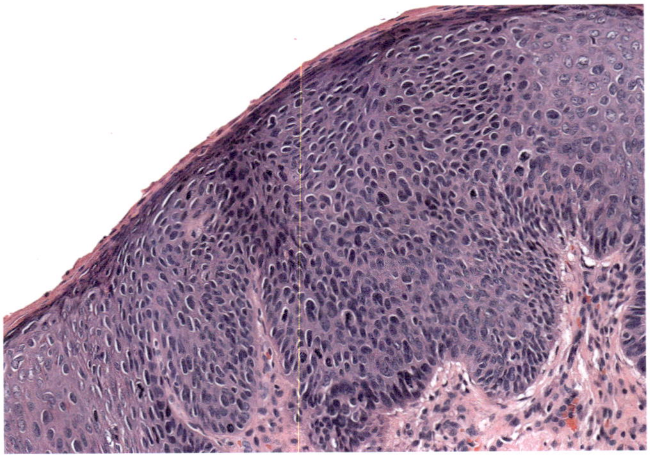

Fig. 7.4 High-grade squamous intraepithelial lesion (HSIL)

term "carcinoma in situ" is not recommended, as it implies a more advanced biological entity than AIN 2/3, which is not supported by our current understanding of these lesions [1].

7.2 Squamous Cell Carcinomas

Squamous cell carcinomas range from those that are very well differentiated and difficult to distinguish from benign lesions, to those that are poorly differentiated and difficult to qualify as squamous. Figure 7.5 shows a moderately differentiated carcinoma that is seen to arise from overlying severe dysplasia, with invasion of the adjacent lamina propria and glandular mucosa by infiltrative nests of cells [1].

Invasion can at times be difficult to identify at the junction between the basaloid dysplastic epithelium and the lamina propria. As in other sites, so-called paradoxical differentiation can be a clue as to the presence of invasion. In Fig. 7.6, paradoxical differentiation consists of larger polygonal cells with more abundant eosinophilic cytoplasm [1].

A desmoplastic reaction (Fig. 7.7) is sometimes present and can help establish a diagnosis of invasive carcinoma.

Combined-modality therapy is the standard of care for most anal squamous cell carcinomas, but it has associated morbidity. Minimally invasive cancers have had good outcomes and are potentially amenable to conservative therapy. The term "superficially invasive squamous cell carcinoma" (SISCCA) of the anal canal has been proposed in an attempt to prospectively identify those patients in whom conservative management is appropriate (Fig. 7.8). Care should involve evaluation by an expert experienced with high-resolution anoscopy and anal canal cancer. The term "SISCCA of the anal canal" is suggested when a carcinoma has an invasive depth of ≤ 3 mm from the basement membrane of the point of origin, with a horizontal spread of ≤ 7 mm in maximal extent, and it has been completely excised [1].

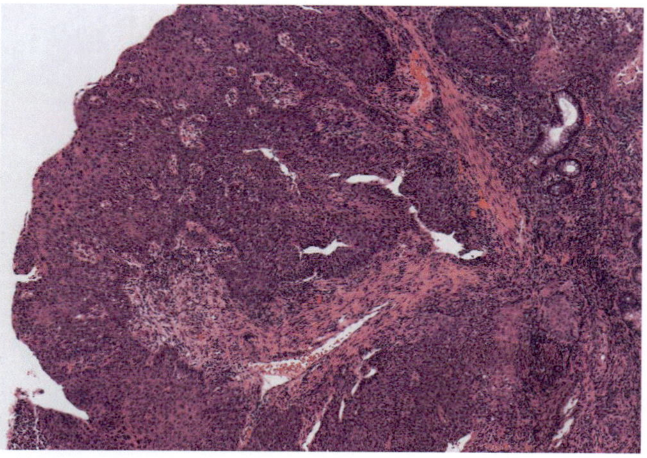

Fig. 7.5 Invasive squamous cell carcinoma (moderately differentiated)

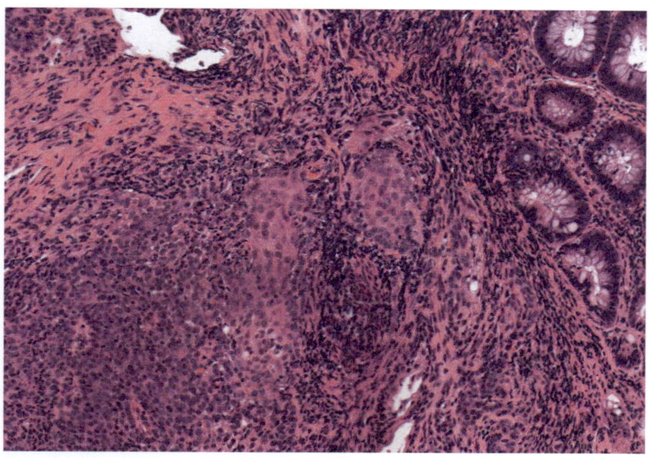

Fig. 7.6 Invasive squamous cell carcinoma, with paradoxical differentiation

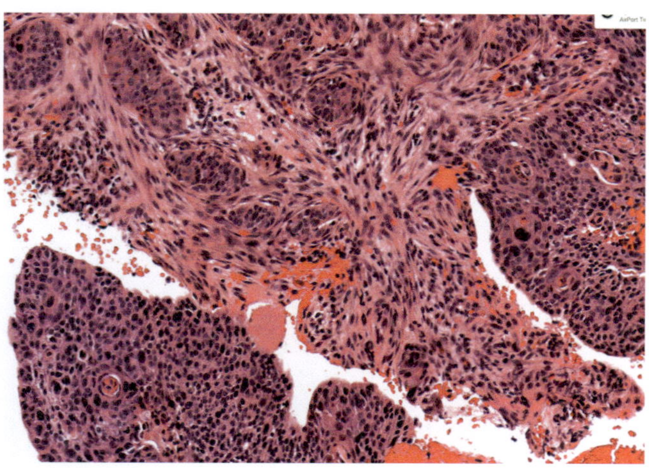

Fig. 7.7 Invasive squamous cell carcinoma, with desmoplastic reaction

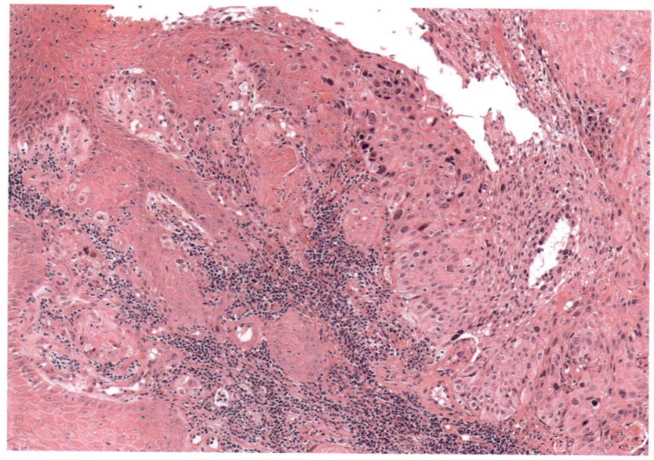

Fig. 7.8 Superficially invasive squamous cell carcinoma (SISCCA)

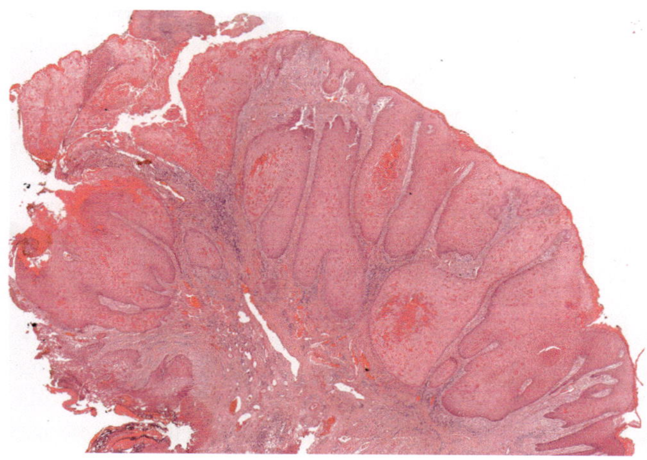

Fig. 7.9 Verrucous carcinoma

Verrucous carcinoma is a subtype of extremely well-differentiated, non–HPV-associated squamous cell carcinoma. The invasive nature of the lesion can sometimes only be appreciated at low power, with the infiltration of the lamina propria by nests of neoplastic cells (Fig. 7.9). Superficial biopsies of this entity may not always be diagnostic of neoplasia, requiring correlation with clinical findings and excision for definitive diagnosis. At higher power, the malignant nature of this carcinoma is difficult to appreciate. The nests of verrucous carcinoma show minimal to absent atypia and mitotic activity. These lesions can be locally destructive, but metastatic behavior is exceptional [5].

Basaloid squamous cell carcinoma (Fig. 7.10) is a variant characterized by a monomorphous proliferation of cells with minimal cytoplasm. Peripheral palisading around the nests of neoplastic cells is common. Mitotic activity is brisk, and areas of comedo-like necrosis are common. Most, if not all, cases

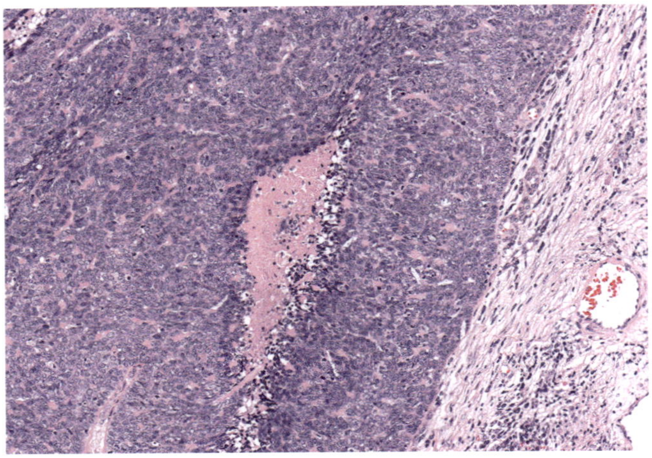

Fig. 7.10 Basaloid squamous cell carcinoma

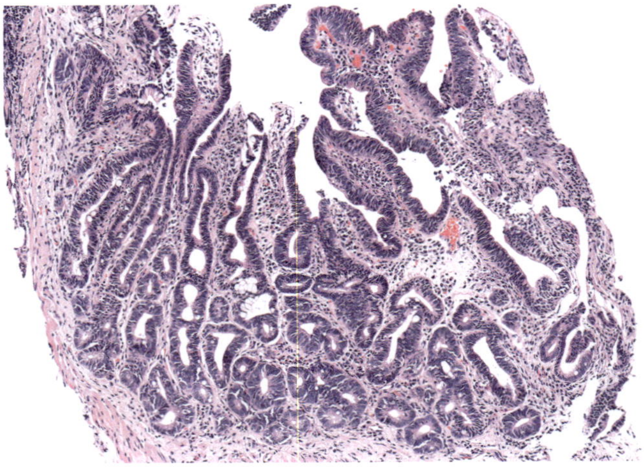

Fig. 7.11 Anal duct adenocarcinoma

show expression of cytokeratin (CK)5/6, overexpression of p16, and presence of high-risk HPV infection. The differential diagnosis includes basal cell carcinoma, melanoma, and neuroendocrine carcinoma. In contrast to basal cell carcinoma, which also expresses CK5/6, atypical mitoses are more frequent and peripheral retraction artefact is absent [6, 7].

7.3 Adenocarcinomas

Anal duct adenocarcinoma (anal gland carcinoma) is a rare variant of adenocarcinoma that is associated with poor prognosis. Because its symptoms overlap with those of benign anal conditions, diagnosis is often delayed. It comprises infiltrative glandular structures lined by cuboidal to short columnar cells (Fig. 7.11). A luminal component is typically absent, and mucin pools may be present [8].

Anal duct carcinomas are more likely to show small tubules and less intracytoplasmic mucin than rectal adenocarcinomas (Fig. 7.12). Extension of proximal primary rectal carcinomas into the anus is much more common and needs to be excluded before a diagnosis of anal duct carcinoma can be made. Immunohistochemistry is often necessary for definitive confirmation, with anal duct carcinomas typically expressing CK7 and lacking expression of CK20 and CDX2 (in contrast to CK7-/CK20+/CD-X2+ rectal carcinomas). Unlike the morphologically similar endocervical adenocarcinoma, they are described as being p16 negative [8].

Colorectal adenocarcinoma with distal extension into the anus (Fig. 7.13) is more commonly seen than anal duct adenocarcinomas. The morphologic features vary, but they generally show more intracytoplasmic mucin, desmoplasia, and dirty necrosis than anal duct carcinomas. Immunostains (as detailed above) are often necessary for a definitive distinction.

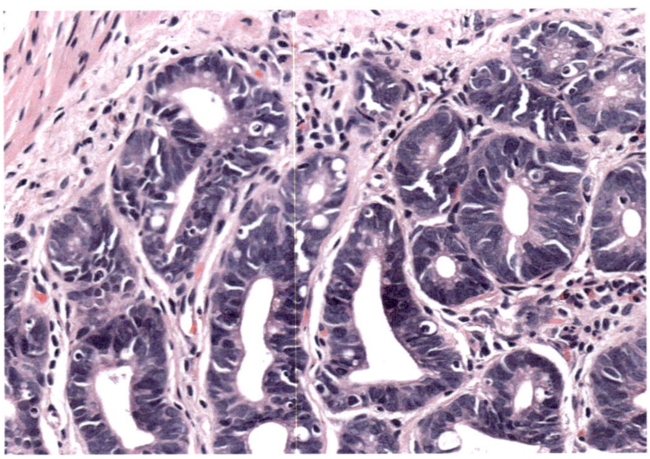

Fig. 7.12 Anal duct adenocarcinoma

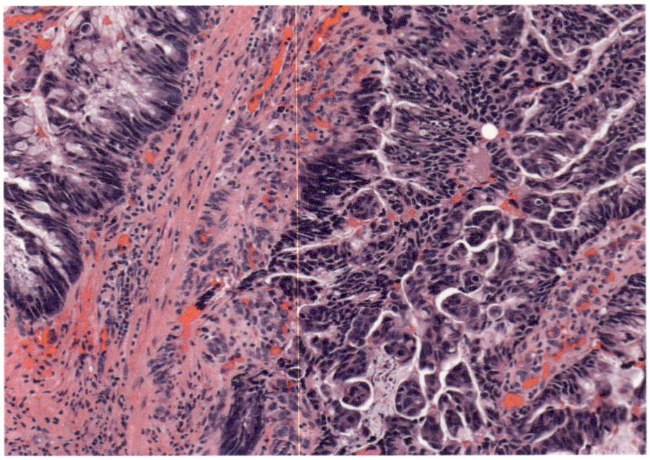

Fig. 7.13 Rectal adenocarcinoma extending into the anus

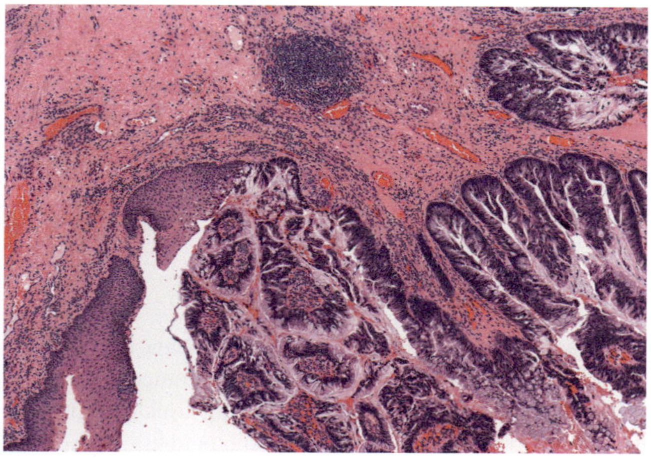

Fig. 7.14 Anal fistula carcinoma

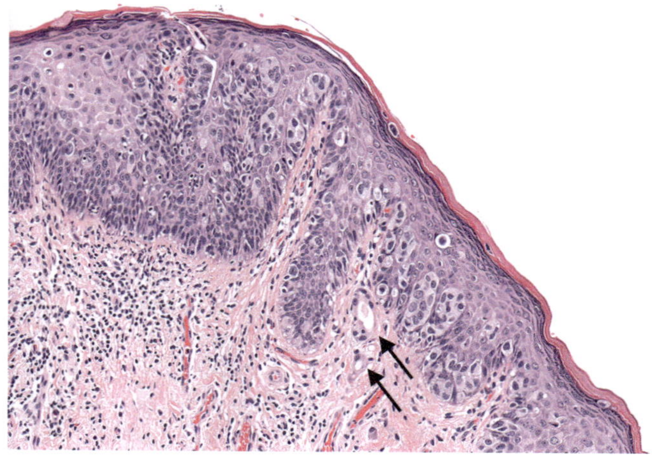

Fig. 7.15 Paget disease. Note the well-formed glands infiltrating through the basement membrane into the superficial lamina propria (*arrows*)

7.4 Anal Fistula Carcinoma

The World Health Organization (WHO) recognizes a separate entity of carcinoma occurring within anal fistulae, often in the setting of Crohn's disease. As in Fig. 7.14, these are most frequently mucinous, but tubular and squamous variants are also seen [9].

7.5 Paget Disease

Extramammary Paget disease refers to a neoplastic proliferation of cells within the epidermal layer of the mucosa. In about half of cases, it represents a proliferation of apocrine-like cells, which are thought to arise from adnexal stem cells [10]. The example in Fig. 7.15 shows the neoplastic cells arranged within the epidermis singly and in small clusters. This proliferation can subsequently become invasive and give rise to an adenocarcinoma.

At higher power (Fig. 7.16), the cells are seen to have enlarged nuclei and variable amounts of pale to eosinophilic cytoplasm. Mitotic figures may be seen, and the cells sometimes have a signet-ring appearance (not shown). The differential diagnosis of extramammary Paget disease includes pagetoid spread by squamous neoplasia (HSIL or squamous cell carcinoma), melanoma, and rectal adenocarcinoma. Thus, an immunohistochemical panel that includes CK7 and CK20, high-molecular-weight keratin, p63, melanoma markers, and gross cystic disease fluid protein 15 (GCDFP-15) is warranted to arrive at a definitive diagnosis [11, 12].

In the other half of cases, extramammary Paget disease represents pagetoid spread of malignant cells from a proximal rectal adenocarcinoma [13, 14]. The example in Fig. 7.17 shows the cells arranged singly and in small clusters, with bland nuclei and abundant foamy cytoplasm. Thus, they appear similar to Paget disease derived from apocrine cells.

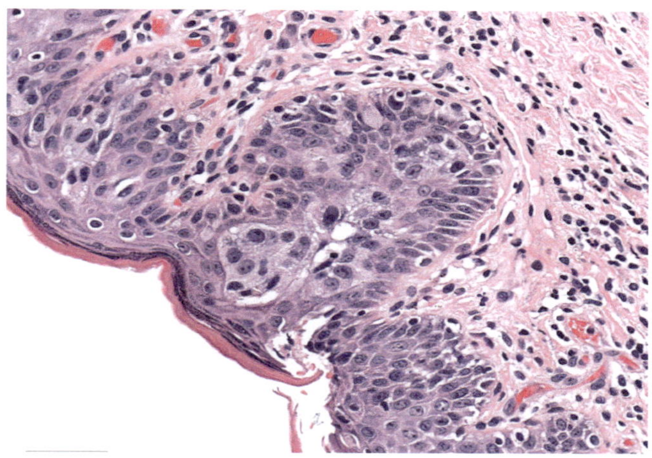

Fig. 7.16 Paget disease, shown at higher-power magnification

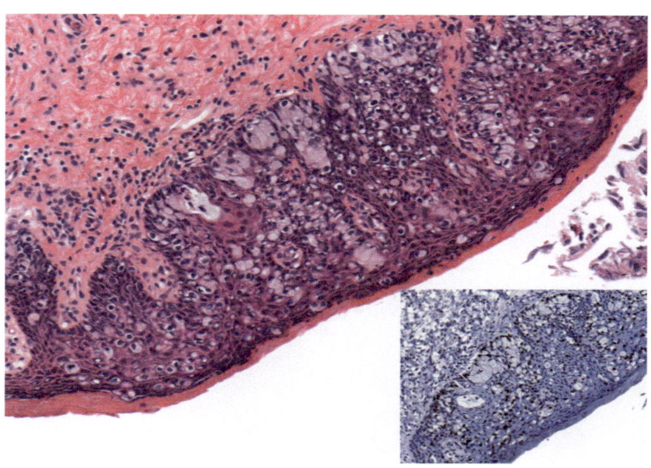

Fig. 7.17 Pagetoid spread by colonic adenocarcinoma; the inset shows CDX2-positive immunohistochemistry

However, immunohistochemistry with CK20(+), CDX2(+), CK7(−), and GCDFP-15(−) confirms origin from the patient's known rectal carcinoma (positive CDX2 inset).

7.6 Hidradenoma Papilliferum

This neoplasm, also known as *mammary-like adenoma*, is likely to be derived from mammary-like anogenital glands. It comprises a maze-like arrangement of anastomosing papillae and branched glands filling cystic spaces. At low power, it is important to appreciate that the edges of the lesion are relatively well-circumscribed. The differential diagnosis includes metastatic adenocarcinoma (colon or breast), endometriosis, and skin adnexal neoplasms (such as apocrine hidradenoma). As in Fig. 7.18, the overlying squamous epithelium is usually normal and not connected to the lesion.

At higher power (Fig. 7.19), two cell layers can be appreciated lining the thin fibrovascular cores of the papillae. The more basal layer is composed of cuboidal cells with clear cytoplasm, whereas the superficial layer comprises columnar cells with eosinophilic cytoplasm. Mild atypia is the norm. Immunohistochemical stains will show expression of myoepithelial markers in the basal layer (p63, smooth muscle actin, myosin, S100, calponin); the superficial layer will express pankeratin, CK5/6, GCDFP-15, ER, PR, and CK7.

7.7 Melanoma

Anal melanomas, a minority of all melanomas, arise from melanocytes native to the anal and perianal mucosa. Grossly, they are often polypoid and can extend proximally to involve the rectum [15, 16]. As in the skin, both epithelioid and desmoplastic variants can occur at this site. The malignant cells grow in asymmetrical, expansile nests within both the epithelium and the lamina propria/dermis (Fig. 7.20).

At higher power, pigment may be visible (as in Fig. 7.21), to suggest a diagnosis of melanoma. The cells are characterized by moderate to severe nuclear atypia, and nucleoli are

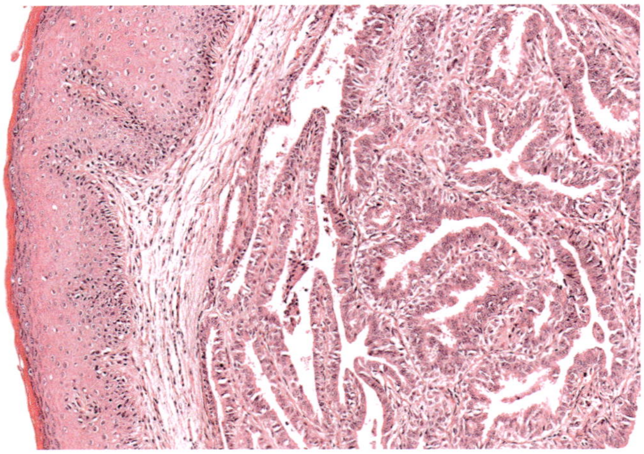

Fig. 7.18 Hidradenoma papilliferum (low-power view)

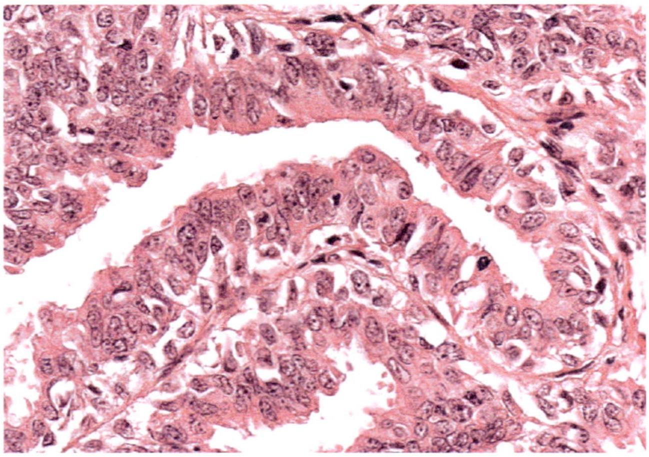

Fig. 7.19 Hidradenoma papilliferum, at higher power

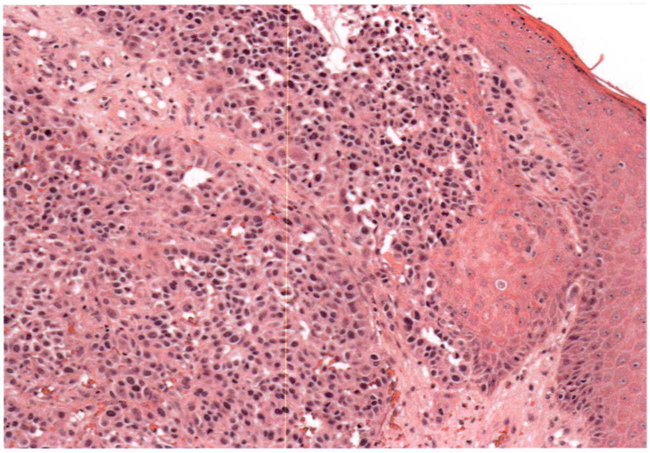

Fig. 7.20 Anal melanoma

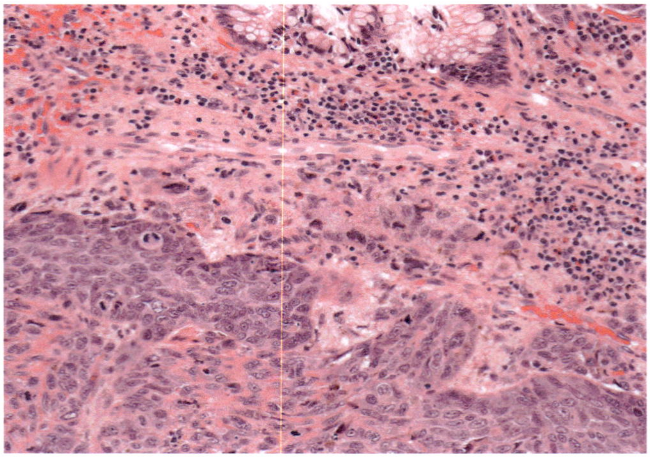

Fig. 7.21 Anal melanoma (higher power view), with visible pigment and brisk mitotic activity

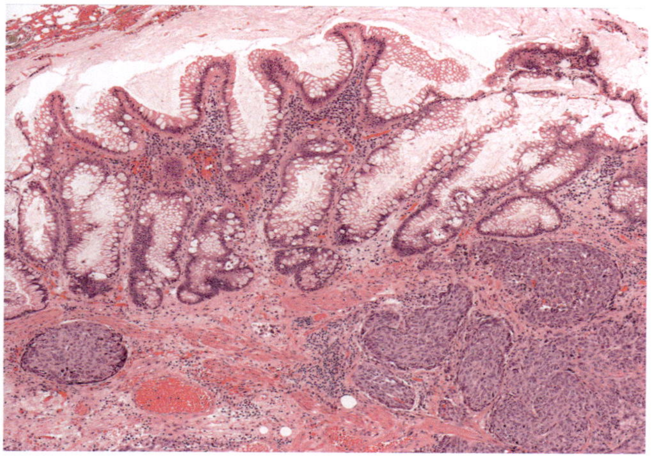

Fig. 7.22 Anal melanoma with colonic hyperplastic changes in the overlying epithelium

often prominent. Mitotic activity is variable, but brisk mitotic activity is more frequently encountered [17].

Melanomas may grow deeply and spread horizontally beneath the overlying epithelium (Fig. 7.22). Hyperplastic changes are often present in the overlying epithelium, either squamous or colonic. Deeper sections may be considered if superficial sampling of a clinically visible mass results only in epithelial hyperplastic or reactive changes.

References

1. Darragh TM, Colgan TJ, Cox JT, Heller DS, Henry MR, Luff RD, Members of LAST Project Work Groups, et al. The lower anogenital squamous terminology standardization project for HPV-associated lesions: background and consensus recommendations from the College of American Pathologists and the American Society for Colposcopy and Cervical Pathology. Arch Pathol Lab Med. 2012;136:1266–97.
2. Lytwyn A, Salit IE, Raboud J, Chapman W, Darragh T, Winkler B, et al. Interobserver agreement in the interpretation of anal intraepithelial neoplasia. Cancer. 2005;103:1447–56.
3. Cotter MB, Kelly ME, O'Connell PR, Hyland J, Winter DC, Sheahan K, Gibbons D. Anal intraepithelial neoplasia: a single centre 19 year review. Color Dis. 2014;16:777–82.
4. Pirog EC, Quint KD, Yantiss RK. P16/CDKN2A and Ki-67 enhance the detection of anal intraepithelial neoplasia and condyloma and correlate with human papillomavirus detection by polymerase chain reaction. Am J Surg Pathol. 2010;34:1449–55.
5. Zidar N, Langner C, Odar K, Hošnjak L, Kamarádová K, Daum O, et al. Anal verrucous carcinoma is not related to infection with human papillomaviruses and should be distinguished from giant condyloma (Buschke-Löwenstein tumour). Histopathology. 2017;70:938–45.
6. Graham RP, Arnold CA, Naini BV, Lam-Himlin DM. Basaloid squamous cell carcinoma of the anus revisited. Am J Surg Pathol. 2016;40:354–60.
7. Patil DT, Goldblum JR, Billings SD. Clinicopathological analysis of basal cell carcinoma of the anal region and its distinction from basaloid squamous cell carcinoma. Mod Pathol. 2013;26:1382–9.
8. Meriden Z, Montgomery EA. Anal duct carcinoma: a report of 5 cases. Hum Pathol. 2012;43:216–20.
9. Thomas M, Bienkowski R, Vandermeer TJ, Trostle D, Cagir B. Malignant transformation in perianal fistulas of Crohn's disease: a systematic review of literature. J Gastrointest Surg. 2010;14:66–73.
10. Regauer S. Extramammary Paget's disease--a proliferation of adnexal origin? Histopathology. 2006;48:723–9.
11. Nowak MA, Guerriere-Kovach P, Pathan A, Campbell TE, Deppisch LM. Perianal Paget's disease: distinguishing primary and secondary lesions using immunohistochemical studies including gross cystic disease fluid protein-15 and cytokeratin 20 expression. Arch Pathol Lab Med. 1998;122:1077–81.
12. Tulchinsky H, Zmora O, Brazowski E, Goldman G, Rabau M. Extramammary Paget's disease of the perianal region. Color Dis. 2004;6:206–9.
13. Battles OE, Page DL, Johnson JE. Cytokeratins, CEA, and mucin histochemistry in the diagnosis and characterization of extramammary Paget's disease. Am J Clin Pathol. 1997;108:6–12.
14. Goldblum JR, Hart WR. Perianal Paget's disease: a histologic and immunohistochemical study of 11 cases with and without associated rectal adenocarcinoma. Am J Surg Pathol. 1998;22:170–9.
15. Bello DM, Smyth E, Perez D, Khan S, Temple LK, Ariyan CE, et al. Anal versus rectal melanoma: does site of origin predict outcome? Dis Colon Rectum. 2013;56:150–7.
16. Nicholson AG, Cox PM, Marks CG, Cook MG. Primary malignant melanoma of the rectum. Histopathology. 1993;22:261–4.
17. Cooper PH, Mills SE, Allen MS Jr. Malignant melanoma of the anus: report of 12 patients and analysis of 255 additional cases. Dis Colon Rectum. 1982;25:693–703.

Index

H. H. Li-Chang et al., *Atlas of Intestinal Pathology*, Atlas of Anatomic Pathology,
https://doi.org/10.1007/978-3-030-12379-6

MIX
Papier aus verantwortungsvollen Quellen
Paper from responsible sources
FSC® C105338

If you have any concerns about our products,
you can contact us on
ProductSafety@springernature.com

In case Publisher is established outside the EU,
the EU authorized representative is:
Springer Nature Customer Service Center GmbH
Europaplatz 3, 69115 Heidelberg, Germany

Printed by Libri Plureos GmbH
in Hamburg, Germany